Insulin-Like Growth Factors in Health and Disease

Guest Editors

CLAIRE M. PERKS, PhD
JEFF M.P. HOLLY, PhD

ENDOCRINOLOGY AND METABOLISM CLINICS OF NORTH AMERICA

www.endo.theclinics.com

Consulting Editor
DEREK LEROITH, MD, PhD

June 2012 • Volume 41 • Number 2

SAUNDERS an imprint of ELSEVIER, Inc.

W.B. SAUNDERS COMPANY
A Division of Elsevier Inc.

1600 John F. Kennedy Boulevard • Suite 1800 • Philadelphia, Pennsylvania 19103-2899

http://www.theclinics.com

ENDOCRINOLOGY AND METABOLISM CLINICS OF NORTH AMERICA Volume 41, Number 2
June 2012 ISSN 0889-8529, ISBN-13: 978-1-4557-3856-4

Editor: Pamela Hetherington

Endocrinology and Metabolism Clinics of North America (ISSN 0889-8529) is published quarterly by Elsevier Inc., 360 Park Avenue South, New York, NY 10010-1710. Months of issue are March, June, September, and December. Periodicals postage paid at New York, NY and additional mailing offices. Subscription prices are USD 313.00 per year for US individuals, USD 536.00 per year for US institutions, USD 158.00 per year for US students and residents, USD 393.00 per year for Canadian individuals, USD 656.00 per year for Canadian institutions, USD 456.00 per year for international individuals, USD 656.00 per year for international institutions, and USD 233.00 per year for international and Canadian and foreign students/residents. To receive student/resident rate, orders must be accompanied by name of affiliated institution, date of term, and the signature of program/ residency coordinator on institution letterhead. Orders will be billed at individual rate until proof of status is received. Foreign air speed delivery is included in all *Clinics* subscription prices. All prices are subject to change without notice. **POSTMASTER:** Send address changes to *Endocrinology and Metabolism Clinics of North America*, Elsevier Health Sciences Division, Subscription Customer Service, 3251 Riverport Lane, Maryland Heights, MO 63043. **Customer Service: Telephone: 1-800-654-2452** (U.S. and Canada); **1-314-447-8871** (outside U.S. and Canada). **Fax: 1-314-447-8029. E-mail: journalscustomerservice-usa@elsevier.com** (for print support); **journalsonlinesupport-usa@elsevier.com** (for online support).

Reprints. For copies of 100 or more, of articles in this publication, please contact the Commercial Rights Department, Elsevier Inc., 360 Park Avenue South, New York, NY 10010-1710; phone: (+1) 212-633-3813; fax: (+1) 212-462-1935; e-mail: reprints@elsevier.com.

Endocrinology and Metabolism Clinics of North America is covered in *MEDLINE/PubMed (Index Medicus), EMBASE/Excerpta Medica, Current Contents/Clinical Medicine, Current Contents/Life Sciences, Science Citation Index, ISI/BIOMED, BIOSIS,* and *Chemical Abstracts*.

Printed in the United States of America.

Contributors

CONSULTING EDITOR

DEREK LEROITH, MD, PhD
Chief, Division of Endocrinology, Metabolism, and Bone Diseases, Department of Medicine, Mount Sinai School of Medicine, New York, New York

GUEST EDITORS

CLAIRE M. PERKS, PhD
School of Clinical Sciences, University of Bristol, IGFs & Metabolic Endocrinology Group, Southmead Hospital, Bristol, United Kingdom

JEFF M.P. HOLLY, PhD
Professor, School of Clinical Sciences, University of Bristol, IGFs & Metabolic Endocrinology Group, Southmead Hospital, Bristol, United Kingdom

AUTHORS

MARTIN L. ADAMO, PhD
Department of Biochemistry, University of Texas Health Science Center, San Antonio, Texas

PHILIPPE F. BACKELJAUW, MD
Professor of Pediatrics, Department of Pediatrics, Cincinnati Children's Hospital Medical Center, University of Cincinnati College of Medicine, Cincinnati, Ohio

STEVEN D. CHERNAUSEK, MD
Professor of Pediatrics, Edith Kinney Gaylord Chair, Department of Pediatrics, University of Oklahoma Health Sciences Center, Oklahoma City, Oklahoma

DAVID R. CLEMMONS, MD
Kenan Professor of Medicine, Division of Endocrinology, Department of Medicine, School of Medicine, University of North Carolina, Chapel Hill, North Carolina

EVA L. FELDMAN, MD, PhD
Russell N. DeJong Professor of Neurology, Department of Neurology, University of Michigan, Ann Arbor, Michigan

ROBERT A. FROST, PhD
Associate Professor, Department of Cellular and Molecular Physiology, Pennsylvania State University College of Medicine, Hershey, Pennsylvania

A. GARTEN, PhD
Department of Women and Child Health, Hospital for Children and Adolescents, Center for Pediatric Research Leipzig (CPL), University Hospitals, Leipzig, Germany

PAUL HALUSKA, MD, PhD
Associate Professor, Division of Medical Oncology, Department of Oncology, Mayo Clinic College of Medicine, Rochester, Minnesota

JEFF M.P. HOLLY, PhD
Professor, School of Clinical Sciences, University of Bristol, IGFs & Metabolic Endocrinology Group, Southmead Hospital, Bristol, United Kingdom

MASANOBU KAWAI, MD, PhD
Department of Bone and Mineral Research, Osaka Medical Center and Research Institute for Maternal and Child Health, Izumi, Osaka, Japan

DANIELA KIEPE, MD
Department of Pediatrics I, University Children's Hospital Heidelberg, Heidelberg, Germany

W. KIESS, MD
Department of Women and Child Health, Hospital for Children and Adolescents, Center for Pediatric Research Leipzig (CPL), University Hospitals, Leipzig, Germany

JOHN F. KUEMMERLE, MD
Professor of Medicine, and Physiology and Biophysics, Vice Chair of Gastroenterology, Hepatology and Nutrition, Departments of Medicine, and Physiology and Biophysics, Medical College of Virginia Campus, Virginia Commonwealth University, Richmond, Virginia

CHARLES H. LANG, PhD
Professor and Vice Chairman, Department of Cellular and Molecular Physiology, Pennsylvania State University College of Medicine, Hershey, Pennsylvania

CLAIRE M. PERKS, PhD
School of Clinical Sciences, University of Bristol, IGFs & Metabolic Endocrinology Group, Southmead Hospital, Bristol, United Kingdom

CLIFFORD J. ROSEN, MD
Center for Translational Research, Maine Medical Center Research Institute, Scarborough, Maine

STACEY A. SAKOWSKI, PhD
Deputy Managing Director, A. Alfred Taubman Medical Research Institute, University of Michigan, Ann Arbor, Michigan

S. SCHUSTER
Department of Women and Child Health, Hospital for Children and Adolescents, Center for Pediatric Research Leipzig (CPL), University Hospitals, Leipzig, Germany

IGNACIO TORRES ALEMAN, PhD
Department of Functional and Systems Neuroscience, Cajal Institute, Ciberned, Madrid, Spain

S. JOHN WEROHA, MD, PhD
Fellow, Department of Oncology, Mayo Clinic College of Medicine, Rochester, Minnesota

BURKHARD TÖNSHOFF, MD, PhD
Department of Pediatrics I, University Children's Hospital Heidelberg, Heidelberg, Germany

SHOSHANA YAKAR, PhD
Department of Basic Science and Craniofacial Biology, David B. Kriser Dental Center, New York University College of Dentistry, New York, New York

Contents

mediator of preadipocyte proliferation, differentiation, and survival. Results from clinical studies on GH treatment in patients with GH deficiency or GH insensitivity syndrome can be used to dissect GH and IGF as well as IGF-binding protein (IGFBP) actions in vivo. In this article, changes of the GH/IGF system during adipocyte differentiation in vitro as well as related signaling pathways and their impact on adipose tissue growth and function are discussed. Clinical considerations include the effects of GH and IGF-I on adipose tissue during treatment of GH deficiency, differences in the IGF system between visceral and subcutaneous adipose tissue depots as well as the recently emerging role for adipose tissue in the regulation of glucose homeostasis.

This review describes the current literature on the interaction between insulin-like growth factors, endocrine hormones, and branched-chain amino acids on muscle physiology in healthy young individuals and during select pathologic conditions. Emphasis is placed on the mechanism by which physical and hormonal signals are transduced at the cellular level to either grow or atrophy skeletal muscle. The key role of the mammalian target of rapamycin and its ability to respond to hypertrophic and atrophic signals informs our understanding how a combination of physical, nutritional, and pharmacologic therapies may be used in tandem to prevent or ameliorate reductions in muscle mass.

The insulin-like growth factor (IGF) regulatory system is critical for skeletal growth and maintenance. Initially there was great hope that the recombinant IGFs might be used clinically for disorders ranging from short stature to fracture repair and osteoporosis. Although this potential was not realized, basic and translational studies have continued, providing significant insights into the role of this family of growth factors in skeletal homeostasis and the pathophysiology of several bone disorders. This article reviews the importance of the IGF regulatory system in skeletal growth and maintenance.

Insulin-like growth factor (IGF) plays an important role in tissue growth and development. Several studies have demonstrated the association between circulating levels of IGF-1 and -2 and cancer risk, and the IGF system has been implicated in the oncogenesis of essentially all solid and hematologic malignancies. The optimal strategy for targeting IGF signaling in patients with cancer is not clear. The modest benefits reported thus far underscore the need for a better understanding of IGF signaling, which would enable clinicians to identify the subset of patients with the greatest likelihood of attaining benefit from this targeted approach.

IGF-I to patients with extreme insulin resistance results in improvement in glycemic control, and IGF-I is associated with lowering glucose and enhancing insulin sensitivity in Type 1 and Type 2 diabetes. However, patients with diabetes are also sensitive to stimulation of side effects in response to IGF-I. IGF-I coordinately links growth hormone and insulin actions and has direct effects on intermediary metabolism.

ENDOCRINOLOGY AND METABOLISM CLINICS OF NORTH AMERICA

NOW AVAILABLE FOR YOUR iPhone and iPad

Foreword

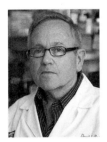

Derek LeRoith, MD, PhD
Consulting Editor

There has been a dramatic intensification of research interest in the insulin-like growth factors (IGFs) over the past decade or so, due to our understanding of their importance in normal physiological functions as well as in pathological processes. Drs Perks and Holly have assembled a remarkable number of authors who describe the latest information on these topics.

In their article on the use of animal models to study the physiological effects of IGF-1, Drs Yakar and Adamo describe the effects of IGFs on body size, skeletal acquisition, muscle gain and maintenance, reproduction, metabolism, and longevity. Circulating and local IGF-1 have effects on bone growth, skeletal acquisition, and muscle size, although the mechanisms are quite complex and the use of mouse models of gene-deletion and transgenic approaches have been helpful in understanding these mechanisms. Both circulating and local IGF-1 may influence the female and male reproductive systems, in both animal tissues and human-derived cells; however, the therapeutic advantages are yet to be defined. Metabolic effects of the GH/IGF-1 axis are quite involved, with GH acting as an anti-insulin hormone, whereas IGF-1 can actually produce opposite effects; these effects of GH and IGF-1 are usually independent of each other. In the case of longevity, studies in rodents have not always reproduced the initial studies in Caenorhabditis elegans that demonstrated caloric restriction with reduced insulin/IGF-1 signaling was associated with longevity.

The article by Drs Perks and Holly introduces the reader to the complexity of the IGF system, with ligands (IGF-1 and IGF-2), six binding proteins (IGFBPs) and two functional receptors, the insulin receptor, and the IGF-1 receptor. The so-called IGF-2 receptor is the mannose-6-phosphate receptor that does not have signaling properties. They then describe some differences between human and experimental models especially in the case of IGF-2 that circulates at very high concentrations in humans but is virtually absent from rodent postnatal serum. IGF-2 is considered more mitogenic than IGF-1 probably since it activates the mitogenic insulin recptor (IR-A) in addition to the IGF-1R, whereas IGF-1 only activates the IGF-1R. This function of IGF-2 may also explain fetal growth in utero where IGF-2 is expressed as are the IR-A receptors. On the other hand, IGF-1 seems to be affected by nutrient intake in both humans and rodents, although its effect on nutrient balance is as yet poorly defined.

Endocrinol Metab Clin N Am 41 (2012) xi–xiii
doi:10.1016/j.ecl.2012.04.022
0889-8529/12/$ – see front matter **endo.theclinics.com**

The IGF system is critical for normal growth and development. Drs Backeljauw and Chernausek define the term "primary IGF-deficiency" to describe those cases of short stature with low IGF-1 levels and normal or elevated GH levels. These are in contrast to GH receptor-deficient, STAT5b-deficient, patients with IGF-1 or ALS mutations or IGF-1 receptor mutations, all of whom have specifically defined genetic causations. The authors describe the value and pitfalls of using serum IGF-1 levels for diagnostic purposes as well as for monitoring response to therapy using GH, for example. Furthermore, they discuss the use of IGF-1 therapy either alone or in combination with IGFBP-3 and describe the responses seen in Laron dwarfs as well as the safety of rhIGF-1 usage.

As discussed in the article by Drs Garten, Schuster, and Kiess, the GH and IGF-1 system has a complicated role in adipocyte physiology. While GH induces lipolysis and FFA release in vivo, in vitro it has been shown to stimulate preadipocyte proliferation but inhibit adipocyte differentiation. On the other hand, IGF-1 plays a role in preadipocyte proliferation and differentiation into mature adipocytes. Furthermore, adipocytes are a major source of endogenous IGF-1, second only to the liver. Finally, there are clinical effects on adipocytes and fat deposits when rhGH or rhIGF-1 are used therapeutically; GH-deficit children have increased adiposity and rhGH reduces fat deposits. Thus while there is substantial in vitro and in vivo evidence for their distinct roles in adipocyte physiology and pathology, many questions remain unanswered.

Bone growth and development have long been known to depend on the IGF system. Furthermore, bone homeostasis and fracture repair are critically dependent on the system. These effects are mediated by both circulating forms of the IGF system as well as local production by bone cells. Drs Kawai and Rosen describe the experimental and clinical studies that demonstrate the importance of the IGF system on bone. Human studies using recombinant IGF-1 have demonstrated a degree of efficacy in patients with osteoporosis, although the risk-benefit ratio given the potential hypoglycemic side effect doesn't bode well for therapeutic usage.

As described by Drs Weroha and Haluska, the IGF system has long been known to be involved in cancer. The IGF system stimulates cellular proliferation and inhibits apoptosis. These effects are mediated primarily via activation of the IGF-1 receptor but also via the insulin receptor, both of which are tyrosine kinase receptors and very similar in amino-acid composition and tertiary structure. Experiments in cell culture and animal models showed that inhibition of the system could retard tumor growth and led to multiple companies developing inhibitors of the IGF-1 receptor, both humanized monoclonal IGF-1 receptor-specific antibodies and small molecule tyrosine kinase inhibitors (TKIs). While the preclinical and early human studies in various types of cancers were very promising, more complete studies, especially with the antibodies, were less convincing due to either compensation by other tyrosine kinase receptors such as the insulin receptor or unacceptable side effects. Nevertheless, studies continue with the TKIs as well and the inhibition of the IGF-1 (and/or IR) may yet prove useful when used with signaling inhibitors such as PI3'K and mTOR.

In a article titled, "IGFs in normal and diseased kidney," Drs Kiepe and Tönshoff describe the heterogeneity of expression of the IGF system in the kidney. They describe how each component of the IGF system plays an important role in kidney development both prenatally and postnatally, the renal handling of IGFs derived from the circulation, the effects of the IGFs on renal glomerular hemodynamics, tubular functions, and the role of IGFs in specific renal disorders such as acute renal failure, chronic renal failure, nephrotic syndrome, and diabetic nephropathy. Finally, they discuss the potential for the use of IGF-1 treatment in some of these common conditions.

As described in the article by Drs Sakowski and Feldman, IGFs play an important role in the growth, development, and survival of the peripheral nervous system (PNS), in addition to their function in the central nervous system. These effects are clearly mediated by both paracrine and autocrine mechanisms. They also describe how the IGF system may involve protection from neurodegenerative disorders and injury to the PNS. Finally, they discuss the clinical role of rhIGF-1 in treating many of these disorders including ALS, where the outcomes have been disappointing and may require reassessment of the mode of delivery, namely, more directly to the target tissue of interest.

Dr Torres Aleman describes how IGF-1 is neuroprotective and how reduced IGF-1 levels may lead to neurodegeneration, at least in the animal models studied. These effects maybe mediated by oxidative stress, inflammation, or excitotoxicity-induced IGF-1 resistance in neural tissues. On the other hand, studies have suggested that Alzheimers may be adversely affected by IGF-1. In his article, Dr Aleman deals with this seeming paradox very scholarly and develops a theme that suggests that IGF-1 may still be a valuable therapeutic option for certain neurodegenerative disorders depending on whether IGF-1 resistance or IGF-1 deficiency is present.

The IGF system is expressed in most tissues including the gastrointestinal tract. Dr Kuemmerle describes the expression of the components in various compartments of the gastrointestinal tract and the potential role of the IGFs in normal growth as well as in pathological conditions. Thus both GH and IGF-1 have proliferative effects on the intestinal mucosa; however, they are also involved in fibrotic conditions as disorders such as colitis and potentially colonic carcinogenesis.

The metabolic effects of IGF-1 are described in the article by Dr Clemmons in the context of both normal physiology and diabetes. Under physiological circumstances IGF-1 stimulates protein synthesis in muscle and free fatty acid utilization in tissues. It suppresses GH and at high concentrations may inhibit pancreatic insulin secretion. In Type 1 diabetics it is often reduced due to GH resistance. In Type 2 diabetics the increased GH secretion enhances insulin resistance and may worsen insulin resistance. Thus, when administered pharmacologically to diabetic patients, glucose homeostasis may improve due to inhibited GH release as well as inhibited glucagon release. In addition, it may mimic insulin effects at various target tissues such as muscle. While IGF-1 treatment of the severe insulin-resistant patient has proven very effective, concerns over its side effects have tempered interest in its clinical use.

Undoubtedly, the reader will find many interesting aspects of the IGF system in this issue, both as an update on the topic and also in considering further areas of exploration. For this, we are grateful to the issue editors and the experts who have contributed their knowledge and time to make this an outstanding issue.

Derek LeRoith, MD, PhD
Division of Endocrinology, Metabolism, and Bone Diseases
Department of Medicine
Mount Sinai School of Medicine
One Gustave L. Levy Place
Box 1055, Altran 4-36
New York, NY 10029, USA

E-mail address:
derek.leroith@mssm.edu

Preface

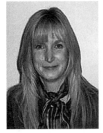 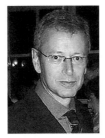

Claire M. Perks, PhD   Jeff M.P. Holly, PhD
Guest Editors

In the 1950s Salmon and Daughaday discovered that growth hormone did not directly stimulate the incorporation of sulfate into cartilage, but rather acted through a serum factor, termed "sulfation factor." The activity of this "sulfation factor" has since become recognized as a complex system that comprises two growth factors, cell surface receptors, six specific high-affinity binding proteins, and insulin-like growth factor binding proteins (IGFBP) proteases. Insulin-like growth factors (IGFs) play a role both pre- and postnatally in mediating the effects of nutrition on cell growth and metabolism and have a plethora of important cellular actions. They are produced by almost every cell in the body and circulate in more than 1000-fold higher concentrations than most other peptide hormones, such as insulin. The IGFBPs are expressed in a tissue-specific manner and they confer specificity to these pluripotential growth factors. This issue of *Endocrinology and Metabolism Clinics* highlights the key roles that the IGFs play in normal physiology and situations where normal physiology is disturbed. We describe the important functions of the IGFs in a variety of different tissues and how they become deregulated in the development and progression of multiple disease states. As a consequence of their role in the disease processes, compounds targeting the IGF axis have become an area of intense preclinical and clinical research that is also covered in this issue of *Endocrinology and Metabolism Clinics*. We thank all the authors who have contributed to this issue and hope it provides an up-to-date summary of what is currently known but

Endocrinol Metab Clin N Am 41 (2012) xv–xvi
doi:10.1016/j.ecl.2012.04.021
0889-8529/12/$ – see front matter © 2012 Elsevier Inc. All rights reserved.

endo.theclinics.com

hope it more importantly highlights questions and issues that still need to be addressed.

Claire M. Perks, PhD
Jeff M.P. Holly, PhD

School of Clinical Sciences
University of Bristol
IGFs & Metabolic Endocrinology Group
Learning & Research Building, 2nd Floor
Southmead Hospital
Bristol BS10 5NB, UK

E-mail addresses:
Claire.M.Perks@bristol.ac.uk (C.M. Perks)
Jeff.Holly@bristol.ac.uk (J.M.P. Holly)

Insulin-Like Growth Factor-1 Physiology: Lessons from Mouse Models

Shoshana Yakar, PhD[a],*, Martin L. Adamo, PhD[b]

KEYWORDS

- Insulin-like growth factor-1 • Physiology • Mouse models • IGF-1

KEY POINTS

- The GH/IGF axis is a key regulator of body size and musculoskeletal acquisition.
- The interplay between the GH/IGF axis and the insulin pathways plays key roles in carbohydrate and lipid metabolism, thus affecting the individual health-span.

INTRODUCTION

Insulin-like growth factor-1 (IGF-1) belongs to a small family of secreted single chain polypeptides that play important roles in growth, development, and metabolism. This family includes proinsulin, insulin, IGF-1, and IGF-2, which show high amino acid sequence homology and share similar ternary structure. IGF-1 and IGF-2 are derived from 2 separate genes and transcribed by virtually all cells. Because these factors play pivotal roles in cellular proliferation, differentiation, and function, they are tightly regulated at the transcriptional and posttranscriptional levels.

IGF-1 acts in an autocrine/paracrine and endocrine modes and is therefore secreted to the serum and delivered to distant tissues. Hepatocytes are the major source of secreted IGF-1, producing 75% of serum IGF-1.[1] In the liver *igf-1* gene expression is regulated mainly by pituitary gland-derived growth hormone (GH), although nutrition and insulin also affect its expression.[2] In turn, endocrine/serum IGF-1 regulates pituitary GH production through a negative feedback loop.[2] In extrahepatic tissues, *igf-1* gene expression is regulated by tissue-specific factors or by GH.[2] Igf-2 gene expression is GH-independent and is tightly regulated by parental imprinting.[3] In humans, igf-1 and igf-2 genes are expressed throughout life. However, although serum IGF-1 levels decrease after puberty, IGF-2 levels in serum remain high throughout adulthood and are 3.5-fold higher than IGF-1 levels.[2] In contrast, in rodents, IGF-2 is transcribed predominantly during fetal growth and its expression in the adult animal is hardly detectable, whereas IGF-1 is the major circulating ligand and does not decline in the adult animal.

[a] Department of Basic Science and Craniofacial Biology, David B. Kriser Dental Center, New York University College of Dentistry, New York, NY 10010-4086, USA; [b] Department of Biochemistry, University of Texas Health Science Center, San Antonio, TX 78229, USA
* Corresponding author.
E-mail address: sy1007@nyu.edu

Endocrinol Metab Clin N Am 41 (2012) 231–247
doi:10.1016/j.ecl.2012.04.008
0889-8529/12/$ – see front matter © 2012 Elsevier Inc. All rights reserved.

endo.theclinics.com

The effects of IGF-1 and IGF-2 on cellular behavior are mediated by the type 1 IGF receptor (IGF-1R), which conveys survival and mitogenic signals to the cell through a complex network of signaling mechanisms.[3] The IGF-1R is a membrane-bound tyrosine kinase heterotetramer. The intracellular domains convey adenosine triphosphate binding sites and are able to autophosphorylate tyrosine residues, which serve as the docking site for intracellular proteins, important for signal transduction.

IGF-1R shares 60% homology with the insulin receptors A and B (IR-A, IR-B) but differs in ligand specificity and affinity as well as in transmission of downstream signals.[4] Because both the IGF-1R and IR are closely related, they can form hybrid heterodimeric receptors consisting each of an insulin and IGF-IR α-β dimer, which mediate mainly IGF signaling.[4] The role of the hybrid receptors is not fully understood.

Binding of the IGFs to the IGF-1R results in autophosphorylation of tyrosines on the intracellular portion of the β-subunit. The phosphorylated tyrosines serve as docking sites for several substrates, including the IR substrates (IRS) 1 to 4 and Shc, which initiate phosphorylation cascades. IRS-1 activates the p85 regulatory subunit of phosphatidylinositol 3-kinase (PI3-K). leading to subsequent increase in membrane-bound phospholipid phosphatidyl insositol-3, 4, 5-triphosphate and the recruitment of phosphoinositide-dependent kinase 1 and Akt (or protein kinase B) to the membrane. There are 3 central effectors to the downstream signaling events triggered by Akt: the mammalian target of rapamycin (mTOR) complex 1 (mTORC1), forkhead transcription factors (FOXO), and glycogen synthase kinase 3 (GSK3). Activation of mTORC1 plays an important role in cell growth and survival by promoting nutrient uptake, storage of energy, and protein translation. This pathway has also been associated with IGF-1–mediated cell survival, proliferation, hypertrophy, and cell migration.[5–7] The FOXO proteins promote cell cycle arrest, apoptosis, oxidative stress, and the activation of gluconeogenic enzymes. Their phosphorylation and cytoplasmic retention is mediated by Akt and implicated in IGF-I–induced cell proliferation, survival, and hypertrophy.[6,8–10] The GSK3 protein, which is inhibited by Akt, increases glycogenesis and is also involved in the Wnt signaling pathway. Studies also suggest that GKS3 is involved in IGF-I–induced antiapoptotic and hypertrophic effects.[6,11,12] Apart from these pathways, Akt can also promote cell survival via the inactivating phosphorylation of the apoptotic protein Bad, and procaspase 9.[13,14]

The bioactivity of IGF is modulated by IGF-binding proteins (IGFBPs), which facilitate their stability in serum and extracellular matrices.[15,16] To date, 6 high-affinity IGFBPs have been characterized.[15,16] The expression and distribution of the IGFBPs are tissue dependent and modified with exercise,[17] surgery, pregnancy,[18] nutrition,[19] and aging.[20] During intrauterine growth, IGFs are found in binary complexes with IGFBPs, in which IGFBP-2 is the predominant binding protein in serum. However, during postnatal growth, 85% of the IGF pool is found in ternary complexes with IGFBP-3 and the acid-labile subunit (ALS), a protein that further stabilizes IGFs in serum.[15,16] Only a few (5%) of the IGFs are found free in serum and their roles are yet unclear. At target tissues, IGFBPs can either reduce or facilitate IGF-1 bioactivity.[15,16] On one hand, IGFBPs can limit access of IGF-1 to cell-surface IGF-1R, because IGFBPs have higher affinity for IGF-1 than the receptor. On the other hand, IGFBPs can act as reservoirs that slowly release the IGFs, allowing prolonged IGF action in local microenvironments. It has been reported that some IGFBPs have IGF-1–independent effects on cells.[15,16]

IGF-1 SYSTEM IN NORMAL PHYSIOLOGY

IGF-1 plays a pivotal role in fetal development, adolescent growth, and adult tissue homeostasis. Together with insulin and GH, IGFs regulate glucose and lipid metabolism, and thereby regulate body composition. Imbalance in IGF production or function is associated with various pathologic conditions, including short stature, insufficient skeletal acquisition, alterations in body composition (lean and fat mass), impairments in reproduction, reduced mental and physical capacity associated with aging, and metabolic disorders. With the development of gene-targeting approaches in animals in the last 2 decades, the roles of the IGF system in normal physiology and disease have become more explicable. The next sections review the effects of the IGF system on musculoskeletal development, reproduction, metabolism, and longevity, as learned from mouse models of IGFs.

Body Size

Animal models of IGF deficiency have confirmed its critical role in embryogenesis and postnatal growth. IGF-1 null mice show marked growth retardation in utero and post-natally. These mice are 65% of normal weight at birth and most die shortly after birth.[21–23] Survivors do not undergo a peripubertal growth spurt and have only 30% of the body weight of wild-type animals as adults. IGF-2 null mice are also growth impaired but their growth retardation occurs exclusively in utero, whereas their post-natal growth is normal,[21] indicating that in mice only IGF-1 is critical postnatally. Like-wise, IGF-1 receptor null mice weigh 55% of wild-type littermates and die within a few hours after birth because of respiratory failure. These mice show organ hypoplasia,[21] lung, skin, bone, and neurologic defects.[21,23] Taken together, the IGF-1R null mice established this receptor as an essential regulator of organogenesis. Contrary to models of IGF deficiency, IGF-1 transgenic mice showed significant increases in body weight and organomegaly caused by tissue hyperplasia.

Studies in mice lacking the different IGFBPs show modest deficiencies in somatic growth (10%–20% decreases in body weight), mostly attributed to decreased IGF levels in serum and decreases in IGF stability in tissues. A triple knockout of IGFBP-3, IGFBP-4, and IGFBP-5, the main IGFBPs present in serum, resulted in only 22% reductions in body weight, despite 65% decreases in serum IGF-1 levels.[24] Similarly, gene inactivation of the ALS, which stabilizes the binary complex of IGF-1 and IGFBP-3 or IGFBP-5, resulted in a ~10% to 20% decrease in body weight.[25,26] Reduced IGF-1 bioavailability was reported in transgenic mice with ubiquitous expression of IGFBPs and the ALS. Overexpression of ALS resulted in reduced body weight gains during the first 3 weeks of growth and significantly reduced body weights through puberty.[27] Global overexpression of IGFBP-1, IGFBP-2, IGFBP-3, or IGFBP-5 also resulted in growth retardation.[24,28–32] A study published by Stratikopoulos and colleagues[33] showed that serum IGF-1 contributes to approximately 30% of the adult body size; therefore the inhibitory effect seen in the IGFBP transgenic mice likely result from inhibition of IGF action in both serum and tissues.

In conjunction with IGF mutagenesis studies, 2 IGF analogues that have a significant reduction in affinity for the IGFBPs but retain normal affinity for the IGF-1 receptor were described: R3-IGF-1[34–36] and Des1-3-IGF-1.[37–40] The R3-IGF-1 mutant has a Glu to Arg substitution at position 3 of the IGF-1 peptide and the Des1-3-IGF-1, has a 3 amino acid truncation at the amino terminus. Both mutants have several times lower affinity to IGFBP-3 than native IGF-1 and show greatly reduced binding to all other IGFBPs.[41–44] Introduction of these 2 mutations to mouse models via knockin resulted in enhanced somatic growth, which was attributed to increased IGF-1 bioavailability in tissues.[45,46] Together, studies of IGFBP knockout and the Des/R3 knockin mouse models support the notion that IGFBPs serve as reservoirs that release and control IGF action in tissues.

Skeletal Acquisition

Growth of long bones occurs at the growth plate, which is a highly complex, spatially polarized structure. GH and IGF-1 regulate longitudinal bone growth via their action on chondrocytes within the growth plate.[47] Excess of GH or IGF accelerates chondrogenesis, enhances linear growth, and inactivates mutations in the GH, IGF, or the GH receptor (GHR), in both human and animal models, retard linear bone growth.[48] In Snell dwarf (dw/dw) mice, deletion of the *pit-1* transcription factor resulted in a loss of GH production and reduced bone length as a result of reductions in cartilage hypertrophy and delayed epiphyseal ossification.[49–51] Likewise, in the Ames dwarf mouse (dt/dt), deletion of the prop-1, an upstream regulator of pit-1, resulted in reductions in lean mass, bone area, and bone mineral content.[52,53] GH binds to its receptor, the GHR, which mediates its effects via the Janus kinase/signal transducer and activator of transcription 5 (STAT5) pathway. Ablation of STAT5 in mice led to reduced bone length in a manner similar to Ames and Snell dwarf mice, although this effect was mainly apparent in male mice.[54] Similarly, total inactivation of the *igf-1* gene resulted in a severe bone phenotype with shortened femoral length, increased chondrocyte apoptosis, and 25% reduction in cortical bone size.[55] IGF-1 actions on the skeleton are mediated via the IGF-1R, the main effectors of which are the insulin-receptor substrate 1 and 2 (IRS-1, IRS-2). IRS-1 or IRS-2 null mice showed growth retardation, low bone mineral density (BMD), reduced cortical and trabecular thickness, and low bone formation rates.[56]

Skeletal acquisition depends not only on the total levels of IGF-1 but also on its bioavailability. Overexpression of the different IGFBPs[24,28–32] or the ALS protein[27] resulted in decreases in cortical bone density, cortical bone volume, cortical thickness, and decreases in cancellous bone. Ablation of IGFBP-2[57] or IGFBP-4,[24] or the ALS protein,[25] also resulted in osteopenic phenotype, likely because of increases in IGF-1 degradation and consequent reductions in its bioavailability.

IGF-1 exerts its effects on skeletal acquisition in an endocrine and autocrine/paracrine manner. Studies from inbred mouse strains showed correlations between serum IGF-1 levels and skeletal acquisition. Mouse strains with low IGF-1 (C57BL/6J) have reduced total BMD and cortical thickness, whereas mice with higher serum IGF-1 levels (C3H/HeJ) show increased total BMD and femoral cortical thickness.[58] In addition, congenic mice (B6.C3H.6T) with a 40% reduction in serum IGF-I also had reduced BMD and delayed development.[59] We have generated a mouse model in which the *igf-1* gene was ablated specifically in the liver.[60] Liver IGF-1–deficient (LID) mice had 75% decreases in serum IGF-1 levels, with minor decreases (~5%) in body length. Skeletal characterization of the LID mice throughout development revealed no alterations in cancellous bone, but significant decreases in femoral total area and cortical area, resulting in slender bones with reduced stiffness and reduced strength in bending.[61] Thus, reductions in serum IGF-1 tended to target cortical bone by preventing periosteal apposition during growth. Marrow area was not altered during early growth and decreased relative to controls from 16 to 32 weeks of age (endosteal infilling). In contrast, increased IGF-1 levels in serum in mice expressing hepatocyte-specific rat IGF-1 transgene (HIT) led to increases in body weight, body length, and femoral length, as well as femoral total area, cortical area, cortical thickness, and robustness.[45,46]

To better understand the role of IGF-1 in bone accrual and maintenance, a tissue-specific gene-targeting approach was used. Ablation of the *igf-1* gene in chondrocytes resulted in significant reductions in body weight, body length, total BMD, and femoral width and length beginning at 4 weeks of age in both genders.[62] Similarly, conditional deletion of IGF-1 in cells expressing type 1 α_2 collagen (skeletal muscle and bone) resulted in 35% reductions in body weight, and ~20% reductions in femur areal BMD.[63] In addition, mineralization was reduced starting at embryonic development as a result of impaired osteoblast function.[63] Tissue-specific modulation of IGF-1 action was also achieved by expression of IGFBPs. IGFBP-4 overexpression in osteoblasts resulted in decreased femoral cortical density, cortical thickness, and periosteal circumference in both genders.[64] Mice expressing IGFBP-5 under the osteocalcin promoter showed decreased BMD, trabecular bone volume, and bone formation as well as mineralization defects indicated by a reduced mineral/matrix ratio in cortical bone and reduced collagen maturity in secondary ossification centers.[65] Because IGF-1 exerts its effects in an endocrine and autocrine/paracrine manner, to better understand its role in osteoblast and osteoclast function, it was necessary to ablate the IGF-1 receptor (rather than the ligand) in a cell-specific manner, to avoid its activation regardless of the IGF-1 source. When IGF-1 receptor was disrupted specifically in osteoblasts, no alterations in body size or femoral length were noted, but matrix mineralization was impaired, as shown by increased osteoid volume and osteoid surface.[66] This study was crucial to establishing the role of IGF-1 in bone mineralization. In contrast, increased expression of IGF-1 specifically in osteoblasts increased femur length, cortical width, and cross-sectional area and enhanced bone formation and mineralization.[67]

Animal models have established that IGF-1 has a fundamental role in determination of bone accrual.[68] We now know that loss of serum IGF-1 affects mainly postpubertal bone accrual. Specifically, serum IGF-1 regulates transversal bone growth and periosteal bone apposition. In contrast, loss of tissue IGF-1 affects early postnatal and prepubertal growth. These studies also showed that the IGF-1 axis in osteoblasts is a strong regulator of bone mineralization.

Muscle Gain and Maintenance

IGF-1 and IGF-2 play key roles in skeletal muscle accrual during development, muscle maintenance, and aging, as well as during muscle injury. Mice deficient in IGF-2 or the IGF-1R show muscle hypoplasia, whereas mice with transgenic IGF-1 expression specifically in muscle display increased muscle mass and enhanced muscle strength.[69] Accordingly, mice that overexpress a skeletal-muscle–specific, dominant negative IGF-IR (MKR mice) have impaired muscle growth, reduced fiber cross-sectional area, and muscle wet weights, relative to control mice.[70]

In vivo studies have shown that IGF-1–induced muscle hypertrophy results from activation and proliferation of muscle satellite cells. IGFs ameliorated the aging/dystrophic muscle phenotype of the *mdx* mice,[71] likely because of increased satellite cell proliferation. Furthermore, in aged mice overexpressing IGF-1, centralized nuclei expressing neonatal myosin heavy chain (an indication of regenerating myofibers) have been identified.[72] The roles of IGF-1 in regulation of cell cycle have been established in various cell lines. Studies have shown that IGF-1 stimulates progression from G1 to S phase via downregulation of the p27Kip1 inhibitor. Accordingly, satellite cells harvested from the muscle of transgenic mice overexpressing IGF-1 under the α-actin promoter showed a 5-fold increase in proliferative capacity, relative to that of controls.[73] Furthermore, administration of IGF-1 to muscle of aged mice inhibited p27Kip1 in satellite cells.[73]

The cellular and molecular mechanisms by which IGFs facilitate muscle growth, differentiation, and maintenance were shown in experimental systems of muscle regeneration. After acute muscle injury, local IGF-1 production is increased (with no alterations in systemic IGF-1 levels) and promotes muscle repair via stimulation of myogenic cell proliferation and survival through activation of the phosphatidylinositol 3-kinase (PI3K) and the mitogen-activated protein kinase (MAPK) pathways.[74] In addition, IGF-1 promotes nerve sprouting and has a protective effect against nerve degeneration.[75–78] Thus, improved outcomes of IGF-1–induced muscle regeneration may also result from its effects on muscle reinnervation during the repair process. Likewise, aged mice treated with IGF-1 have thicker neurons with increased branches compared with those of aged controls.[79]

Paradoxically, IGF stimulates two mutually exclusive cellular responses, namely mitogenesis and myogenesis (differentiation), through activation of the IGF-1R. The intuitive question that arises is: how do cells select their response to IGF signal? A recent study with primary myocytes and the C2C12 muscle cell line showed that IGF-1 mediates different cellular responses under normoxic and hypoxic conditions.[80] Under normoxia, IGF activates the Akt-mTOR, p38, and extracellular signal-regulated kinase (Erk1/2) MAPK pathways. However, hypoxia suppresses basal and IGF-induced Akt-mTOR and p38 activity and enhances and prolongs IGF-induced Erk1/2 activation in a hypoxia-inducible factor 1-dependent fashion. This finding implies that during acute injury and hypoxic conditions, IGF-1 induces satellite cell proliferation, an early response important in the regenerative process. Physiologically, it is suggested that cells integrate IGF-1R activation with oxygen availability and respond accordingly.

IGF-1 in muscle plays a critical in promoting hypertrophy as well as in the response to muscle damage and subsequent regeneration. IGF-1 signals to both satellite cells and myofibers, and its distinct effects in muscle likely depend on oxygen tension.

Reproduction

Female reproduction in mammals is a complex process, which involves many developmental steps and cell-cell communication. Endocrine, paracrine, and autocrine action of steroid hormones and growth factors from systemic or local origin coordinate the primary follicle, preantral, and antral follicle development and ovulation.[81] IGF-1 plays an important role in cellular differentiation and reproductive function.[82]

Studies in animal models have shown that IGFs and insulin augment the action of gonadotropins in the control of ovarian steroidogenesis and follicular maturation. In synergy with gonadotropins and other growth factor families such as TGF (transforming growth factor) superfamily members, the IGF system participates in the selection of the dominant follicle[83] and subsequent development into the Graafian follicle,[84–86] as well as in the processes of ovulation,[87] corpus luteum formation,[88] and atresia of nondominant follicles.[89] Animal studies have shown the interaction between intraovarian/intrafollicular IGF system and follicle-stimulating hormone (FSH) action in granulosa cells. IGF-1 regulates antrum formation and synergizes FSH action by increasing the aromatase activity in granulosa cells.[90–93]

IGF-1 is selectively expressed in the granulosa cells of developing follicles and is critical for normal reproductive function in mice,[94,95] whereas the IGF-1R is expressed in both the granulosa cells and in oocytes of murine and human follicles, suggesting a potential paracrine action of IGF-1.[93,96] IGF-1 stimulates the proliferation and differentiation of granulosa cells[97] and promotes maturation of follicles and denuded human and mouse oocytes in vitro.[98] Ablation of the igf-1 -gene in mice leads to infertility characterized by follicular arrest at the late preantral stage,[93,99] suggesting an essential role of IGF-1 during folliculogenesis.

IGF bioavailability in the ovary is regulated by IGFBPs,[100] which have inhibitory roles in regulating IGF-1 actions.[101–103] Mice overexpressing the IGFBP-1 under the control of the α1-antitrypsin promoter show reduced ovulation rate, possibly associated with impairment in IGF-1 action on follicular cells as well as altered gonadotropin-releasing hormone and luteinizing hormone (LH) secretions.[101] In addition, transgenic mice that overexpress IGFBP-5,[103] IGFBP-3[102] driven by the mouse phosphoglycerate kinase I, or the cytomegalovirus (CMV) promoters show reduced litter size. Likewise, transgenic mice that overexpress the ALS driven by CMV promoter show significant reductions in litter size,[27] likely as a result of sequestration of IGF-1 and severe reductions in its bioavailability. Knockout of the pregnancy-associated plasma protein-A, a metalloprotease that cleaves the IGFBP4 in the ovary, showed an overall reduction in litter size, reduced number of ovulated oocytes, and reduced expression of ovarian steroidogenic enzyme.[104]

IGF and insulin signaling pathways in the central nervous system (CNS) have been also implicated in female reproductive function, and specific ablation of their cognitive receptors (in nestin-positive cells) showed impaired follicular maturation, likely because of hypothalamic dysregulation of LH.[105] However, oocyte-specific ablation of the IR, IGF-1R, or both[98] showed normal female reproductive functions reflected by normal estrous cyclicity, oocyte development and maturation, parturition frequency, and litter size. IGF-1 and IRs in the CNS regulate the gonadotroph axis, whereas in the ovary their presence in granulosa cells plays a major role in oocyte function. Studies have suggested that intrafollicular IGF-1 is a determinant of follicular selection and dominance, and it is the net bioavailability of intrafollicular IGF-1 that may distinguish follicles destined to ovulate from those that succumb to atresia.[85,93]

Metabolic Homeostasis

Insulin is the principle regulator of carbohydrate and lipid metabolism.[106] However, its interactions with the GH/IGF axis also contribute to metabolic homeostasis. The interplay between GH and insulin is well documented[48] and is not within the scope of this review. GH antagonizes insulin action in liver and peripheral tissues, and it increases hepatic glucose production via stimulation of gluconeogenesis and glycogenolysis. Moreover, GH decreases glucose uptake by muscle, and stimulates lipolysis and free fatty acid secretion, which subsequently antagonize insulin action. In animal models with reduced IGF-1 in serum, such as the LID mice, GH is increased because of an impaired negative feedback at the level of the pituitary, leading to hyperinsulinemia, deterioration of insulin action, and impaired carbohydrate metabolism.[107,108]

In the early 1990s, with the availability of recombinant IGF-1, various groups studied the potency of recombinant IGF-1 to cure patients with severe insulin resistance.[109] These studies showed that a bolus injection of recombinant IGF-1 could reduce both insulin and blood glucose levels. IGF-1 therapy lasted for 1 to 16 months,[110–114] and although it consistently reduced glucose and insulin levels, the very high doses of IGF-1 caused adverse complications such as muscle pain, fluid retention, benign intercranial hypertension, and worsening retinopathy. Also, because of the tight regulation of the GH/IGF-1 axis, interpretation of the results from these studies is difficult because, in addition to its insulin-like effects, IGF-1 also inhibits GH secretion. Yet, with the development of tissue-specific gene targeting, we were able to show that in a mouse model with decreased serum IGF-1 and increased GH (LID mouse), inhibition of GH restored insulin sensitivity, suggesting that GH (and not IGF-1) plays a major role in modulating insulin action.[107,108] In addition, in a mouse model with 2-fold to 3-fold increases in serum IGF-1 levels (HIT mice), in which GH levels were similar to those of control mice, we found that insulin sensitivity was not enhanced but was comparable with controls.[115] Nonetheless, in a clinical study with acromegalic patients treated with a GH antagonist (pegvisomant), insulin sensitivity was improved, but further improvement was observed when a combined treatment of pegvisomant and IGF-1 was given,[116] suggesting that IGF-1 exerts additional effects on insulin sensitivity that are not mediated by suppression of GH secretion.

IGF-1R is not expressed in adult liver or adipose tissue and therefore IGF-1–mediated metabolic effects originate from other insulin-responsive tissues. Likewise, disruption of the IGF-1R in β cells resulted in a defect in insulin secretion and subsequent insulin resistance.[117,118] Similarly, IGF-1 plays important roles in the central control of peripheral metabolism. Intracerebroventricular infusion of exogenous IGF-1 increases liver sensitivity to insulin.[119] Nonetheless, neuronal-specific IGF-1R inactivation in mice shows no metabolic phenotype, but showed low serum GH levels.[120] Muscle-specific IGF-1R inactivation did not result in metabolic phenotype, although inactivation of cardiac IGF-1R resulted in impaired exercise-induced cardiac hypertrophy.[121] However, inactivation of both IGF-1R and IRs in muscle via overexpression of a dominant negative IGF-1R resulted in adverse insulin resistance and diabetes.[122]

Insulin, GH, and IGF-1 cointeract to establish controlled carbohydrate and lipid metabolism. IGF-1 has insulin-like effects when given exogenously in high concentrations. However, the role of physiologic IGF-1 is less clear because of its tight regulation by GH.

Insulin/IGF-1 Signaling and the Health Span

One of the most paradoxic recent developments in insulin and IGF-1 signaling (IIS) research has been observations that reduction in IIS extends life span. Studies in Caenorhabditis elegans indicate that down-mutations in daf2 and AGE, which encode orthologs of the mammalian insulin/IGF-1 receptor and PI3K, respectively, extend life span. Moreover, inactivating mutations in daf16, which encode an ortholog of the mammalian FOXO transcription factor, prevent daf2 and AGE mutants from extending life span. PI3K normally phosphorylates and inhibits the activity of FOXO, which promotes the transcription of genes mediating resistance to stress, such as superoxide dismutase, thus providing a mechanistic explanation of how reduced IIS could increase health span.[123] Similar findings have been made in the other major invertebrate model of aging, Drosophila melanogaster.[124]

An obvious question is whether disruption of mammalian IIS produces increased health span by a similar mechanism. Calorie restriction (CR) and deficiency of GH or the GHR produce robust increases in life span and resistance to stress in mice.[125] Because caloric restricted and GH-deficient/GH-resistant dwarfs have decreased levels of serum insulin and IGF-1,[126–128] it has long been postulated that reduced IIS mediates the life-span–extending effects of CR and GH deficiency/resistance. However, recent studies suggest that GH deficiency increases stress resistance via upregulation of the Nrf2 transcription factor,[129] and that serum IGF-1 deficiency impedes expression of Nrf-2,[130] suggesting that increased protection against oxidative stress is a function of reduced GH per se. Moreover, reduced serum IGF-1 in LID mice extends median, but not maximal, life span[131] and thus does not phenocopy CR or GH deficiency/resistance. Studies examining disruption of IIS signaling per se have indicated that loss of the fat cell IR increases life span,[132] as does loss of IRS-1 in female mice,[133] p66 Shc,[134] and p70S6K.[135] However, the mechanisms of these effects are unclear. For example, GH-deficient/GH-resistant mice show enhanced insulin sensitivity, whereas fat cell IR knockouts and whole body p70S6K deficiency results in resistance to obesity.[132,136] IRS-1 null mice show lifelong insulin resistance, but are protected against the development of age-related glucose intolerance presumably because of increased pancreatic insulin content, which could result in increase in insulin secretion to compensate for the insulin resistance.[133] GH-deficient/GH-resistant mice have an opposite metabolic phenotype: they are glucose intolerant as a result of sluggish insulin release, but are more insulin sensitive, which presumably protects them from fasting hyperglycemia.[126,127] Thus, paradoxically, loss of GH/IIS signaling in these models may lead to certain metabolic advantages. Moreover, p66Shc may impede IIS[137]; thus loss of p66Shc may enhance IIS rather than disrupting it.

Disruption of the IGF-1 receptor has yielded mixed results. In 1 study,[138] heterozygous loss of 1 IGF-1R allele extended life span by ~30% in females (significant) and ~16% in males (insignificant). However, the overall survival of the wild-type 129 mice used in this study was 19 months, which is significantly shorter than expected in this strain.[139] When these studies were conducted on the C57Bl/6J background in conditions that resulted in robust (ie, >30 months) median survival of the wild-type control, life span was extended by only 6% in female Igf1r +/− mice and was not increased in males.[140] In both studies, there was evidence for resistance to oxidative stress. Because the IGF-1 heterozygous mutation protects against the development of Alzheimer disease in a mouse model,[141] it is possible that IGF-1R deficiency protects against stressors. However, the Igf1r +/− mouse develops age-related insulin resistance in females, resulting in increased sensitivity to insulin resistance and glucose intolerance induced by a high-fat diet.[142] Moreover, a brain-specific knockout of the IGF-1R produced increased median, but not maximal, life span.[120] Interpretation of these results was confounded by decreased serum GH in this model. Thus, overall, it is unclear to what extent and how reduced IIS may increase mammalian health span.

REFERENCES

1. Adamo ML, Neuenschwander S, LeRoith D, et al. Structure, expression, and regulation of the IGF-I gene. Adv Exp Med Biol 1993;343:1–11.
2. Frystyk J, Skjaerbaek C, Dinesen B, et al. Free insulin-like growth factors (IGF-I and IGF-II) in human serum. FEBS Lett 1994;348:185–91.
3. Werner H, Bruchim I. The insulin-like growth factor-I receptor as an oncogene. Arch Physiol Biochem 2009;115:58–71.
4. Werner H, Weinstein D, Bentov I. Similarities and differences between insulin and IGF-I: structures, receptors, and signalling pathways. Arch Physiol Biochem 2008;114:17–22.
5. Finlay D, Cantrell D. Phosphoinositide 3-kinase and the mammalian target of rapamycin pathways control T cell migration. Ann N Y Acad Sci 2010;1183: 149–57.
6. Leger B, Cartoni R, Praz M, et al. Akt signalling through GSK-3beta, mTOR and Foxo1 is involved in human skeletal muscle hypertrophy and atrophy. J Physiol 2006;576:923–33.
7. Park IH, Erbay E, Nuzzi P, et al. Skeletal myocyte hypertrophy requires mTOR kinase activity and S6K1. Exp Cell Res 2005;309:211–9.
8. Burgering BM, Medema RH. Decisions on life and death: FOXO forkhead transcription factors are in command when PKB/Akt is off duty. J Leukoc Biol 2003;73:689–701.
9. Elia L, Contu R, Quintavalle M, et al. Reciprocal regulation of microRNA-1 and insulin-like growth factor-1 signal transduction cascade in cardiac and skeletal muscle in physiological and pathological conditions. Circulation 2009;120: 2377–85.
10. Stitt TN, Drujan D, Clarke BA, et al. The IGF-1/PI3K/Akt pathway prevents expression of muscle atrophy-induced ubiquitin ligases by inhibiting FOXO transcription factors. Mol Cell 2004;14:395–403.

11. Schakman O, Kalista S, Bertrand L, et al. Role of Akt/GSK-3beta/beta-catenin transduction pathway in the muscle anti-atrophy action of insulin-like growth factor-I in glucocorticoid-treated rats. Endocrinology 2008;149:3900–8.

12. Vyas DR, Spangenburg EE, Abraha TW, et al. GSK-3beta negatively regulates skeletal myotube hypertrophy. Am J Physiol Cell Physiol 2002;283:C545–51.

13. Pang Y, Zheng B, Fan LW, et al. IGF-1 protects oligodendrocyte progenitors against TNFalpha-induced damage by activation of PI3K/Akt and interruption of the mitochondrial apoptotic pathway. Glia 2007;55:1099–107.

14. Tseng YH, Ueki K, Kriauciunas KM, et al. Differential roles of insulin receptor substrates in the anti-apoptotic function of insulin-like growth factor-1 and insulin. J Biol Chem 2002;277:31601–11.

15. Baxter RC. Insulin-like growth factor (IGF)-binding proteins: interactions with IGFs and intrinsic bioactivities. Am J Physiol Endocrinol Metab 2000;278:E967–76.

16. Mohan S, Baylink DJ. IGF-binding proteins are multifunctional and act via IGF-dependent and -independent mechanisms. J Endocrinol 2002;175:19–31.

17. Wakai K, Suzuki K, Ito Y, et al. Time spent walking or exercising and blood levels of insulin-like growth factor-I (IGF-I) and IGF-binding protein-3 (IGFBP-3): a large-scale cross-sectional study in the Japan Collaborative Cohort study. Asian Pac J Cancer Prev 2009;10(Suppl):23–7.

18. Forbes K, Westwood M. The IGF axis and placental function. A mini review. Horm Res 2008;69:129–37.

19. Kaaks R. Nutrition, insulin, IGF-1 metabolism and cancer risk: a summary of epidemiological evidence. Novartis Found Symp 2004;262:247–60 [discussion: 260–8].

20. Frystyk J. Aging somatotropic axis: mechanisms and implications of insulin-like growth factor-related binding protein adaptation. Endocrinol Metab Clin North Am 2005;34:865–76, viii.

21. Baker J, Liu JP, Robertson EJ, et al. Role of insulin-like growth factors in embryonic and postnatal growth. Cell 1993;75:73–82.

22. Liu JL, Grinberg A, Westphal H, et al. Insulin-like growth factor-I affects perinatal lethality and postnatal development in a gene dosage-dependent manner: manipulation using the Cre/loxP system in transgenic mice. Mol Endocrinol 1998;12:1452–62.

23. Powell-Braxton L, Hollingshead P, Warburton C, et al. IGF-I is required for normal embryonic growth in mice. Genes Dev 1993;7:2609–17.

24. Ning Y, Schuller AG, Bradshaw S, et al. Diminished growth and enhanced glucose metabolism in triple knockout mice containing mutations of insulin-like growth factor binding protein-3, -4, and -5. Mol Endocrinol 2006;20:2173–86.

25. Courtland HW, DeMambro V, Maynard J, et al. Sex-specific regulation of body size and bone slenderness by the acid labile subunit. J Bone Miner Res 2010;25:2059–68.

26. Yakar S, Rosen CJ, Bouxsein ML, et al. Serum complexes of insulin-like growth factor-1 modulate skeletal integrity and carbohydrate metabolism. FASEB J 2009;23:709–19.

27. Silha JV, Gui Y, Modric T, et al. Overexpression of the acid-labile subunit of the IGF ternary complex in transgenic mice. Endocrinology 2001;142:4305–13.

28. Ben Lagha N, Seurin D, Le Bouc Y, et al. Insulin-like growth factor binding protein (IGFBP-1) involvement in intrauterine growth retardation: study on IGFBP-1 overexpressing transgenic mice. Endocrinology 2006;147:4730–7.

29. Eckstein F, Pavicic T, Nedbal S, et al. Insulin-like growth factor-binding protein-2 (IGFBP-2) overexpression negatively regulates bone size and mass, but not

density, in the absence and presence of growth hormone/IGF-I excess in transgenic mice. Anat Embryol (Berl) 2002;206:139–48.

30. Hoeflich A, Wu M, Mohan S, et al. Overexpression of insulin-like growth factor-binding protein-2 in transgenic mice reduces postnatal body weight gain. Endocrinology 1999;140:5488–96.

31. Salih DA, Mohan S, Kasukawa Y, et al. Insulin-like growth factor-binding protein-5 induces a gender-related decrease in bone mineral density in transgenic mice. Endocrinology 2005;146:931–40.

32. Silha JV, Mishra S, Rosen CJ, et al. Perturbations in bone formation and resorption in insulin-like growth factor binding protein-3 transgenic mice. J Bone Miner Res 2003;18:1834–41.

33. Stratikopoulos E, Szabolcs M, Dragatsis I, et al. The hormonal action of IGF1 in postnatal mouse growth. Proc Natl Acad Sci U S A 2008;105:19378–83.

34. Coolican SA, Samuel DS, Ewton DZ, et al. The mitogenic and myogenic actions of insulin-like growth factors utilize distinct signaling pathways. J Biol Chem 1997;272:6653–62.

35. Flint DJ, Tonner E, Beattie J, et al. Several insulin-like growth factor-I analogues and complexes of insulin-like growth factors-I and -II with insulin-like growth factor-binding protein-3 fail to mimic the effect of growth hormone upon lactation in the rat. J Endocrinol 1994;140:211–6.

36. McCusker RH, Kaleko M, Sackett RL. Multivalent cations and ligand affinity of the type 1 insulin-like growth factor receptor on P2A2-LISN muscle cells. J Cell Physiol 1998;176:392–401.

37. Ballard FJ, Francis GL, Ross M, et al. Natural and synthetic forms of insulin-like growth factor-1 (IGF-1) and the potent derivative, destripeptide IGF-1: biological activities and receptor binding. Biochem Biophys Res Commun 1987;149:398–404.

38. Ballard FJ, Ross M, Upton FM, et al. Specific binding of insulin-like growth factors 1 and 2 to the type 1 and type 2 receptors respectively. Biochem J 1988;249:721–6.

39. Ross M, Francis GL, Szabo L, et al. Insulin-like growth factor (IGF)-binding proteins inhibit the biological activities of IGF-1 and IGF-2 but not des-(1-3)-IGF-1. Biochem J 1989;258:267–72.

40. Szabo L, Mottershead DG, Ballard FJ, et al. The bovine insulin-like growth factor (IGF) binding protein purified from conditioned medium requires the N-terminal tripeptide in IGF-1 for binding. Biochem Biophys Res Commun 1988;151:207–14.

41. Bayne ML, Applebaum J, Underwood D, et al. The C region of human insulin-like growth factor (IGF) I is required for high affinity binding to the type 1 IGF receptor. J Biol Chem 1989;264:11004–8.

42. Gillespie C, Read LC, Bagley CJ, et al. Enhanced potency of truncated insulin-like growth factor-I (des(1-3)IGF-I) relative to IGF-I in lit/lit mice. J Endocrinol 1990;127:401–5.

43. King R, Wells JR, Krieg P, et al. Production and characterization of recombinant insulin-like growth factor-I (IGF-I) and potent analogues of IGF-I, with Gly or Arg substituted for Glu3, following their expression in *Escherichia coli* as fusion proteins. J Mol Endocrinol 1992;8:29–41.

44. Lemmey AB, Martin AA, Read LC, et al. IGF-I and the truncated analogue des-(1-3)IGF-I enhance growth in rats after gut resection. Am J Physiol 1991; 260:E213–9.

45. Elis S, Courtland HW, Wu Y, et al. Elevated serum levels of IGF-1 are sufficient to establish normal body size and skeletal properties even in the absence of tissue IGF-1. J Bone Miner Res 2010;25:1257–66.

46. Elis S, Wu Y, Courtland HW, et al. Unbound (bioavailable) IGF1 enhances somatic growth. Dis Model Mech 2011;4:649–58.

47. Nilsson O, Marino R, De Luca F, et al. Endocrine regulation of the growth plate. Horm Res 2005;64:157–65.

48. List EO, Sackmann-Sala L, Berryman DE, et al. Endocrine parameters and phenotypes of the growth hormone receptor gene disrupted (GHR-/-) mouse. Endocr Rev 2011;32:356–86.

49. Li S, Crenshaw EB 3rd, Rawson EJ, et al. Dwarf locus mutants lacking three pituitary cell types result from mutations in the POU-domain gene pit-1. Nature 1990;347:528–33.

50. Lighten AD, Hardy K, Winston RM, et al. IGF2 is parentally imprinted in human preimplantation embryos. Nat Genet 1997;15:122–3.

51. van Buul-Offers S, Smeets T, Van den Brande JL. Effects of growth hormone and thyroxine on the relation between tibial length and the histological appearance of the proximal tibial epiphysis in Snell dwarf mice. Growth 1984;48:166–75.

52. Andersen B, Pearse RV 2nd, Jenne K, et al. The Ames dwarf gene is required for Pit-1 gene activation. Dev Biol 1995;172:495–503.

53. Heiman ML, Tinsley FC, Mattison JA, et al. Body composition of prolactin-, growth hormone, and thyrotropin-deficient Ames dwarf mice. Endocrine 2003; 20:149–54.

54. Udy GB, Towers RP, Snell RG, et al. Requirement of STAT5b for sexual dimorphism of body growth rates and liver gene expression. Proc Natl Acad Sci U S A 1997;94:7239–44.

55. Wang Y, Nishida S, Sakata T, et al. Insulin-like growth factor-I is essential for embryonic bone development. Endocrinology 2006;147:4753–61.

56. DeMambro VE, Kawai M, Clemens TL, et al. A novel spontaneous mutation of Irs1 in mice results in hyperinsulinemia, reduced growth, low bone mass and impaired adipogenesis. J Endocrinol 2010;204:241–53.

57. DeMambro VE, Clemmons DR, Horton LG, et al. Gender-specific changes in bone turnover and skeletal architecture in igfbp-2-null mice. Endocrinology 2008;149:2051–61.

58. Bouxsein ML, Rosen CJ, Turner CH, et al. Generation of a new congenic mouse strain to test the relationships among serum insulin-like growth factor I, bone mineral density, and skeletal morphology in vivo. J Bone Miner Res 2002;17:570–9.

59. Turner CH, Sun Q, Schriefer J, et al. Congenic mice reveal sex-specific genetic regulation of femoral structure and strength. Calcif Tissue Int 2003;73:297–303.

60. Yakar S, Liu JL, Stannard B, et al. Normal growth and development in the absence of hepatic insulin-like growth factor I. Proc Natl Acad Sci U S A 1999;96:7324–9.

61. Yakar S, Canalis E, Sun H, et al. Serum IGF-1 determines skeletal strength by regulating subperiosteal expansion and trait interactions. J Bone Miner Res 2009;24:1481–92.

62. Govoni KE, Lee SK, Chung YS, et al. Disruption of insulin-like growth factor-I expression in type IIalpha1 collagen-expressing cells reduces bone length and width in mice. Physiol Genomics 2007;30:354–62.

63. Govoni KE, Wergedal JE, Florin L, et al. Conditional deletion of insulin-like growth factor-I in collagen type 1alpha2-expressing cells results in postnatal lethality and a dramatic reduction in bone accretion. Endocrinology 2007;148:5706–15.

64. Zhang M, Faugere MC, Malluche H, et al. Paracrine overexpression of IGFBP-4 in osteoblasts of transgenic mice decreases bone turnover and causes global growth retardation. J Bone Miner Res 2003;18:836–43.

65. Atti E, Boskey AL, Canalis E. Overexpression of IGF-binding protein 5 alters mineral and matrix properties in mouse femora: an infrared imaging study. Calcif Tissue Int 2005;76:187–93.
66. Zhang M, Xuan S, Bouxsein ML, et al. Osteoblast-specific knockout of the insulin-like growth factor (IGF) receptor gene reveals an essential role of IGF signaling in bone matrix mineralization. J Biol Chem 2002;277: 44005–12.
67. Jiang J, Lichtler AC, Gronowicz GA, et al. Transgenic mice with osteoblast-targeted insulin-like growth factor-I show increased bone remodeling. Bone 2006;39:494–504.
68. Yakar S, Courtland HW, Clemmons D. IGF-1 and bone: new discoveries from mouse models. J Bone Miner Res 2010;25:2543–52.
69. Mathews LS, Hammer RE, Behringer RR, et al. Growth enhancement of transgenic mice expressing human insulin-like growth factor I. Endocrinology 1988; 123:2827–33.
70. Kim H, Barton E, Muja N, et al. Intact insulin and insulin-like growth factor-I receptor signaling is required for growth hormone effects on skeletal muscle growth and function in vivo. Endocrinology 2005;146:1772–9.
71. Schertzer JD, van der Poel C, Shavlakadze T, et al. Muscle-specific overexpression of IGF-I improves E-C coupling in skeletal muscle fibers from dystrophic mdx mice. Am J Physiol Cell Physiol 2008;294:C161–8.
72. Musaro A, McCullagh K, Paul A, et al. Localized Igf-1 transgene expression sustains hypertrophy and regeneration in senescent skeletal muscle. Nat Genet 2001;27:195–200.
73. Chakravarthy MV, Abraha TW, Schwartz RJ, et al. Insulin-like growth factor-I extends in vitro replicative life span of skeletal muscle satellite cells by enhancing G1/S cell cycle progression via the activation of phosphatidylinositol 3'-kinase/Akt signaling pathway. J Biol Chem 2000;275:35942–52.
74. Milasincic DJ, Calera MR, Farmer SR, et al. Stimulation of C2C12 myoblast growth by basic fibroblast growth factor and insulin-like growth factor 1 can occur via mitogen-activated protein kinase-dependent and -independent pathways. Mol Cell Biol 1996;16:5964–73.
75. Chen L, Lund PK, Burgess SB, et al. Growth hormone, insulin-like growth factor I, and motoneuron size. J Neurobiol 1997;32:202–12.
76. Dobrowolny G, Giacinti C, Pelosi L, et al. Muscle expression of a local Igf-1 isoform protects motor neurons in an ALS mouse model. J Cell Biol 2005;168: 193–9.
77. Messi ML, Delbono O. Target-derived trophic effect on skeletal muscle innervation in senescent mice. J Neurosci 2003;23:1351–9.
78. Parsons SA, Banks GB, Rowland JA, et al. Genetic disruption of the growth hormone receptor does not influence motoneuron survival in the developing mouse. Int J Dev Biol 2003;47:41–9.
79. Caroni P, Grandes P. Nerve sprouting in innervated adult skeletal muscle induced by exposure to elevated levels of insulin-like growth factors. J Cell Biol 1990;110:1307–17.
80. Ren H, Accili D, Duan C. Hypoxia converts the myogenic action of insulin-like growth factors into mitogenic action by differentially regulating multiple signaling pathways. Proc Natl Acad Sci U S A 2010;107:5857–62.
81. Kwintkiewicz J, Giudice LC. The interplay of insulin-like growth factors, gonadotropins, and endocrine disruptors in ovarian follicular development and function. Semin Reprod Med 2009;27:43–51.

82. LeRoith D, Yakar S. Mechanisms of disease: metabolic effects of growth hormone and insulin-like growth factor 1. Nat Clin Pract Endocrinol Metab 2007;3:302–10.

83. Ginther OJ, Gastal EL, Gastal MO, et al. Critical role of insulin-like growth factor system in follicle selection and dominance in mares. Biol Reprod 2004;70:1374–9.

84. Balasubramanian K, Lavoie HA, Garmey JC, et al. Regulation of porcine granulosa cell steroidogenic acute regulatory protein (StAR) by insulin-like growth factor I: synergism with follicle-stimulating hormone or protein kinase A agonist. Endocrinology 1997;138:433–9.

85. LaVoie HA, Garmey JC, Veldhuis JD. Mechanisms of insulin-like growth factor I augmentation of follicle-stimulating hormone-induced porcine steroidogenic acute regulatory protein gene promoter activity in granulosa cells. Endocrinology 1999;140:146–53.

86. Santiago CA, Voge JL, Aad PY, et al. Pregnancy-associated plasma protein-A and insulin-like growth factor binding protein mRNAs in granulosa cells of dominant and subordinate follicles of preovulatory cattle. Domest Anim Endocrinol 2005;28:46–63.

87. Wuertz S, Nitsche A, Jastroch M, et al. The role of the IGF-I system for vitellogenesis in maturing female sterlet, *Acipenser ruthenus* Linnaeus, 1758. Gen Comp Endocrinol 2007;150:140–50.

88. Hourvitz A, Kuwahara A, Hennebold JD, et al. The regulated expression of the pregnancy-associated plasma protein-A in the rodent ovary: a proposed role in the development of dominant follicles and of corpora lutea. Endocrinology 2002;143:1833–44.

89. Arraztoa JA, Monget P, Bondy C, et al. Expression patterns of insulin-like growth factor-binding proteins 1, 2, 3, 5, and 6 in the mid-cycle monkey ovary. J Clin Endocrinol Metab 2002;87:5220–8.

90. Adashi EY, Resnick CE, Hurwitz A, et al. The intra-ovarian IGF system. Growth Regul 1992;2:10–5.

91. Adashi EY, Rohan RM. Intraovarian regulation: peptidergic signaling systems. Trends Endocrinol Metab 1992;3:243–8.

92. Baker J, Hardy MP, Zhou J, et al. Effects of an Igf1 gene null mutation on mouse reproduction. Mol Endocrinol 1996;10:903–18.

93. Zhou J, Kumar TR, Matzuk MM, et al. Insulin-like growth factor I regulates gonadotropin responsiveness in the murine ovary. Mol Endocrinol 1997;11: 1924–33.

94. Bondy CA, Werner H, Roberts CT Jr, et al. Cellular pattern of insulin-like growth factor-I (IGF-I) and type I IGF receptor gene expression in early organogenesis: comparison with IGF-II gene expression. Mol Endocrinol 1990;4:1386–98.

95. Hernandez ER, Roberts CT Jr, LeRoith D, et al. Rat ovarian insulin-like growth factor I (IGF-I) gene expression is granulosa cell-selective: 5′-untranslated mRNA variant representation and hormonal regulation. Endocrinology 1989; 125:572–4.

96. Zhou J, Chin E, Bondy C. Cellular pattern of insulin-like growth factor-I (IGF-I) and IGF-I receptor gene expression in the developing and mature ovarian follicle. Endocrinology 1991;129:3281–8.

97. Cara JF, Rosenfield RL. Insulin-like growth factor I and insulin potentiate luteinizing hormone-induced androgen synthesis by rat ovarian thecal-interstitial cells. Endocrinology 1988;123:733–9.

98. Pitetti JL, Torre D, Conne B, et al. Insulin receptor and IGF1R are not required for oocyte growth, differentiation, and maturation in mice. Sex Dev 2009;3:264–72.

99. Liu JP, Baker J, Perkins AS, et al. Mice carrying null mutations of the genes encoding insulin-like growth factor I (Igf-1) and type 1 IGF receptor (Igf1r). Cell 1993;75:59–72.

100. Chandrashekar V, Zaczek D, Bartke A. The consequences of altered somatotropic system on reproduction. Biol Reprod 2004;71:17–27.

101. Froment P, Seurin D, Hembert S, et al. Reproductive abnormalities in human IGF binding protein-1 transgenic female mice. Endocrinology 2002;143: 1801–8.

102. Modric T, Silha JV, Shi Z, et al. Phenotypic manifestations of insulin-like growth factor-binding protein-3 overexpression in transgenic mice. Endocrinology 2001;142:1958–67.

103. Salih DA, Tripathi G, Holding C, et al. Insulin-like growth factor-binding protein 5 (Igfbp5) compromises survival, growth, muscle development, and fertility in mice. Proc Natl Acad Sci U S A 2004;101:4314–9.

104. Nyegaard M, Overgaard MT, Su YQ, et al. Lack of functional pregnancy-associated plasma protein-A (PAPPA) compromises mouse ovarian steroidogenesis and female fertility. Biol Reprod 2010;82(6):1129–38.

105. Bruning JC, Gautam D, Burks DJ, et al. Role of brain insulin receptor in control of body weight and reproduction. Science 2000;289:2122–5.

106. Kahn CR. Knockout mice challenge our concepts of glucose homeostasis and the pathogenesis of diabetes. Exp Diabesity Res 2003;4:169–82.

107. Yakar S, Liu JL, Fernandez AM, et al. Liver-specific igf-1 gene deletion leads to muscle insulin insensitivity. Diabetes 2001;50:1110–8.

108. Yakar S, Setser J, Zhao H, et al. Inhibition of growth hormone action improves insulin sensitivity in liver IGF-1-deficient mice. J Clin Invest 2004;113:96–105.

109. McDonald A, Williams RM, Regan FM, et al. IGF-I treatment of insulin resistance. Eur J Endocrinol 2007;157(Suppl 1):S51–6.

110. Kuzuya H, Matsuura N, Sakamoto M, et al. Trial of insulinlike growth factor I therapy for patients with extreme insulin resistance syndromes. Diabetes 1993; 42:696–705.

111. Moses AC, Morrow LA, O'Brien M, et al. Insulin-like growth factor I (rhIGF-I) as a therapeutic agent for hyperinsulinemic insulin-resistant diabetes mellitus. Diabetes Res Clin Pract 1995;28(Suppl):S185–94.

112. Schoenle EJ, Zenobi PD, Torresani T, et al. Recombinant human insulin-like growth factor I (rhIGF I) reduces hyperglycaemia in patients with extreme insulin resistance. Diabetologia 1991;34:675–9.

113. Vestergaard H, Rossen M, Urhammer SA, et al. Short- and long-term metabolic effects of recombinant human IGF-I treatment in patients with severe insulin resistance and diabetes mellitus. Eur J Endocrinol 1997;136:475–82.

114. Zenobi PD, Glatz Y, Keller A, et al. Beneficial metabolic effects of insulin-like growth factor I in patients with severe insulin-resistant diabetes type A. Eur J Endocrinol 1994;131:251–7.

115. Wu Y, Sun H, Yakar S, et al. Elevated levels of insulin-like growth factor (IGF)-I in serum rescue the severe growth retardation of IGF-I null mice. Endocrinology 2009;150:4395–403.

116. O'Connell T, Clemmons DR. IGF-I/IGF-binding protein-3 combination improves insulin resistance by GH-dependent and independent mechanisms. J Clin Endocrinol Metab 2002;87:4356–60.

117. Kulkarni RN, Holzenberger M, Shih DQ, et al. beta-Cell-specific deletion of the Igf1 receptor leads to hyperinsulinemia and glucose intolerance but does not alter beta-cell mass. Nat Genet 2002;31:111–5.

118. Xuan S, Kitamura T, Nakae J, et al. Defective insulin secretion in pancreatic beta cells lacking type 1 IGF receptor. J Clin Invest 2002;110:1011–9.

119. Muzumdar RH, Ma X, Yang X, et al. Central resistance to the inhibitory effects of leptin on stimulated insulin secretion with aging. Neurobiol Aging 2006;27: 1308–14.

120. Kappeler L, De Magalhaes Filho C, Dupont J, et al. Brain IGF-1 receptors control mammalian growth and lifespan through a neuroendocrine mechanism. PLoS Biol 2008;6:e254.

121. Kim J, Wende AR, Sena S, et al. Insulin-like growth factor I receptor signaling is required for exercise-induced cardiac hypertrophy. Mol Endocrinol 2008;22: 2531–43.

122. Le Roith D, Kim H, Fernandez AM, et al. Inactivation of muscle insulin and IGF-I receptors and insulin responsiveness. Curr Opin Clin Nutr Metab Care 2002;5: 371–5.

123. Samuelson AV, Carr CE, Ruvkun G. Gene activities that mediate increased life span of C. elegans insulin-like signaling mutants. Genes Dev 2007;21:2976–94.

124. Hwangbo DS, Gershman B, Tu MP, et al. Drosophila dFOXO controls lifespan and regulates insulin signalling in brain and fat body. Nature 2004;429:562–6.

125. Brown-Borg HM. Longevity in mice: is stress resistance a common factor? Age (Dordr) 2006;28:145–62.

126. Dominici FP, Arostegui Diaz G, Bartke A, et al. Compensatory alterations of insulin signal transduction in liver of growth hormone receptor knockout mice. J Endocrinol 2000;166:579–90.

127. Dominici FP, Hauck S, Argentino DP, et al. Increased insulin sensitivity and upregulation of insulin receptor, insulin receptor substrate (IRS)-1 and IRS-2 in liver of Ames dwarf mice. J Endocrinol 2002;173:81–94.

128. Sonntag WE, Lynch CD, Cefalu WT, et al. Pleiotropic effects of growth hormone and insulin-like growth factor (IGF)-1 on biological aging: inferences from moderate caloric-restricted animals. J Gerontol A Biol Sci Med Sci 1999;54:B521–38.

129. Sun LY, Bokov AF, Richardson A, et al. Hepatic response to oxidative injury in long-lived Ames dwarf mice. FASEB J 2011;25:398–408.

130. Bailey-Downs LC, Mitschelen M, Sosnowska D, et al. Liver-specific knockdown of IGF-1 decreases vascular oxidative stress resistance by impairing the Nrf2-dependent antioxidant response: a novel model of vascular aging. J Gerontol A Biol Sci Med Sci 2012;67:313–29.

131. Svensson J, Sjogren K, Faldt J, et al. Liver-derived IGF-I regulates mean life span in mice. PLoS One 2011;6:e22640.

132. Bluher M, Michael MD, Peroni OD, et al. Adipose tissue selective insulin receptor knockout protects against obesity and obesity-related glucose intolerance. Dev Cell 2002;3:25–38.

133. Selman C, Lingard S, Choudhury AI, et al. Evidence for lifespan extension and delayed age-related biomarkers in insulin receptor substrate 1 null mice. FASEB J 2008;22:807–18.

134. Menini S, Amadio L, Oddi G, et al. Deletion of p66Shc longevity gene protects against experimental diabetic glomerulopathy by preventing diabetes-induced oxidative stress. Diabetes 2006;55:1642–50.

135. Selman C, Tullet JM, Wieser D, et al. Ribosomal protein S6 kinase 1 signaling regulates mammalian life span. Science 2009;326:140–4.

136. Um SH, Frigerio F, Watanabe M, et al. Absence of S6K1 protects against age- and diet-induced obesity while enhancing insulin sensitivity. Nature 2004;431: 200–5.

137. Xi G, Shen X, Clemmons DR. p66shc negatively regulates insulin-like growth factor I signal transduction via inhibition of p52shc binding to Src homology 2 domain-containing protein tyrosine phosphatase substrate-1 leading to impaired growth factor receptor-bound protein-2 membrane recruitment. Mol Endocrinol 2008;22:2162–75.

138. Holzenberger M, Dupont J, Ducos B, et al. IGF-1 receptor regulates lifespan and resistance to oxidative stress in mice. Nature 2003;421:182–7.

139. Smith GS, Walford RL, Mickey MR. Lifespan and incidence of cancer and other diseases in selected long-lived inbred mice and their F 1 hybrids. J Natl Cancer Inst 1973;50:1195–213.

140. Bokov AF, Garg N, Ikeno Y, et al. Does reduced IGF-1R signaling in Igf1r+/- mice alter aging? PLoS One 2011;6:e26891.

141. Cohen E, Paulsson JF, Blinder P, et al. Reduced IGF-1 signaling delays age-associated proteotoxicity in mice. Cell 2009;139:1157–69.

142. Garg N, Thakur S, McMahan CA, et al. High fat diet induced insulin resistance and glucose intolerance are gender-specific in IGF-1R heterozygous mice. Biochem Biophys Res Commun 2011;413:476–80.

Insulin-Like Growth Factor Physiology

What we have Learned from Human Studies

Jeff M.P. Holly, PhD*, Claire M. Perks, PhD

KEYWORDS

- Insulin-like growth factor I • Insulin-like growth factor II
- Insulin-like growth factor binding protein • Insulin-like growth factor receptors

KEY POINTS

- Although very similar to insulin and its receptor; the modus operandi of the insulin-like growth factors (IGFs) within the body is very different from that of the traditional peptide hormone.
- In the tissues the IGFs are important regulators of cell survival, growth, metabolism, and differentiated function; the complex system of interacting proteins may confer some specificity to these actions.
- The IGFs play an important role in metabolic regulation. Many of the major health issues that are increasingly common in our societies relate to the energy imbalance associated with a modern lifestyle and the consequent metabolic disturbance.

BACKGROUND

The insulin-like growth factors (IGF-I and IGF-II) were originally described in the late 1950s as skeletal growth factors that were produced in the liver in response to pituitary growth hormone (GH) and appeared to mediate the effects on whole-body somatic growth, and hence were called somatomedins.[1] The IGFs were independently discovered as "insulin-like" activity that was present in serum and could not be blocked by very specific insulin antibodies, which was termed nonsuppressible insulin-like activity.[2] When these peptides were subsequently characterized structurally[3] it was realized that they shared considerable homology with proinsulin and hence were given their present names. Accumulating evidence indicated that in addition to production in the liver, both IGF-I and IGF-II were produced in most, if not all, tissues. It also became clear that in addition to their metabolic and growth-promoting actions, the IGFs were also able to regulate cell survival, adhesion, motility, differentiation, and

School of Clinical Sciences, University of Bristol, IGFs & Metabolic Endocrinology Group, Learning & Research Building, 2nd Floor, Southmead Hospital, Bristol BS10 5NB, UK
* Corresponding author.
E-mail address: Jeff.holly@bristol.ac.uk

Endocrinol Metab Clin N Am 41 (2012) 249–263
doi:10.1016/j.ecl.2012.04.009
0889-8529/12/$ – see front matter © 2012 Elsevier Inc. All rights reserved.

most differentiated cell functions. With their ubiquitous presence and pluripotential actions, the IGFs have been purported to play important roles in a wide variety of human abnormalities, many of which are the topic of the other articles in this issue. This article concentrates on studies that have indicated how the IGF system operates and its role in normal human physiology, and focuses on aspects that are different from those revealed in animal models or have yet to be examined in such experimental models.

SYSTEMIC MODUS OPERANDI

The growth factors IGF-I and IGF-II share a high degree of homology with proinsulin, and their actions on cells are mediated by a classic transmembrane tyrosine kinase cell-surface receptor that is also remarkably similar to the insulin receptor, particularly in the tyrosine kinase domain. These receptors each exist as dimers within the cell surface, and they are so similar that in cells where both are expressed there is substantial heterodimerization, forming hybrid IGF-I/insulin receptors. These hybrids appear to act more like IGF-I receptors in vitro, but their physiologic role in vivo is poorly understood. All of these receptors share considerable overlap in their intracellular signaling capability.[4] There is also an IGF-II receptor, a single large transmembrane protein that is completely unrelated to the IGF-I and insulin receptors. The IGF-II receptor does not appear to act as a traditional signaling receptor in response to IGF-II binding. In relation to IGF function it is thought to act as a clearance receptor for IGF-II, because disruption of gene expression in mice resulted in elevated IGF-II levels and overgrowth. These receptors therefore appear to provide an additional safeguard to control the amount of IGF-II to which a cell is exposed in addition to all of the IGF-binding proteins (IGFBPs) that will control both IGF-I and IGF-II. These receptors, however, are clearly multifunctional. Their most well characterized role is as mannose-6-phosphate receptors involved in the targeting of lysosomal enzymes to the lysosomes within the cell. However, they also bind latent transforming growth factor β and enable its activation on the cell surface, and also bind to retinoids, urokinase receptors, and many other proteins. The potential functional consequences of interactions between IGF-II and all the other possible ligands of the IGF-II receptor are far from clear.[5]

Despite the remarkable similarities between the IGFs and insulin and their signaling receptors, they have evolved in mammals to operate in a very different way as communication systems within the body. Insulin expression is very restricted, principally just to the β cells of the pancreatic islets. It is stored there in secretory granules within the cells and secreted via the regulated secretory pathway from these cells in response to stimuli, primarily glucose fluctuations. Regulated secretion from the pancreas is therefore the primary determinant of insulin activity throughout the body. By contrast, the IGFs are expressed widely and in many cell types in tissues throughout the body. Furthermore, like most other cytokines, the IGFs are not stored within secretory granules within cells but are secreted as they are produced, via the constitutive secretory pathway. Insulin therefore acts in a classic endocrine manner; it is secreted from the pancreas into the circulation and is carried around the body until it encounters a cell receptor in a target tissue. By contrast, when the IGFs are secreted they then immediately associate with soluble high-affinity binding proteins, the IGFBPs, which are present in excess. The IGFBPs sequester the IGFs and considerably slow their clearance; enabling very high concentrations of IGFs to accumulate. In the circulation 2 of the IGFBPs, IGFBP-3 and IGFBP-5, are bound to a further large glycoprotein, the acid-labile subunit (ALS) that is present in excess. This ternary complex formation slows clearance even more such that in adult humans the total IGF-I and IGF-II concentration in the circulation is around 100 nM. This concentration is around 1000 times higher than that of insulin, and whereas insulin levels fluctuate acutely in response to metabolic requirements, the levels of IGFs are very stable because of their slow clearance. At the cellular level, optimal regulation of the IGF receptor is achieved with concentrations of just 1 to 2 nM, indicating that there is vast excess in the circulation. In the tissues IGF concentrations are less than 20% of that in the circulation,[6] which is still a large excess over that needed for cell regulation. Therefore, although the IGFs are not stored within cells, the IGFBP complexes maintain a large extracellular store. Hence, whereas the activity of insulin throughout the body is largely determined by the rate of secretion from the pancreas, by contrast the constitutive secretion of the IGFs within any tissue is just one component that determines the total amount of IGF that the cells are exposed to, and control of activity is much more complex. The IGFs are bound to the IGFBPs with higher affinity than to the IGF-I receptor, so most of the IGF in the body is relatively unavailable for receptor activation. Activity in a tissue is therefore not necessarily determined by secretion rate of IGFs and not necessarily determined by total IGF concentration. It is also not safe to assume that IGFBPs just bind IGFs and reduce their availability for receptor activation. There is considerable evidence that IGFBPs not only can sequester IGFs away from cell receptors and restrict activity but also can enhance activity at the cellular level via a variety of mechanisms,[7] and also enhance delivery of IGFs to specific tissue compartments.[8]

The 6 binding proteins are unrelated to the cell-surface receptors but are structurally very closely related to each other, although they are each products of distinct genes and they all have very distinct functional properties.[7] In terms of physiology, there is still very limited understanding of the exact role of each of the IGFBPs. In humans IGFBP-3 clearly acts as the main circulating carrier protein, but it is also expressed extensively in many tissues and obviously has many additional local functions. One of these IGFBPs, IGFBP-1, is more restricted in its sites of expression; the IGFBP-1 that is present in the circulation is predominantly derived from the liver where its expression is under the dynamic control of insulin, which suppresses its production. In the circulation IGFBP-1 levels undergo a circadian variation as a result of this dynamic insulin regulation, which seems to provide an additional acute control to ensure that IGF activity is modulated appropriate to prevailing metabolic conditions.[9]

With large soluble stores of IGFs that are maintained in association with the high-affinity IGFBPs, it is clear that there must be mechanisms for lowering the affinity of these interactions to make the IGF available for cellular actions in the tissues. In the circulation, the majority of IGF is associated with IGFBP-3 and the ALS. The ALS binds to a C-terminal region of IGFBP-3 that also binds to proteoglycans present on cell surfaces and in the extracellular matrix (ECM). It is therefore possible that proteoglycans on the surface of the capillary endothelium compete for binding to IGFBP-3 and displace the ALS, generating a binary complex from the ternary complex.[10] The binary complex would then be more able to cross the endothelium and transport the IGF into the tissue. There is, however, another mechanism for controlling delivery of IGF from the circulatory reservoir. A circulating protease that acts specifically on IGFBP-3 has been described in many different conditions.[11] This protease results in limited cleavage of IGFBP-3. The cleaved IGFBP-3 still retains IGF in the ternary complex, but is bound with a lower affinity. Even a small decrease in affinity could result in a shift in the complex equilibrium that must exist in vivo, with the IGF reequilibrating to other IGFBPs that are present and which are generally not cleaved by the same protease. These other IGFBPs only form binary complexes and therefore have greater ability to transport the IGFs out into target tissues. Indeed, some of these binary complexes differentially deliver IGFs to specific tissues.[8] There have been many studies documenting increases in IGFBP-3 proteolysis in the circulation in pregnancy and many other conditions, especially catabolic states whereby an increase in the availability of these anabolic IGFs may be an advantage.[11] In addition to the IGFBP-3 protease, it has become clear that each of the IGFBPs appears to be subject to specific proteolysis. In humans, proteases capable of cleaving IGFBP-3 appear to be ubiquitously present in both the circulation and extravascular fluids. In the normal healthy individual there is little detectable IGFBP-3 protease activity in serum, because of the presence of inhibitors that protect the IGFBP-3 from proteolysis.[11] Increases in proteolysis that are observed in different conditions appear to be due to a decrease in these inhibitors rather than an increase in levels of proteases.[12] Outside of the circulation in the tissues where the IGFs are destined to act, this system operates in a slightly different manner. The protease inhibitors appear to be restrained to within the circulation, whereas proteases that can cleave IGFBP-3 are present in extravascular interstitial fluids; consequently, IGFBP-3 proteolysis is relatively unopposed and hence much more extensive in the tissues, presumably making the IGF more available for cell receptors. This system in the tissues is disturbed in inflammatory conditions, whereby an increase in capillary permeability enables the circulating protease inhibitors access to the extravascular space and IGFBP-3 proteolysis is then suppressed.[12] The authors have investigated this situation in patients with psoriasis for whom skin interstitial fluid from affected and nonaffected areas of skin were sampled along with blood samples,[13] and in patients with rheumatoid arthritis for whom synovial fluid from affected knee joints were sampled along with circulating blood samples.[14] In the normal tissue the levels of IGFs were relatively low, and most of the IGFBP-3 was present in binary complexes (92.3%) and was found to be predominantly proteolytically cleaved. In the inflamed tissue, however, increased levels of IGFs, IGFBP-3, and ALS were observed, but the majority of the IGFBP-3 was then in ternary complexes (65.4%), and was intact and not cleaved.[14] The authors have investigated the effect of inflammation and vascular permeability in a further 9 patients with rheumatoid arthritis during an intervention study in which the patients received intra-articular injections of glucocorticoids to reduce the inflammation. Following the steroid administration to the inflamed joint, the synovial fluid levels of IGF-I, IGFBP-3, and ALS all decreased down to levels approaching those in normal synovial fluid and the reductions in these levels correlated with reductions in serum levels of C-reactive protein, indicating a relationship with reduced inflammation. The reduced levels of IGFBP-3 and ALS were accompanied by increased IGFBP-3 proteolysis, and the majority of IGFBP-3 was then again proteolyzed, resembling that in normal tissue (**Fig. 1**). The observations from this intervention trial are consistent with the increased proteolysis of IGFBP-3 observed in normal tissues resulting from the inhibitors that are present in the circulation being absent in tissues; however, in inflamed tissues the resulting increase in capillary permeability leads to leakage of these inhibitors into the tissue, resulting in the reduced proteolysis observed, which can then be normalized by local steroid administration. The changes in capillary permeability are reflected by the amount of ALS detected in the extravascular fluid, and parallel the changes in IGFBP-3 proteolysis.

All of the IGF that is present in the body is effectively present in IGFBP complexes, and there is clearly a very complex system with 6 IGFBPs, each of which exists in several functionally distinct forms attributable to various posttranslational modifications including limited cleavage and phosphorylation. There are proteases and accompanying inhibitors for each of the individual IGFBPs; the best characterized being the

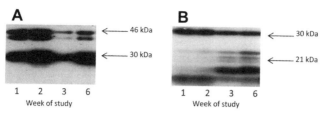

Fig. 1. (A) Western immunoblot showing the pattern of IGFBP-3 isoforms present in synovial fluid aspirated from a knee joint (suprapatellar bursa) from a patient with rheumatoid arthritis at weeks 1 and 2 before an intra-articular injection of 40 mg triamcinolone (a long-acting corticosteroid) and then at weeks 3 and 6 (which correspond to 1 and 4 weeks following the steroid injection). A considerable proportion of intact IGFBP-3 is present in the 2 differentially glycosylated forms at 42 to 44 kDa before the steroid injection. Following the steroid injection at weeks 3 and 6, the pattern of IGFBP-3 isoforms reverts to that seen in normal synovial fluid in subjects without arthritis, with most of the IGFBP-3 being in the form of the 30-kDa proteolytic fragment. (B) Autoradiographs of the same synovial fluid samples analyzed in an IGFBP-3 protease assay. Samples were preincubated with radioiodinated recombinant IGFBP-3 for 4 hours at 37°C before electrophoretic separation, blotting, and autoradiography to reveal proteolytic fragmentation of the intact nonglycosylated IGFBP-3 seen at 30 kDa. The results show an increase in IGFBP-3 protease activity in the samples taken following the intra-articular steroid injection, as revealed by a reduction in the intact band at 30 kDa and an increase in the bands corresponding to smaller fragments resulting from proteolysis. The increased protease activity following the steroid injection then resembled the activity observed in synovial fluid from subjects without inflammatory conditions.

PAPP-A system for cleaving IGFBP-4.[15] It has also become clear that each of the IGFBPs interacts with high affinity with many other proteins, particularly in the ECM and on the cell surface. The pattern of expression of all of these interacting components varies between tissues, and within any tissue varies with developmental stage and pathology. This sophisticated complexity of interacting components for controlling IGF availability and actions provides an insight into how some specificity could be conferred on this pluripotential system. With the IGFs ubiquitously present in vast excess and potentially able to regulate virtually every cell function, the sophisticated interplay of multiple components seems to provide a means of conferring specificity such that their actions can be very finely controlled in a tissue-specific manner.

DISTINCTIONS BETWEEN HUMANS AND EXPERIMENTAL MODELS

Studies of normal physiology in living humans are limited by obvious constraints regarding invasive access to tissues and the extent that the system can be manipulated and challenged, and much of what we have learned about physiology has been derived from the use of laboratory animals. The advent of molecular techniques that enable individual genes to be overexpressed or switched off within live animals has led to major advances in our understanding of specific pathways such as that for the IGFs (as reviewed elsewhere in this issue by Yakar). There are, however, some limitations to the use of rodent models for advancing our understanding of the role that the IGF system plays in human physiology and pathology. One clear limitation relates to the major species difference in how IGF-II is expressed in humans compared with rodents, described in the next section. There are also some more general concerns: the IGFs are implicated as playing an important role in many of the major health issues that now confront us. The nutritionally dependent IGF system has evolved to regulate tissue growth and development according to metabolic conditions, enabling the organism to adapt to its environment. Many of the major health conditions that we now face arise from our modern lifestyle and its consequent energy imbalance, therefore it is not surprising that the IGFs may be involved. In addition to the major epidemics of obesity and diabetes, which are clear manifestations of metabolic imbalance, metabolic disturbances will soon overtake smoking as the main avoidable cause of cancer and have also been implicated in other chronic disorders such as dementia. Genome-wide association studies have failed to find common genetic variants that contribute in a major way to most of these chronic disorders, and it is widely considered that multiple genes may be involved and that many of these conditions are a consequence of maladaptations to our modern lifestyle due to gene-environment interactions. The conventional experimental approach to investigate pathology in the laboratory is to use genetically homogeneous rodent colonies; however, this approach examines the effect of exposures on a single genotype. Human populations, by contrast, comprise infinitely varied genotypes, each of which can respond in many different ways to the same exposures: even in the most obesogenic environment only some individuals become obese. Gene knock-out and knock-in experiments in laboratory animals can reveal large effects, but these experiments involve large changes in one gene against a homogeneous genetic background in a colony of animals. Human population studies, however, generally examine small changes attributable to genetic variance against an extremely heterogeneous genetic background and, unsurprisingly, frequently reveal only very small effects. In addition, the standard rodent experiment compares an intervention group with an untreated control group. These control animals, however, live a sedentary life with continuous access to food, within confined containers in standardized conditions with constant day-night cycles, and hence no environmental stimuli. As a result these control animals are inactive, relatively overweight, insulin resistant, and live much shorter lives than normal rodents living in their natural habitats that exercise considerably more and feed intermittently.[16] Interventions that are perceived to induce metabolic advantage in such experiments are in many cases just correcting these abnormalities already present in the control animals. This experimental paradigm may have had many unwitting and unrecognized consequences. For example, many new cancer therapies exhibit efficacy in animal studies but then prove to be ineffective in human clinical trials. Could this be due to tumor development being different in the metabolically moribund animals used in the preclinical trials? Similarly, most cell-culture experiments are traditionally performed in very hyperglycemic media that can alter many cell responses.

In relation to the role that the IGF system may play in cancer, there is a further important distinction between most experimental models and actual clinical cancers in human populations. Screening and autopsy studies of human populations have consistently and clearly established that in the elderly there is a high prevalence of small neoplasias in tissues such as the breast, prostate, and colorectum. The prevalence increases gradually with age, reaching a very high level in the elderly; around 50% of people have a neoplasia in their colorectum by the age of 80 years[17] and up to 80% of men older than 90 years have a neoplasia in their prostate.[18] The prevalence of these neoplasias is far higher than the incidence of the corresponding clinical cancer within the population, presumably because most of the neoplasias detected at autopsy are slow, indolent lesions that would not develop into a clinical cancer before the individual dies of other causes. These observations indicate that most individuals would probably be harboring at least one subclinical neoplasia by the age of 70 years. There is limited evidence to indicate that variations in IGF-I may initiate the oncogenic process, and in elderly human populations the interesting questions relate to how the activity of IGF-I, and potential manipulations of this, will affect the development of the neoplastic lesions that are already present in most elderly people. Studies in experimental animals are generally in young animals that are still growing, and studies that have examined whether raised GH/IGF-I levels cause cancer are not relevant to the elderly human population in which most individuals will already harbor latent occult preclinical neoplasias. The risk of initiating new cancers is a major concern but the impact on these pre-existing neoplasias is a much bigger concern. Manipulations of IGF-I in rodent models also have to be interpreted with the knowledge that any alterations in IGF-I occur in the context of the almost complete absence of systemic IGF-II levels; this is very different from the human situation whereby variations in IGF-I levels are always in the context of the presence of a relative excess of IGF-II.

Until these experimental issues are overcome, there are still many aspects of human IGF pathophysiology that can only be learned from studies of humans.

IGF-II AND METABOLISM

In terms of abundance within the body, IGF-II is by far the most prevalent IGF present throughout the life span in humans, but such is not the case in rodents. For many years it was thought that IGF-I and IGF-II activate the same cell-surface IGF-I receptor, and the clear distinctions in their physiology raised puzzling questions. The distinction between the two IGFs is most clear in early development. IGF-II plays a very important role in fetal and early neonatal growth and development, and this role appears to be conserved in humans similarly to that defined in rodent models. In utero IGF-II has an important role in placental function and in the control of nutrient partitioning.[19] Both IGF-II and the IGF-II receptor are imprinted genes. This imprinting appears to have evolved to balance the genetic conflict between parents. The paternal imprinted genes enhance nutrient extraction from the mother and growth of the fetus to ensure the survival and development of the father's offspring. This process is facilitated by paternal imprinting of the IGF-II gene in the mouse fetus, and this paternal imprinting appears to have been conserved in humans. By contrast, the mother needs to constrain the fetal development and balance nutrient extraction for the fetus to ensure her own survival and reproductive competence for future potential fetuses, with potentially different fathers. This process is facilitated by maternal imprinting of the IGF-II receptor gene in the mouse,[20] although this does not seem to have been conserved in humans in whom the expression of this gene does not appear to be imprinted.[21] As the pituitary develops and takes control of the endocrine system, pituitary GH drives systemic IGF-I production, which then plays a more dominant role in growth and development. In rodents there is a clear switch at weaning, when the expression of IGF-II virtually ceases and there is an obvious end to the major systemic role played by IGF-II. In higher mammals this switch does not occur, and in humans IGF-II remains the most prevalent IGF throughout life. In adult humans there are around 4-fold higher levels of IGF-II than IGF-I in the circulation, and it is still unclear as to why or what role IGF-II then plays throughout adult life. In rodents there is virtually no IGF-II in the adult circulation, therefore these experimental models are not informative regarding the role of IGF-II in the adult human. This major species difference is also a significant confounding factor in the use of these experimental models for examining interventions targeting the IGF system for the treatment of pathologic conditions in adult humans.

Unlike the large body of literature documenting large variations in IGF-I levels with age, nutrition, and different physiologic conditions and pathologies, studies of IGF-II levels have found very little variation in any conditions.[22] There are, however, several strands of evidence indicating potential roles for IGF-II in adult human physiology, and many of these consistently suggest a role in metabolic regulation. Early observations of the systemic consequences of tumors associated with excess production of these growth factors suggested distinctions in pathophysiology between IGF-I and IGF-II. There have not been reports of common tumors that produce sufficient IGF-I to increase circulating levels, but systemic levels are increased in acromegaly because of pituitary tumors of the GH-producing cells that then result in stimulation of hepatic production of IGF-I. The symptoms of this condition reflect the growth-promoting actions of IGF-I: gigantism if presenting in childhood, whereas in adulthood, after the growth plates have fused, the manifestation of growth stimulation is restricted to the soft cartilaginous tissues apparent in changed facial features, particularly enlargement of the nose and hands (an increase in ring size is often the first apparent symptom). By contrast, there is a clinical syndrome associated with overproduction of IGF-II directly from tumors, called non–islet cell tumor induced hypoglycemia. The systemic symptoms of this condition are not associated with tissue growth but with disturbed metabolism, principally severe episodic hypoglycemia. Consistent with this evidence from classic endocrinology, more recent evidence has emerged from genetic epidemiology investigating associations between variance within IGF-II-linked genes and common chronic diseases in human populations, which have also suggested that IGF-II has an important role in metabolic regulation. The IGF-II gene is located on chromosome 11 next to the insulin gene, and several cohort studies have found associations between interindividual variations in this region and body weight and obesity,[23,24] and with abdominal and visceral fat.[25] That these genetic variants have functional consequences is supported by reports that circulating IGF-II concentrations are also associated with weight, weight-hip ratio, and weight gain in cohorts.[26–28] Abnormal circulating levels of the shed extracellular domain of the IGF-II receptor have also been observed in patients with obesity and type 2 diabetes.[29] In addition, serum levels of IGFBP-2 have been associated with measures of fat mass, central adiposity, and insulin resistance,[28] and with the metabolic syndrome and cardiovascular risk factors[30] in human populations. Further evidence has also emerged from genome-wide association studies, which have consistently found associations between the risk of type 2 diabetes and a polymorphism in the IGF2BP2 gene (which encodes for a binding protein that binds to IGF-II mRNA within the cell, rather than IGFBP-2, which binds to the secreted IGF-peptides),[31,32] and this polymorphism has also been associated with fasting insulin levels and measures of impaired β-cell function.[33]

A report of a clinical case with a chromosomal breakpoint upstream of the IGF-II gene separating the gene from some of its telomeric enhancers has also been reported to result in intrauterine growth retardation (consistent with the recognized role of IGF-II in fetal development) but also the development of atypical diabetes diagnosed at the age of 23 years, associated with insulin resistance and a marked increase in abdominal adiposity.[34] This case would also be consistent with an important role for IGF-II in metabolic regulation, especially adiposity and insulin resistance.

Another line of evidence has emerged from a completely different area of research, investigations of structure-function relationships of the cell-surface receptors. It has been known for many years that the insulin receptor exists in two distinct isoforms, IR-A and IR-B, which are derived from alternative splicing of the insulin receptor gene. This fact was originally considered to have little consequence, as the two receptor isoforms varied very little in their response to insulin. Recent studies, however, have established that the IR-A isoform has a high affinity for IGF-II, approaching the affinity with which it binds to insulin.[35] As IGF-II and insulin bind with similar affinities to the IR-A but with IGF-II being present in humans at around a 1000-fold higher concentration than insulin, this means that in reality IGF-II would be the predominant ligand activating this receptor, and recent studies have shown that compared with insulin, IGF-II triggers different cell signaling and responses.[36–38] Although much has still to be learned regarding the physiology of these receptors, this does begin to help explain how IGF-II may have such different physiology to IGF-I and, if IGF-II acts via an isoform of the insulin receptor rather than the IGF-I receptor, this may help explain its role in metabolic regulation. Ultimately, all of this accumulating evidence may eventually help to explain why such high levels of IGF-II are maintained throughout life in humans.

IGF-I AND NUTRITIONAL PROGRAMMING

Interest in endocrine programming has increased considerably since the seminal work of David Barker raised the concept that many chronic conditions that are now common in human populations originated because of adaptations to exposures early in life. Initially observations that the risk of death due to ischemic heart disease was related to an individual's birth weight[39] were extended to similar associations with the incidence of stroke, type 2 diabetes, and dyslipidemia. This proposal led to the concept that exposures during fetal development, for which birth weight was thought to serve as a proxy, may predispose individuals to many of the chronic diseases experienced later in adult life; this was termed the fetal origins hypothesis (or often just the Barker hypothesis). Further evidence also linked birth weight to a range of other chronic disorders including osteoporosis, depression, and cognitive decline,[40] and the hypothesis was broadened to become the Developmental Origins of Adult Health and Disease (DOHaD) hypothesis.[41] The DOHaD hypothesis was that fetal nutrition and other exposures resulted in adaptations of placental and fetal hormones, and that when this occurred during critical periods during gestation it could result in the reprogramming of key metabolic hormones such as insulin, IGFs, and GH, with long-term consequences on metabolic and cardiovascular health in later adult life.[42] Many direct intervention studies in animal models generally confirmed the basic concepts of the hypothesis, and provided further evidence for developmental programming.[43,44]

The role for IGF-I in mediating the effects of nutrition on growth and development appears to have been retained throughout evolution. The importance of IGF-I for many childhood growth disorders is reviewed in an article by Backeljauw & Chernausek elsewhere in this issue. That IGF-I levels relate to subsequent growth in normal children has been confirmed in longitudinal cohort studies,[45] and these levels of IGF-I have been related to nutritional intake in the same children,[46] consistent with IGF-I mediating the effects of nutrition on growth. Cross-sectional studies examining the nutritional determinants of IGF-I in children have confirmed the importance of protein intake,[47] and milk consumption, which is one of the main sources of protein intake in childhood, has consistently been reported to be the strongest determinant of IGF-I levels.[48–53] In addition to the direct effect of protein intake on hepatic IGF-I production,[47] milk also stimulates GH levels and induces a potent increase in insulin,[54] and GH and insulin then also both enhance IGF-I production.[55]

The acute effects of nutrition promoting systemic IGF-I levels are well established and conserved in all species investigated. Several cross-sectional studies and intervention trials in children, however, have revealed a long-term programming effect of nutrition in childhood that affects IGF-I levels much later in life, and this effect is opposite to the recognized short-term effects. These new findings establish that in humans nutritional exposures, not just in utero and in early infancy but throughout childhood, have very long-term consequences on IGF-I levels throughout the rest of the life span. Infants consuming formula-feed have higher circulating IGF-I levels compared with infants who are breastfed, because of the higher animal protein content of formula compared with human breast milk[56,57]; however, by the age of 7.5 years children who were formula fed as infants had markedly lower serum IGF-I concentrations,[58] indicating that the long-term effect was opposite to the acute effect. These findings were confirmed and extended in a second small observational study from Copenhagen that found lower IGF-I levels in infants at 2 months who were breastfed compared with those who were exclusively formula fed; however, by age 17 years those who were breastfed subsequently had higher IGF-I levels, and there was a negative association between IGF-I levels at 9 months and at 17 years.[59] Further evidence of a long-term programming effect came in a long-term follow-up of a randomized trial of milk supplementation given during pregnancy and throughout infancy up to the age of 5 years. When serum IGF-I levels were measured in the subjects from this trial 20 years after the end of the supplementation, those receiving the extra milk had reduced levels of IGF-I.[60] Evidence of an even more long-term effect was obtained in a follow-up of the Boyd-Orr Study cohort. Subjects from families with high milk consumption in the 1930s (average age 6.5 years) had lower circulating IGF-I levels measured 65 years later.[61] The only other evidence linking nutrition in early life with IGF-I levels measured much later in adulthood was from a natural experiment involving the long-term follow-up of people exposed to the 1944-1945 Dutch famine,[62] which again provided evidence for a paradoxic enduring effect opposite to the well-known short-term effect of nutrition. Consistent with this short-term effect, children who are malnourished have markedly reduced IGF-I levels,[63] but in the follow-up of the Dutch famine cohort those girls who were seriously deprived of food for almost 6 months at a median age of 12 years had higher levels of serum IGF-I when measured 51 years later.[62] These data again indicated that nutritional exposures in childhood are able to reprogram IGF-I levels with an effect that is detectable many decades later, and also indicated that such exposures even in late childhood/early adolescence could still have these long-term programming effects. Childhood lasts longer in humans than in any other species and it seems that this plasticity in the endocrine system allowing adaptation to environmental exposures is maintained throughout the duration of human childhood. Increased serum IGF-I levels feed back to suppress pituitary GH secretion,[64] and it is possible that nutrition-induced increases in IGF-I in childhood result in effects on the hypothalamic-pituitary system leading to a lasting resetting of this axis and reducing GH secretion as the child adapts to increased nutrition, but with the effect that IGF-I levels are then lower throughout subsequent adult life.

There has been considerable interest in early-life programming of chronic adult diseases, with an emphasis on maternal and infant nutrition. The new observations described here, however, indicate that hormonal systems retain plasticity throughout childhood and that nutritional exposures in late childhood have long-term programming effects on hormone levels that can be detected 50 to 65 years later in life. This finding may be very important in relation to the current global epidemic of childhood obesity that indicates excess nutrition as being common among children. This nutritional imbalance could have profound long-term effects because it may reset IGF-I levels with potential consequences on many common chronic diseases later in life that are affected by IGF-I, as outlined in the subsequent articles in this issue.

AGING AND THE ELDERLY

With better living standards and the control of many infectious diseases, many more people are living longer to much older ages, which naturally increases the prevalence of all conditions associated with aging. Until recently aging was generally considered to be largely a passive process involving cumulative wear-and-tear and tissue damage, resulting in a gradual decline in function. Studies from experimental genetics, however, have now clearly demonstrated that the aging process is actually regulated by hormonal pathways, and that longevity can be dramatically extended by manipulations of these pathways.[65,66]

The extrapolation of these findings from the genetic models to humans, however, is not entirely straightforward. In flies, worms, and even in rodents, life span is tightly linked to reproductive competence. When the organism is no longer able to reproduce, it is then in competition for food with the next generation that will carry the species forward, and therefore there is evolutionary benefit for the rapid death of the postreproductive individuals. As mammals evolved, however, there became a stage when there was an advantage for young individuals to learn survival skills from the wisdom accrued by the longest surviving individuals, at which point evolution favored maintaining the older generation beyond its reproductive life span. The regulation of aging in this postreproductive stage is less well understood, and the experimental models employing lower species are of limited value. The limitations on human life span in the postreproductive, aged population are generally chronic conditions such as cardiovascular disease and cancer; these may be very different from the limitations on life span in nematodes, flies, and even rodents.

Despite these caveats there is substantial evidence from genetic studies indicating that the relationship between the IGF pathway and longevity has been conserved in humans, much the same as that defined in many lower species.[67,68]

For most humans, however, the problems of aging are not the constraints of ultimate longevity after a life spent under perfectly controlled conditions, but are the problems of frailty encountered after a life exposed to many environmental insults. The evidence from clinical studies of conditions related to frailty in the elderly raises an interesting paradox because much of this evidence suggests that frailty relates to the decline in GH and IGF-I with age, and implies that strategies that result in increased levels of IGF-I may be of therapeutic benefit in the elderly.[69] Frailty is associated with the gradual loss of muscle mass and function (sacropenia), loss of bone mass (osteoporosis), and cognitive decline. These degenerative processes are associated with the age-related decline in the anabolic activity of the GH/IGF-I axis,[70] and there has been much debate about potential therapeutic strategies to manipulate the axis to counter age-related frailty. Indeed, there is considerable unapproved and unlicensed use of GH as an anti-aging therapy despite the current expert advice.[71] Unlike the problems addressed in the experimental models, the real problem to be addressed with human aging is how the IGF system has an impact on the balance between quantity of life and quality of life, and this promises to be an interesting research question for some time to come.

REFERENCES

1. Daughaday WH, Salmon WD Jr. The origins and development of the somatomedin hypothesis. Totowa (NJ): Humana Press; 1999.
2. Froesch ER, Buergi H, Ramseier EB, et al. Antibody-suppressible and nonsuppressible insulin-like activities in human serum and their physiologic significance. An insulin assay with adipose tissue of increased precision and specificity. J Clin Invest 1963;42:1816–34.
3. Rinderknecht E, Humbel RE. Amino-terminal sequences of two polypeptides from human serum with nonsuppressible insulin-like and cell-growth-promoting activities: evidence for structural homology with insulin B chain. Proc Natl Acad Sci U S A 1976;73(12):4379–81.

4. Kim JJ, Accili D. Signalling through IGF-I and insulin receptors: where is the specificity? Growth Horm IGF Res 2002;12(2):84–90.
5. Ghosh P, Dahms NM, Kornfeld S. Mannose 6-phosphate receptors: new twists in the tale. Nature reviews. Mol Cell Biol 2003;4(3):202–12.
6. Xu S, Cwyfan-Hughes SC, van der Stappen JW, et al. Insulin-like growth factors (IGFs) and IGF-binding proteins in human skin interstitial fluid. J Clin Endocrinol Metab 1995;80(10):2940–5.
7. Holly J, Perks C. The role of insulin-like growth factor binding proteins. Neuroendocrinology 2006;83(3–4):154–60.
8. Bar RS, Clemmons DR, Boes M, et al. Transcapillary permeability and subendothelial distribution of endothelial and amniotic fluid insulin-like growth factor binding proteins in the rat heart. Endocrinology 1990;127(3):1078–86.
9. Holly JM. The physiological role of IGFBP-1. Acta Endocrinol 1991;124(Suppl 2): 55–62.
10. Payet LD, Firth SM, Baxter RC. The role of the acid-labile subunit in regulating insulin-like growth factor transport across human umbilical vein endothelial cell monolayers. J Clin Endocrinol Metab 2004;89(5):2382–9.
11. Maile LA, Holly JM. Insulin-like growth factor binding protein (IGFBP) proteolysis: occurrence, identification, role and regulation. Growth Horm IGF Res 1999;9(2): 85–95.
12. Maile LA, Xu S, Cwyfan-Hughes SC, et al. Active and inhibitory components of the insulin-like growth factor binding protein-3 protease system in adult serum, interstitial, and synovial fluid. Endocrinology 1998;139(12):4772–81.
13. Xu S, Savage P, Burton JL, et al. Proteolysis of insulin-like growth factor-binding protein-3 by human skin keratinocytes in culture in comparison to that in skin interstitial fluid: the role and regulation of components of the plasmin system. J Clin Endocrinol Metab 1997;82(6):1863–8.
14. Whellams EJ, Maile LA, Fernihough JK, et al. Alterations in insulin-like growth factor binding protein-3 proteolysis and complex formation in the arthritic joint. J Endocrinol 2000;165(3):545–56.
15. Chen BK, Overgaard MT, Bale LK, et al. Molecular regulation of the IGF-binding protein-4 protease system in human fibroblasts: identification of a novel inducible inhibitor. Endocrinology 2002;143(4):1199–205.
16. Martin B, Ji S, Maudsley S, et al. "Control" laboratory rodents are metabolically morbid: why it matters. Proc Natl Acad Sci U S A 2010;107(14):6127–33.
17. Renehan AG, Bhaskar P, Painter JE, et al. The prevalence and characteristics of colorectal neoplasia in acromegaly. J Clin Endocrinol Metab 2000;85(9):3417–24.
18. Sheldon CA, Williams RD, Fraley EE. Incidental carcinoma of the prostate: a review of the literature and critical reappraisal of classification. J Urol 1980; 124(5):626–31.
19. Gluckman PD, Pinal CS. Regulation of fetal growth by the somatotrophic axis. J Nutr 2003;133(5 Suppl 2):1741S–6S.
20. Reik W, Constancia M, Fowden A, et al. Regulation of supply and demand for maternal nutrients in mammals by imprinted genes. J Physiol 2003;547(Pt 1):35–44.
21. Vu TH, Jirtle RL, Hoffman AR. Cross-species clues of an epigenetic imprinting regulatory code for the IGF2R gene. Cytogenet Genome Res 2006;113(1–4): 202–8.
22. Holly JM. The IGF-II enigma. Growth Horm IGF Res 1998;8(3):183–4.
23. O'Dell SD, Miller GJ, Cooper JA, et al. ApaI polymorphism in insulin-like growth factor II (IGF2) gene and weight in middle-aged males. Int J Obes Relat Metab Disord 1997;21(9):822–5.

24. Rodriguez S, Gaunt TR, O'Dell SD, et al. Haplotypic analyses of the IGF2-INS-TH gene cluster in relation to cardiovascular risk traits. Hum Mol Genet 2004;13(7): 715–25.

25. Rice T, Chagnon YC, Perusse L, et al. A genomewide linkage scan for abdominal subcutaneous and visceral fat in black and white families: the HERITAGE Family Study. Diabetes 2002;51(3):848–55.

26. Sandhu MS, Gibson JM, Heald AH, et al. Low circulating IGF-II concentrations predict weight gain and obesity in humans. Diabetes 2003;52(6):1403–8.

27. Heald AH, Karvestedt L, Anderson SG, et al. Low insulin-like growth factor-II levels predict weight gain in normal weight subjects with type 2 diabetes. Am J Med 2006;119(2):167.e9–167.e15.

28. Martin RM, Holly JM, Davey Smith G, et al. Associations of adiposity from childhood into adulthood with insulin resistance and the insulin-like growth factor system: 65-year follow-up of the Boyd Orr Cohort. J Clin Endocrinol Metab 2006;91(9):3287–95.

29. Jeyaratnaganthan N, Hojlund K, Kroustrup JP, et al. Circulating levels of insulin-like growth factor-II/mannose-6-phosphate receptor in obesity and type 2 diabetes. Growth Horm IGF Res 2010;20(3):185–91.

30. Heald AH, Kaushal K, Siddals KW, et al. Insulin-like growth factor binding protein-2 (IGFBP-2) is a marker for the metabolic syndrome. Exp Clin Endocrinol Diabetes 2006;114(7):371–6.

31. Zhao Y, Ma YS, Fang Y, et al. IGF2BP2 genetic variation and type 2 diabetes: a global meta-analysis. DNA Cell Biol 2011. [Epub ahead of print].

32. Jia H, Yu L, Jiang Z, et al. Association between IGF2BP2 rs4402960 polymorphism and risk of type 2 diabetes mellitus: a meta-analysis. Arch Med Res 2011;42(5):361–7.

33. Rodriguez S, Eiriksdottir G, Gaunt TR, et al. IGF2BP1, IGF2BP2 and IGF2BP3 genotype, haplotype and genetic model studies in metabolic syndrome traits and diabetes. Growth Horm IGF Res 2010;20(4):310–8.

34. Murphy R, Baptista J, Holly J, et al. Severe intrauterine growth retardation and atypical diabetes associated with a translocation breakpoint disrupting regulation of the insulin-like growth factor 2 gene. J Clin Endocrinol Metab 2008;93(11): 4373–80.

35. Denley A, Bonython ER, Booker GW, et al. Structural determinants for high-affinity binding of insulin-like growth factor II to insulin receptor (IR)-A, the exon 11 minus isoform of the IR. Mol Endocrinol 2004;18(10):2502–12.

36. Pandini G, Conte E, Medico E, et al. IGF-II binding to insulin receptor isoform A induces a partially different gene expression profile from insulin binding. Ann N Y Acad Sci 2004;1028:450–6.

37. Sacco A, Morcavallo A, Pandini G, et al. Differential signaling activation by insulin and insulin-like growth factors I and II upon binding to insulin receptor isoform A. Endocrinology 2009;150(8):3594–602.

38. Morcavallo A, Genua M, Palummo A, et al. Insulin and insulin-like growth factor II differentially regulate endocytic sorting and stability of the insulin receptor isoform A. J Biol Chem 2012;287(14):11422–36.

39. Barker DJ, Winter PD, Osmond C, et al. Weight in infancy and death from ischaemic heart disease. Lancet 1989;2(8663):577–80.

40. Kajantie E. Early-life events. Effects on aging. Hormones (Athens) 2008;7(2): 101–13.

41. Barker DJ. The developmental origins of adult disease. J Am Coll Nutr 2004; 23(Suppl 6):588S–95S.

42. Barker DJ, Gluckman PD, Godfrey KM, et al. Fetal nutrition and cardiovascular disease in adult life. Lancet 1993;341(8850):938–41.
43. Symonds ME, Gardner DS. Experimental evidence for early nutritional programming of later health in animals. Curr Opin Clin Nutr Metab Care 2006;9(3):278–83.
44. Langley-Evans SC. Nutritional programming of disease: unravelling the mechanism. J Anat 2009;215(1):36–51.
45. Rogers I, Metcalfe C, Gunnell D, et al. Insulin-like growth factor-I and growth in height, leg length, and trunk length between ages 5 and 10 years. J Clin Endocrinol Metab 2006;91(7):2514–9.
46. Rogers IS, Gunnell D, Emmett PM, et al. Cross-sectional associations of diet and insulin-like growth factor levels in 7- to 8-year-old children. Cancer Epidemiol Biomarkers Prev 2005;14(1):204–12.
47. Thissen JP, Ketelslegers JM, Underwood LE. Nutritional regulation of the insulin-like growth factors. Endocr Rev 1994;15(1):80–101.
48. Rogers I, Emmett P, Gunnell D, et al. Milk as a food for growth? The insulin-like growth factors link. Public Health Nutr 2006;9(3):359–68.
49. Hoppe C, Udam TR, Lauritzen L, et al. Animal protein intake, serum insulin-like growth factor I, and growth in healthy 2.5-y-old Danish children. Am J Clin Nutr 2004;80(2):447–52.
50. Hoppe C, Molgaard C, Juul A, et al. High intakes of skimmed milk, but not meat, increase serum IGF-I and IGFBP-3 in eight-year-old boys. Eur J Clin Nutr 2004; 58(9):1211–6.
51. Zhu K, Du X, Cowell CT, et al. Effects of school milk intervention on cortical bone accretion and indicators relevant to bone metabolism in Chinese girls aged 10-12 y in Beijing. Am J Clin Nutr 2005;81(5):1168–75.
52. Larnkjaer A, Hoppe C, Molgaard C, et al. The effects of whole milk and infant formula on growth and IGF-I in late infancy. Eur J Clin Nutr 2009;63(8):956–63.
53. Rich-Edwards JW, Ganmaa D, Pollak MN, et al. Milk consumption and the prepubertal somatotropic axis. Nutr J 2007;6:28.
54. Ostman EM, Liljeberg Elmstahl HG, Bjorck IM. Inconsistency between glycemic and insulinemic responses to regular and fermented milk products. Am J Clin Nutr 2001;74(1):96–100.
55. Brismar K, Fernqvist-Forbes E, Wahren J, et al. Effect of insulin on the hepatic production of insulin-like growth factor-binding protein-1 (IGFBP-1), IGFBP-3, and IGF-I in insulin-dependent diabetes. J Clin Endocrinol Metab 1994;79(3): 872–8.
56. Chellakooty M, Juul A, Boisen KA, et al. A prospective study of serum insulin-like growth factor I (IGF-I) and IGF-binding protein-3 in 942 healthy infants: associations with birth weight, gender, growth velocity, and breastfeeding. J Clin Endocrinol Metab 2006;91(3):820–6.
57. Savino F, Fissore MF, Grassino EC, et al. Ghrelin, leptin and IGF-I levels in breast-fed and formula-fed infants in the first years of life. Acta Paediatr 2005;94(5): 531–7.
58. Martin RM, Holly JM, Smith GD, et al. Could associations between breastfeeding and insulin-like growth factors underlie associations of breastfeeding with adult chronic disease? The Avon Longitudinal Study of Parents and Children. Clin Endocrinol 2005;62(6):728–37.
59. Larnkjaer A, Ingstrup HK, Schack-Nielsen L, et al. Early programming of the IGF-I axis: negative association between IGF-I in infancy and late adolescence in a 17-year longitudinal follow-up study of healthy subjects. Growth Horm IGF Res 2009; 19(1):82–6.

60. Ben-Shlomo Y, Holly J, McCarthy A, et al. Prenatal and postnatal milk supplementation and adult insulin-like growth factor I: long-term follow-up of a randomized controlled trial. Cancer Epidemiol Biomarkers Prev 2005;14(5):1336–9.
61. Martin RM, Holly JM, Middleton N, et al. Childhood diet and insulin-like growth factors in adulthood: 65-year follow-up of the Boyd Orr Cohort. Eur J Clin Nutr 2007;61(11):1281–92.
62. Elias SG, Keinan-Boker L, Peeters PH, et al. Long term consequences of the 1944-1945 Dutch famine on the insulin-like growth factor axis. Int J Cancer 2004;108(4):628–30.
63. Soliman AT, Hassan AE, Aref MK, et al. Serum insulin-like growth factors I and II concentrations and growth hormone and insulin responses to arginine infusion in children with protein-energy malnutrition before and after nutritional rehabilitation. Pediatr Res 1986;20(11):1122–30.
64. Holly JM, Amiel SA, Sandhu RR, et al. The role of growth hormone in diabetes mellitus. J Endocrinol 1988;118(3):353–64.
65. Barzilai N, Bartke A. Biological approaches to mechanistically understand the healthy life span extension achieved by calorie restriction and modulation of hormones. J Gerontol A Biol Sci Med Sci 2009;64(2):187–91.
66. Kenyon CJ. The genetics of ageing. Nature 2010;464(7288):504–12.
67. Fontana L, Partridge L, Longo VD. Extending healthy life span—from yeast to humans. Science 2010;328(5976):321–6.
68. Ziv E, Hu D. Genetic variation in insulin/IGF-1 signaling pathways and longevity. Ageing Res Rev 2011;10(2):201–4.
69. Ceda GP, Dall'Aglio E, Morganti S, et al. Update on new therapeutic options for the somatopause. Acta Biomed 2010;81(Suppl 1):67–72.
70. Perrini S, Laviola L, Carreira MC, et al. The GH/IGF1 axis and signaling pathways in the muscle and bone: mechanisms underlying age-related skeletal muscle wasting and osteoporosis. J Endocrinol 2010;205(3):201–10.
71. Thorner MO. Statement by the Growth Hormone Research Society on the GH/IGF-I axis in extending health span. J Gerontol A Biol Sci Med Sci 2009;64(10):1039–44.

The Insulin-Like Growth Factors and Growth Disorders of Childhood

Philippe F. Backeljauw, MD[a], Steven D. Chernausek, MD[b],*

KEYWORDS

- Growth hormone • Insulin-like growth factor • Short stature • GH receptor deficiency
- Recombinant human insulin-like growth factor treatment

KEY POINTS

- Insulin-like growth factors (IGFs) are the dominant regulators of human growth.
- Measures of circulating IGF-I are useful in diagnosing growth disorders in childhood and in evaluating response to growth hormone therapy.
- Recombinant human IGF-I is an effective treatment of severe primary IGF deficiency.

INTRODUCTION

Homologues of the insulin-like growth factor (IGF) system function in species as primitive as *Caenorhabditis elegans* and growth is IGF-dependent for all vertebrate species. For humans, the IGFs are the dominant regulators of somatic growth. In this article, the clinical manifestations of specific growth disorders of children caused by defects in the growth hormone (GH)/IGF pathway are described and how they reveal specific aspects of IGF biology is shown. Measurement of IGF-I in blood and the usefulness of such determinations in the medical care of children are reviewed. The use of recombinant human IGF-I (rhIGF-I) for the treatment of IGF deficiency (IGFD) is discussed. Potential future developments in IGF-I are highlighted.

We have elected to use the term IGFD because it describes a common feature of many growth disorders that putatively involve the GH/IGF axis. We also refer to primary IGFD, a term recently introduced into literature that has caused controversy

Disclosures: SDC is a paid consultant for Ipsen, which manufactures and markets recombinant human insulin-like growth factor I. PFB receives grant funding from and has participated in advisory boards for Ipsen.

[a] Department of Pediatrics, Cincinnati Children's Hospital Medical Center, University of Cincinnati College of Medicine, 3333 Burnett Avenue, Cincinnati, OH 45229, USA;
[b] Department of Pediatrics, University of Oklahoma Health Sciences Center, 1200 Children's Avenue, Suite 4500, Oklahoma City, OK 73104-4600, USA
* Corresponding author.
E-mail address: Steven-Chernausek@OUHSC.edu

Endocrinol Metab Clin N Am 41 (2012) 265–282
doi:10.1016/j.ecl.2012.04.010
0889-8529/12/$ – see front matter © 2012 Elsevier Inc. All rights reserved.

endo.theclinics.com

because of its connection with the US Food and Drug Administration (FDA) approval of rhIGF-I for treatment of GH insensitivity syndromes.[1] Despite this situation, we find the term useful for several reasons. First, it emphasizes the central role of IGF-I in human growth. Second, it is analogous to other primary endocrine deficiencies such as primary hypothyroidism in which the target gland fails to produce adequate amounts of its primary hormone (thyroxine) with reciprocal increases in the pituitary trophic hormone (thyroid-stimulating hormone [TSH]). The term indicates the approved therapeutic use for rhIGF-I.

GROWTH DISORDERS CAUSED BY GH/IGF PATHWAY DEFECTS
Primary IGFD

Primary IGFD is a condition found in adequately nourished, short-statured patients who have low serum IGF-I concentrations in the setting of normal or increased GH secretion (**Table 1**). This condition is distinct from abnormalities of the hypothalamus and pituitary gland that lead to insufficient secretion of GH and result in secondary IGF-I deficiency. Primary IGFD results from defects at or beyond the level of the GH receptor (GHR) (**Fig. 1**). The following sections discuss different causes of primary IGFD.

GHR deficiency

The human GHR is a transmembrane protein belonging to the superfamily of cytokine receptors. The *GHR* gene, located on chromosome 5p13.1-p12, contains 10 exons, of which exons 3 to 7 encode the extracellular GH binding domain.[2] After GH associates with this constitutively homodimeric receptor, recruitment/phosphorylation of Janus-family tyrosine kinase 2 (JAK2) activates post-GHR signaling mechanisms involving mitogen-activated protein kinase-extracellular signal-regulated kinase 1 and 2, phosphatidylinositol 3-kinase, and signal transducer and activator of transcription (STAT) pathways. Of special importance are the STATs,[3] with STAT5b constituting a critical element for *IGF1* gene transcription and mediating most GH effects on skeletal growth.

The first GHR defects delineated involved large deletions encoding the extracellular domain of the *GHR* gene, providing a molecular basis for the severe growth failure associated with GH insensitivity (Laron syndrome). A variety of molecular defects affecting the GHR have subsequently been identified. These defects include mutations of *GHR* giving rise to abnormal GH binding, defective GHR dimerization, abnormal anchoring in the cell membrane, or defective signal transduction. Abnormalities involving the extracellular domain are the most common, with more than 60 such mutations described to date.[4] Most disrupt GH binding and therefore are associated with low concentrations of GH binding protein (GHBP, a circulating form of the GHR extracellular domain). Such loss of GH binding typically results in the classic phenotype of Laron syndrome accompanied by low serum concentrations of all GH-dependent peptides: IGF-I, IGF binding protein 3 (IGFBP-3), and the acid-labile subunit (ALS).[5] The statural growth of these children is characterized by relatively normal length at birth, followed by progressive, severe postnatal growth failure. The patients' height standard deviation scores (SDS) vary from −12 to −2.2 (mean −6.1). Clinically, they often have a prominent forehead, midfacial hypoplasia, central adiposity, and acromicria.[4] Hypoglycemia during the early years of life is common.[5]

Although GHBP concentrations are typically low in Laron syndrome, patients have been described with the phenotypic and biochemical features of classic GH insensitivity, but with normal or increased serum GHBP. In these cases, GH binding is retained, but GHR function disrupted. For example, substitution of aspartate residue by histidine at position 152 in the extracellular domain allows GH binding but not receptor dimerization.[6] Other GH-insensitive patients have been found to carry *GHR*

Table 1
Phenotypes of patients with defects in GH/IGF axis

Condition	Affected Gene	Prenatal Growth	Postnatal Growth	GH/IGF Axis	Other Features
GH insensitivity, Laron syndrome	GHR	Normal	↓↓↓	GH ↑ IGF-I ↓ IGFBP-3 ↓	Hypoglycemia common; affected usually homozygous
STAT5b deficiency	STAT5b	Normal	↓↓↓↓	GH ↑ IGF-I ↓ IGFBP-3 ↓	Immune deficiency; affected usually homozygous
IGF-I gene mutation	IGF1	↓↓	↓↓↓↓	GH ↑ IGF-I ↓ IGFBP-3 NI	Deafness, microcephaly, carbohydrate intolerance; affected usually homozygous
Russell-Silver syndrome	IGF2 via abnormal cytosine methylation	↓↓	↓↓↓↓	GH NI IGF-I NI IGFBP-3 NI	Dysmorphic features and body asymmetry; normal IGF-II levels
ALS deficiency	IGFALS	Normal	↓−↓↓	GH NI IGF-I ↓ IGFBP-3 ↓ ALS undetectable	Phenotype similar to constitutional delay of growth and adolescence; affected usually homozygous
IGF resistance	IGF1R	↓↓−↓↓↓	↓↓↓	GH NI-↑ IGF-I NI-↑ IGFBP-3 NI-↑	Variable effect on intellect/mental status; usually hemizygous, heterozygous, or compound heterozygote

Abbreviations: ALS, acid-labile subunit; IGFBP-3, insulin-like growth factor binding protein 3; IGF1R, type I IGF receptor; NI, normal; STAT, signal transducer and activator of transcription.

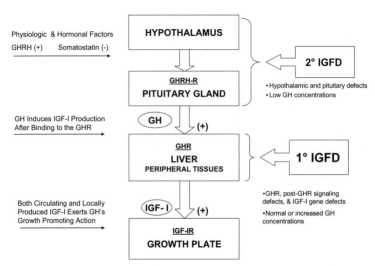

Fig. 1. The GH/IGF-I axis. GHRH, GH-releasing hormone; R, receptor. (*Modified from* Rosenthal S, Cohen P, Clayton P, et al. Treatment perspectives in idiopathic short stature with a focus on IGF-I deficiency. Pediatr Endocrinol Rev 2007;4(2):253.)

splice site mutations that result in the loss of the intracellular domain[7] with defective GHR anchoring in the cell membrane. Several other *GHR* mutations disrupting the intracellular domain have been identified that result in GHR truncation[8] or abnormal phosphorylation with reduced activation of STAT5.[9]

STAT5b deficiency

As mentioned earlier, STAT5b is a major mediator of post-GHR signaling, itself initiating gene transcription. The first human described with STATb deficiency had a clinical phenotype reminiscent of GH insensitivity with severe short stature (height SDS −7.5) and low IGF-I and IGFBP-3 in the face of increased GH concentrations.[10,11] This situation was caused by homozygosity for a missense mutation, which caused a marked reduction of STAT5b phosphorylation and reduced production of IGF-I, IGFBP-3, and ALS. Shortly after this first report, a second patient was identified with similar clinical and biochemical features. Additional individuals with *STAT5b* gene defects have been described since then, with ages from 2 to 31 years. Their height deficit ranged from −5.6 to −9.9 SDS. These patients all had immune defects manifesting variously as hemorrhagic varicella, pulmonary infections, lymphocytic interstitial pneumonia, and pulmonary fibrosis.[12–15] This situation is because STAT5b is involved in the signaling pathway for a variety of cytokines, including interleukin 2 and γ interferon. In addition, because STAT5b is also involved in prolactin signaling, hyperprolactinemia is found in affected patients.[11,12,15,16] Thus, a clinical picture of severe primary IGFD associated with immune dysfunction, interstitial lung disease in particular, and hyperprolactinemia strongly indicates a *STAT5b* mutation.

IGF1 gene mutations

The first individual with an *IGF1* gene deletion was reported in 1996.[17] The patient was a 15-year-old boy who was the product of a consanguineous marriage. He had intrauterine growth retardation (birth length −5.4 SDS), a small head circumference (−4.9 SDS at birth), and severe postnatal short stature (height SDS −6.9), Additional clinical features included severe developmental delay, sensorineural deafness, delayed puberty, and carbohydrate intolerance. The patient was homozygous for a partial deletion within *IGF1*, resulting in the absence of functional IGF-I. As expected, circulating concentrations of IGF-I were undetectable in the face of increased GH concentrations. Three additional cases have been described since this initial report.[18–20] Two patients have homozygous point mutations in the *IGF1* gene, resulting in an IGF-I that is detectable in immunoassays but not biologically active. These patients had normal or increased IGF-I concentrations.[18,20]

All patients with *IGF1* gene deficiency thus far have low birth weight and develop severe postnatal growth failure. Although they all have some degree of mental retardation, not all patients have hearing loss. The addition of prenatal growth impairment to postnatal growth failure clearly differentiates IGF-I gene defects from defects in the GHR or STAT5b, which underscores that IGF-I is a major mediator of both prenatal and postnatal growth, and that IGF-I dependent intrauterine growth is, for the most part, non-GH mediated.[19]

Deficiency of ALS

Domene and colleagues[21] initially described a 17-year-old male with subtle growth retardation associated with ALS deficiency. The patient had normal prenatal growth, no dysmorphic features, and normal general development, but had delayed puberty. The patient had very low blood levels of IGF-I (–5.3 SDS), IGFBP-3 (–9.7 SDS), and undetectable ALS with normal GH secretion. Despite such significant abnormalities of the GH/IGF-I axis, the boy's growth deficit was modest (height SDS –2). His ALS deficiency resulted from a homozygous frameshift mutation in the *IGFALS* gene, which predicted a truncated, inactive protein. Since then, about 20 other patients, most of them males, have been described with homozygous or compound heterozygous mutations of *IGFALS*.[22–28] Their height deficits range from about –0.5 to –4.2 SDS. All show very low IGF-I and IGFBP-3 concentrations, as well as undetectable ALS concentrations. Stimulated GH concentrations are normal or increased, IGF-I does not increase after GH administration, and the growth response to therapy with exogenous GH is poor. The growth impairment in ALS-deficient patients is significantly less than that observed in others with equivalent degrees of IGFD and likely reflects preserved or enhanced GH action and IGF-I production in target tissues. Although the role of ALS deficiency in growth disorders is not clear, emerging data indicate that heterozygous *IGFALS* mutations may explain the height deficit observed in a subset of patients with idiopathic short stature (ISS).[29]

Idiopathic IGFD

Individuals with ISS comprise a heterogeneous group of patients for whom the cause of short stature is unclear, but is likely explained by the presence of a variety of molecular anomalies and environmental circumstances. Assessing the prevalence of IGFD in this group of patients has diagnostic and potentially therapeutic implications. From 20% to 50% of children with ISS have been found to have IGF-I concentrations less than –2 SDS.[30–32] However, there is no obvious cause for IGFD in most patients with ISS. It is possible that some have subtle defects in GH secretion not detected by standard testing. Alternatively, IGFD could be related to the presence of a heterozygous GHR mutation,[33] especially if such a defect behaves in a dominant-negative manner.[4]

Studies by Cohen and colleagues[34] support the suggestion that partial GH insensitivity contributes to the growth deficit in ISS. These investigators showed that patients with ISS, when compared with those with GH deficiency (GHD), require larger doses of GH to achieve equivalent circulating IGF-I concentrations. Also, as noted earlier, some patients with ISS have *IGFALS* mutations. Thus, the proportion of patients left with the unsatisfying diagnosis of ISS should diminish with time as new explanations for growth disorders are discovered and new diagnostic tools become available. The clinician should investigate these patients with all diagnostic tools available to allow for correct diagnosis and an individualized treatment approach.

Russell-Silver Syndrome

Russell-Silver syndrome (RSS) is a genetic disorder characterized by prenatal and postnatal growth retardation accompanied by typical dysmorphic features such as triangular facies, clinodactyly, and micrognathia; body asymmetry is found in approximately 50% of cases.[35] A methylation defect involving the *IGF2* locus (11p15) is present in 40% to 50% of RSS, providing evidence that reduced IGF-II production plays a pathogenic role in these cases. Normally, only the paternal *IGF2* allele is expressed because of imprinting. Hypomethylation suppresses the paternal *IGF2* gene, resulting in IGF-II deficiency, which is believed to explain the growth restriction. The fact that Beckwith-Wiedemann syndrome, a disorder of excessive growth, is caused by hypermethylation at the same loci and presumed biallelic *IGF2* expression supports this postulate, as does the reduced IGF-II production from RSS fibroblasts.[36]

Circulating concentrations of IGF-II are normal in patients with RSS with 11p15 hypomethylation,[37] but this has been explained by the fact that circulating IGF-II is derived primarily from the liver, which uses a nonimprinted promoter for the control of *IGF2* gene expression. Circulating concentrations of IGF-I are also solidly normal in these patients, which is distinct from other short children born small for gestational age who usually have IGF-I levels in the low normal range or below.[38] RSS is the only condition of attenuated growth in humans attributable to IGF-II deficiency.

IGF Resistance Syndrome

In 2003, we reported the first cases of IGF resistance caused by mutations in the type 1 IGF receptor gene (*IGF1R*) in humans.[39] In 1 case, a nonsense mutation led to a 50% reduction in IGF1R expression, whereas the other was a compound heterozygote for missense mutations affecting IGF1R function. Subsequent reports describe additional cases from which emerge typical clinical and laboratory features found in humans harboring *IGF1R* anomalies.[40–46] The clinical picture is dominated by prenatal and postnatal growth deficits, often severe with heights in the –2 to –5 SDS range. The children have neither major dysmorphic features nor organ anomalies, but head circumference is reduced. Mental development has been described as deficient to normal, but extensive, formal testing has not been performed. Hearing seems to be normal in contrast to those with *IGF1* defects. One of the initial cases we reported subsequently developed impaired glucose tolerance,[47] potentially because of the effect of reduced IGF signaling leading to pancreatic β cell dysfunction.[48]

Because IGF-I is a negative regulator of GH secretion, IGF resistance at the somatotroph would be expected to enhance GH output, resulting in increased concentrations of IGF-I and IGFBP-3. This situation has been found in some, but not all, patients described to date. The reason for this variability is unknown, but is perhaps because of differences in IGF sensitivity/signaling among tissues.

These data indicate that IGF1R signaling is a major determinant of growth and that graded reductions in abundance or function of IGF1R affect growth in humans. All of the mutations leading to IGF resistance in cases described to date are compatible with reduced but not absent receptor function. The fact that *IGF1R* null humans have not been identified suggests that the condition may be lethal, as is the case for murine null mutants.[49] Based on this finding, one predicts, as more cases are identified, that a spectrum of growth and metabolic phenotypes will emerge resulting from IGF1R variants of different severities.

IGF IN THE CIRCULATION
IGF-I Assay

The measurement of IGF-I in serum or plasma is valuable in the evaluation of growth disorders and for monitoring of individuals treated with GH. Most IGF-I in plasma is in a ternary complex consisting of IGF-I, IGFBP-3, and the ALS. As a consequence, the half-life of IGF-I is prolonged, resulting in stable blood levels over the course of a day, which, in theory, accurately reflect GH secretion and action. However, several factors complicate both the measurement and interpretation of IGF-I concentrations. Detailed discussion of IGF assay nuances is beyond the scope of this article and can be found elsewhere.[50] Here, we emphasize major points needed for appropriate use and interpretation.

There is a large age-related variation in blood levels of IGF-I, which increase approximately 5-fold between infancy and adolescence.[51] Thus, high-quality normative data over the lifespan are needed when used in the clinical setting. Second, IGFBPs can interfere with measurement depending on the assay used and the condition of the patient. In some cases, the IGF-I is underestimated, in others overestimated. Intuitively, measurement of free IGF-I might seem advantageous, like free T4 determination. Quantifying free IGF-I is cumbersome and no more discriminating than other assay types.[52] Therefore, most IGF assays use some form of IGFBP removal to reduce the untoward effects but still measure total IGF-I. Although IGF-I is produced by multiple tissues, that found in the circulation predominantly reflects hepatic production. Therefore, blood-borne IGF-I represents only part of a large somatic pool and may not always accurately depict tissue levels. Mouse models wherein hepatic production of IGF-I is eliminated show marked reduction in plasma IGF-I levels, but only modest reduction in growth,[53,54] presumably because of preserved production of IGF-I in peripheral tissues. For clinical purposes, one should therefore use assays that have abundant and well-described normative data and that reduce IGFBP interference and consider carefully the clinical context of the patient being evaluated.

IGF-I Blood Levels

Despite the vagaries of IGF-I assays noted earlier, time has shown that measurement of circulating IGF-I in the blood is useful. The important questions are:

1. Can measurement of circulating IGF-I be used to detect GHD?
2. Does the level of IGF-I in the blood predict subsequent response to therapy?
3. What is the usefulness of measuring IGF-I during therapy with GH?

Diagnosing GHD

Measurement of circulating IGF-I by immunoassay is useful in the evaluation of short children, age 3 years and older. Younger than this age, the levels in normal individuals are relatively low and overlap substantially with those children with GHD. Several studies have examined the sensitivity and specificity of IGF-I in detecting GHD in groups of short-statured children.[55] Sensitivities typically range from 70% to 90% and specificities from 50% to 80%. The variations reflect the characteristics of specific assays as well as the difficulty of using other measures to obtain a clear separation of GHD from short stature as a result of other causes. In those individuals with severe GHD caused by central nervous system anomalies or molecular defects in GH secretion, circulating IGF-I is almost always less than −2 SDS for age and sex. However, others with lesser degrees of GHD frequently have IGF-I concentrations in the lower end of the normal range, as do many individuals with ISS. One study found a relatively weak relationship between circulating IGF-I and results of pharmacologic tests of GH release in children, indicating that these tests reflect distinct features of GH biology.[56] Therefore, a reasonable approach is to take IGF-I concentrations less than −2 SDS as strong evidence of GHD if other conditions that decrease IGF-I (**Box 1**) have been excluded. Likewise, circulating concentrations greater than the mean for age and sex eliminate GHD as a diagnostic possibility. The remainder must be judged by carefully weighing clinical and laboratory data. The diagnosis of GHD for many patients is a clinical one and rests on a combination of auxology, measures of GH and IGF-I, and imaging studies such as skeletal age and magnetic resonance imaging of the pituitary and hypothalamus.

Prediction of response

The response to GH treatment among short children is highly variable and judging the effectiveness for an individual takes a minimum of several months of observation. As a consequence, many studies have been conducted to identify predictors, hormonal and auxologic, which could be used at the onset of therapy. Studies that examine the ability of IGF-I to predict subsequent response to GH therapy in some cases show mixed results,[57] although they more often find that that lower circulating levels of IGF-I are associated with a better response to GH in individuals with ISS, short children born small for gestational age, and those with varying degrees of GHD.[58–60] Most studies show that baseline IGF-I level is a better index of GH response than other predictors such as parental height, age at start, and maximal GH value after stimulation. However, the predictive value of IGF-I is not so robust as to be used as a sole criterion for selecting individuals for treatment. In addition, most often studies use a single or a relatively narrow range of GH dosing, which limits generalization.

IGF-I measurements during GH therapy

Assessment of IGF-I blood level during GH therapy can be used to assess compliance with the therapeutic regimen, to avoid an excessive GH dose that might lead to complications, and perhaps to guide therapy in other ways. It has been recommended that circulating concentrations that exceed the +2.5 SDS for age and sex should prompt a reduction of GH dose.[61] However, the evidence that this practice reduces complications or side effects in children is limited. Keeping IGF-I levels within the normal range makes sense for individuals with bona fide GHD, especially when they

---

Box 1
Differential diagnosis of low circulating IGF-I concentration

- GH deficiency
- GHR dysfunction (GH resistance/insensitivity)
- Post-GHR signaling defect (STAT5b)
- *IGF1* gene defect
- ALS deficiency
- Hepatic insufficiency (eg, cirrhosis)
- Malnutrition
- Hypothyroidism
- Delayed puberty
- Poorly controlled diabetes mellitus
- Chronic illness
- Glucocorticoid therapy

have reached normal height percentiles and the purpose of GH treatment is to replace GH and maintain normal growth. For other conditions in which GH is being used as a pharmacologic agent, perhaps to overcome a degree of IGF resistance, the rationale and value are less evident.

Cohen and colleagues[62] have recently examined the usefulness of using circulating concentrations of IGF-I to guide GH dosing in a group of short children. These investigators conducted a randomized, controlled trial adjusting GH dose to achieve IGF-I concentrations either in the normal (average) range or modestly supranormal (+2 SDS) and compared their responses with individuals given standard, weight-based dosing. Those for whom GH dose was adjusted to yield average IGF-I levels grew as well as those given weight-based dosing, but did so with wide variation in GH dose. Those given GH to reach IGF-I levels higher than average grew faster over the 2 years of study. When the patients were segregated based on pretreatment GH testing, the investigators found that those classified as GHD (peak response to stimuli less than 7 ng/mL) seemed more sensitive to GH in terms of growth response and their ability to increase circulating levels of IGF-I than those with normal GH release.[34] This finding suggests that the growth deficit in patients with ISS (ie, short children with low IGF-I and normal GH secretory response) can be explained, in part, by elements of both GH and IGF-I resistance. Thus, measurement of circulating IGF-I may be a valuable supplement in the management of children treated with GH, but clinical response, judged by skeletal growth, should be the main driver of therapeutic decisions.

Concerns about adverse effects of prolonged, high circulating concentrations of IGF-I, in addition to suggesting GH overdose, have arisen because of the associations between IGF-I and malignancy. For example, women with relatively high circulating concentrations of IGF-I have a modestly increased risk for breast cancer[63] and IGF-I–deficient children may have a lower risk of cancer.[64] Furthermore, there is a wealth of additional biologic information indicating that tumor growth can be stimulated by both GH and IGF-I.[65] This finding means that physicians should carefully weigh the pros and cons of treating any short child with GH. For those with clear-cut GHD, GH replacement is recommended and should be considered standard of care in most cases. For others, GH treatment is a therapeutic option that must be considered in the context of anticipated risks and benefits.

TREATMENT OF PRIMARY IGFD
Forms of Drug

rhIGF-I (mecasermin) was approved for the treatment of severe primary IGFD in the United States by the FDA in 2005 and by the European Medicines Agency (EMA) in 2007. In the United States severe primary IGFD is defined by the FDA as height SDS –3.0 or less, basal IGF-I SDS –3.0 or less, and normal or increased GH concentrations. In Europe severe primary IGFD is also defined by a height SDS –3.0 or less, but with basal IGF-I concentrations less than the 2.5th percentile (EMEA/H/C/000704 -II-13). rhIGF-I is also indicated for children who develop growth-attenuating antibodies against GH.

rhIGF-I is administered in a dose range of 40 to 120 μg/kg twice daily via subcutaneous injection. The half-life after a single subcutaneous injection in pediatric patients with severe primary IGFD is estimated to be just less than 6 hours on average. The clearance of the drug is inversely proportional to the IGFBP-3 concentration and is estimated to be 0.04 L/h/kg at an IGFBP-3 concentration of 3 mg/L.[66] The recommended starting dose is 40 to 80 μg/kg twice daily. If well tolerated for at least 1 week, the dose may be increased by 40 μg/kg to a maximum dose of 120 μg/kg twice daily.

rhIGF-I should be given shortly before or after a meal (or snack) to decrease the risk of hypoglycemia.

Mecasermin rinfabate is rhIGF-I complexed with rhIGFBP-3. The longer half-life (approximately 20 hours) allowed once-daily injections.[67] It was believed that use of the complex might reduce the high concentrations of free IGF-I and thereby mitigate some of the adverse effects of IGF-I monotherapy. rhIGF-I/rhIGFBP-3 complex is not available for the treatment of severe primary IGFD or any other short stature indication. Therefore, the sections that follow focus on the efficacy and safety of rhIGF-I and only briefly discuss information obtained from studies with the rhIGF-I/rhIGFBP-3 complex.

Efficacy

Clinical studies on 100 to 150 individuals treated with rhIGF-I for severe primary IGFD have been published over the last 10 years.[68–73] These data indicate that rhIGF-I therapy is effective in promoting statural growth, but that the growth response to rhIGF-I rarely allows these patients to reach an adult height within the normal range. In all the published studies, rhIGF-I was administered subcutaneously in doses ranging from 40 to 120 µg/kg twice daily, except in 1 study in which a once-a-day treatment regimen was used.[72]

Laron and colleagues administered IGF-I once daily subcutaneously before breakfast for 3 to 5 years to 9 children.[72,74] Using dosages as high as 150 µg/kg daily, patients' first-year growth velocities increased from 4.7 cm/y at baseline to 8.2 cm/y; growth velocities the second year averaged 6.0 cm/y. Additional studies further confirmed the statural benefit of IGF-I therapy when compared with placebo.[70,71] These reports underscored the smaller response to IGF-I therapy in patients with GH insensitivity syndrome compared with GH-deficient patients treated with GH.

In the largest study reported to date, 76 children with IGFD caused by GH insensitivity were treated with rhIGF-I for up to 12 years under a predominantly open-label study design.[69] Baseline height velocity increased from 2.8 cm/y on average to 8 cm/y during the first year of treatment, and was dose-dependent. Height velocities were lower during the subsequent years, but remained above baseline for up to 8 years. Results of final or near-final adult height have been reported in a subset of 16 patients.[75] Mean height SDS increased from –7.1 SDS at baseline to –5.1 SDS as a result of IGF-I therapy. This finding translates to an average estimated gain in height of 13.5 cm. There was significant variability in treatment response, with some patients improving their expected final height by more than 20 cm, whereas others improved their expected height by less than 5 cm. Although some patients reached a height within the normal range, most remained short at completion of therapy.

Another 33 patients were treated through the European Multicenter Study on GH Insensitivity Syndromes.[73] They too received 40 to 120 µg rhIGF-I per kg after meals subcutaneously twice daily. In patients treated for 48 months or longer (n = 17), mean height SDS improved from –6.5 ± 1.3 to –4.9 ± 1.9, with younger patients showing the better response. Also noted was a negative relationship between height, IGFBP-3 SDS, and response to rhIGF-I therapy in those treated with IGF-I at 80 µg/kg twice daily.[76] This finding suggests that the more severe the GH/IGF-I axis abnormality, the greater the growth response with rhIGF-I.

The effect of treatment with rhIGF-I/IGFBP-3 complex also has been reported.[77] Compared with rhIGF-I monotherapy trials, a higher daily IGF-I dose equivalent of rhIGF-I/IGFBP-3 was needed to achieve an improvement in height SDS of 0.8 over 2 years of therapy in 8 patients with severe primary IGFD. Although there are theoretic advantages to the complex, the clinical response to treatment with rhIGF-I/IGFBP-3 seems, at best, equal to that of rhIGF-I alone.

Safety

rhIGF-I produces insulin-like effects when administered at therapeutic doses[78] and thus hypoglycemia is a risk for patients treated with rhIGF-I. In trials, hypoglycemia was observed in about half of the patients with severe IGFD reported and was occasionally pronounced (eg, resulting in a seizure).[69] The situation is complicated because GH-insensitive patients frequently show spontaneous hypoglycemia; some hypoglycemic events are likely related to the rhIGF-I treatment, whereas others undoubtedly are not. At least half of the patients who had hypoglycemia reported an adverse event in 1 trial had shown low blood glucose measures before rhIGF-I therapy.[69] Hypoglycemia is primarily a concern in the youngest and smallest patients with IGFD and can be avoided by eating a meal at the time of rhIGF-I injection. Close monitoring of patients before and on IGF-I therapy showed that there was little effect on premeal blood glucose concentrations when adequate quantities of carbohydrates were consumed.

Lipohypertrophy at injection sites (similar to that observed with insulin) has been reported in patients receiving rhIGF-I,[68,69] but is prevented with proper dispersion of the injections. Several other long-term adverse events seem related to lymphoid tissue hypertrophy. Snoring, otitis media, conductive hearing loss, and tonsil/adenoid growth were found in nearly 25% of patients treated for many years. The size of the spleen also increases rapidly during the first couple of years of treatment, but normalizes afterward. Renal size increases to the upper normal range after 6 to 7 years of therapy, but renal function is never compromised. Less common but more serious is the occurrence of intracranial hypertension, reported in several patients with IGFD treated with rhIGF-I. The intracranial hypertension resolves without sequelae after discontinuation of the medication, which usually can then be reinstituted at a lower dose. Transient, mild increases in intracranial pressure may also be responsible for the frequent reports of headaches, occurring most often during the first month of IGF-I therapy. Acromegaloid coarsening of the face, with changes in eyebrows, lips, and nose, has been described in a few patients, particularly in those of pubertal age after several years of rhIGF-I therapy. These changes seem to be reversible, at least in part, after discontinuation of the rhIGF-I therapy after the completion of linear growth.

Despite these safety concerns, rhIGF-I seems to have an overall acceptable safety profile, especially when considering the lack of alternative therapies for severe IGFD. However, continued vigilance is important, because IGF-I has not been used in large numbers of patients over prolonged periods. Most of our clinical experience is in children with severe primary IGFD and the number of patients treated for 10 years or more is limited. Additional safety data are becoming available from the IGFD registry, which monitors commercially treated patients, many of whom are without severe primary IGFD. The registry data affirm that hypoglycemia and headache are the most common adverse events, affecting 7.9% and 5.3% of patients, respectively.[79] Continued acquisition of such safety information is important because it reflects more patients (more than 1000 were registered in the database as of 2010) who seem to be less severely affected than those reported in earlier trials of rhIGF-I.

Patient Selection

The diagnosis of GH insensitivity as a cause of severe primary IGFD is generally straightforward, with patients showing extremely low levels of IGF-I and IGFBP-3 in the face of increased GH secretion. Likewise, the rare patient who develops antibodies sufficient to neutralize GH is usually readily identified; they have severe GHD caused by null lesions in GH gene and become tachyphylactic to GH treatment early on. Patients with more obscure causes of primary IGFD are more challenging and require a detailed search for potential abnormalities of the GH/IGF-I axis. Such evaluation not only includes assessment of the GH secretory status but also examination of the distal part of the GH/IGF-I axis, with measurement of IGF-I, IGFBP-3, GHBP, and ALS. Assessment of GH sensitivity by measuring circulating IGF-I concentrations after multiple daily injections of human GH (the IGF generation test) has been proposed as a method to detect less obvious forms of IGFD.[80] Although these maneuvers do identify patients with extreme forms of classic primary IGFD, they have not been robust at identifying less severely affected patients. The spectrum of GH (in)sensitivity is likely broader than that represented by the small group of patients with severe primary IGFD. For less affected patients, there remain major diagnostic challenges related to the nature and scope of the particular molecular defects causing these milder forms of primary IGFD. Additional, controlled therapeutic trials with rhIGF-I are needed to provide further insight about which patient groups are expected to benefit from rhIGF-I therapy.

Recommendations

Therapy with IGF-I is approved for use in children with significant short stature (more than 3 SD less than the mean), low serum IGF-I (more than 3 SD less than the mean), and normal to increased GH concentrations. The patient groups, after complete assessment of the GH/IGF-I axis, that can therefore be recommended for IGF-I therapy include: severe GH insensitivity (*GHR* mutations, GH signaling defect, or *STAT5b* mutation), IGF-I deficiency (caused by mutation or deletion of IGF-I), patients with *GH1* gene deletion who produce antibodies against exogenous GH, and patients with clinical diagnosis of dysfunctional GH/IGF-I axis resulting in severe primary IGFD. Additional indications (less severe primary IGFD) are under investigation, and therapy should not be initiated for these patients until clinical trial data are available unless they are enrolled in a specific clinical study. The expansion of the use of rhIGF-I beyond these indications remains experimental and is not justified until there is evidence for either superior growth response, improved cost-effectiveness, or a better safety profile when compared with available therapies. The Drugs and Therapeutics Committee of the Pediatric Endocrine Society states, "the use of rhIGF-I is only justified in conditions approved by the FDA. The use of IGF-I outside the FDA recommendations should, therefore, only be investigational."

FUTURE DEVELOPMENTS

The optimal use and appropriate therapeutic targets for rhIGF-I remain to be determined. Following initial studies of rhIGF-I therapy in severe primary IGFD, additional controlled therapeutic trials using rhIGF-I in patients with milder degrees of IGFD have been conducted. These trials include studies treating patients with ISS and IGF-I concentrations less than –2 SDS (but not <–3 SDS) with rhIGF-I given either once or twice daily.[81,82] In prepubertal patients treated with twice-daily IGF-I, first-year height velocity and height SDS increased significantly and was not much different from what is observed when ISS patients are treated with GH. Treatment with twice-daily rhIGF-I was well tolerated, but a study using once-daily rhIGF-I administration at higher doses was prematurely discontinued because of the high prevalence of hypoglycemia.[81]

Another area of exploration has been the combination of rhIGF-I with GH therapy. This approach may have advantages over monotherapy with either rhIGF-I or GH, especially for patients who have milder forms of GH insensitivity or GHD. The direct growth-promoting effects of GH could be enhanced by those of IGF-I, in addition to maintaining normal IGFBP and ALS concentrations, thereby influencing IGF-I half-life, clearance, and distribution. This situation could result in increased tissue levels of IGF-I and induce substantially more anabolic actions than either hormone alone. Moreover, the anti-insulin effects of GH may be counteracted by the insulin-like effects of IGF-I, with a resultant normalization of carbohydrate balance. Preliminary data from controlled studies in patients with short stature using a combination of GH and rhIGF-I yielded encouraging short-term efficacy results. In a study of patients with unexplained short stature (height SDS $\leq$ –2) and relatively low IGF-I concentrations (IGF-I SDS $\leq$ –1), 1 group was treated with 45 µg/kg/d of GH alone (a supraphysiologic dose), whereas the other groups received combined GH and rhIGF-I.[83] The first-year height velocities for patients were 9.2 cm per year for the GH-only group and 12.1 cm per year for those receiving GH and IGF-I at 150 µg/kg/d. Ongoing treatment and monitoring are required to confirm these efficacy data and to determine whether the combination of GH and rhIGF-I is superior to GH or IGF-I alone, in terms of safety and efficacy, and acceptable for treatment in patients with milder forms of growth failure.

Using circulating IGF-I concentrations to guide GH therapy as performed by Cohen and colleagues[62] is an example of individualizing treatment based on additional bio-logic data. The intrinsic differences to GH and IGF sensitivities became apparent through those experiments and suggest that more work is needed in this area to opti-mize care. Still needed is better definition of the causes of IGFD and the ability to quan-tify IGF sensitivity, analogous to the ways in which we now measure insulin secretion and sensitivity. Such knowledge will permit a more personalized approach to patients, allowing physicians to determine the likely response, judge the relative risks and toxic-ities involved, and select the optimal therapy.

The activity of the GH/IGF axis is a major determinant of growth, and many condi-tions that lead to disordered growth involve aberrations along GH/IGF pathways. A recent publication[84] identified 180 genetic loci that influence height in humans, many of which are involved in GH/IGF pathways. IGFD is a frequent concomitant of ISS, yet most times remains unexplained. The ability to scan and identify variations in the genome, epigenome, and proteome in humans will result in better under-standing of disease mechanisms and, when applied to clinical medicine, will diminish the fraction of short children termed idiopathic and lead to better care of children with growth disorders.

REFERENCES

1. Rosenbloom AL. Recombinant human insulin-like growth factor-1 treatment: prime time or timeout? [Commentary on "Recombinant human insulin like growth factor-1 treatment: ready for prime time" by Bright GM, Mendoza JR, Rosenfeld RG, Endocrinol Metab Clin North Am 2009; 38:625–38]. Int J Pediatr Endocrinol 2009;2009:429684.
2. Leung DW, Spencer SA, Cachianes G, et al. Growth hormone receptor and serum binding protein: purification, cloning and expression. Nature 1987;330(6148): 537–43.
3. Waters MJ, Hoang HN, Fairlie DP, et al. New insights into growth hormone action. J Mol Endocrinol 2006;36(1):1–7.
4. Savage MO, Attie KM, David A, et al. Endocrine assessment, molecular charac-terization and treatment of growth hormone insensitivity disorders. Nat Clin Pract Endocrinol Metab 2006;2(7):395–407.

5. Laron Z. Insulin-like growth factor-I treatment of children with Laron syndrome (primary growth hormone insensitivity). Pediatr Endocrinol Rev 2008;5(3):766–71.

6. Duquesnoy P, Sobrier ML, Duriez B, et al. A single amino acid substitution in the exoplasmic domain of the human growth hormone (GH) receptor confers familial GH resistance (Laron syndrome) with positive GH-binding activity by abolishing receptor homodimerization. EMBO J 1994;13(6):1386–95.

7. Woods KA, Fraser NC, Postel-Vinay MC, et al. A homozygous splice site mutation affecting the intracellular domain of the growth hormone (GH) receptor resulting in Laron syndrome with elevated GH-binding protein. J Clin Endocrinol Metab 1996;81(5):1686–90.

8. Milward A, Metherell L, Maamra M, et al. Growth hormone (GH) insensitivity syndrome due to a GH receptor truncated after Box1, resulting in isolated failure of STAT 5 signal transduction. J Clin Endocrinol Metab 2004;89(3):1259–66.

9. Rosenfeld RG, Belgorosky A, Camacho-Hubner C, et al. Defects in growth hormone receptor signaling. Trends Endocrinol Metab 2007;18(4):134–41.

10. Hwa V, Little B, Adiyaman P, et al. Severe growth hormone insensitivity resulting from total absence of signal transducer and activator of transcription 5b. J Clin Endocrinol Metab 2005;90(7):4260–6.

11. Kofoed EM, Hwa V, Little B, et al. Growth hormone insensitivity associated with a STAT5b mutation. N Engl J Med 2003;349(12):1139–47.

12. Fang P, Kofoed EM, Little BM, et al. A mutant signal transducer and activator of transcription 5b, associated with growth hormone insensitivity and insulin-like growth factor-I deficiency, cannot function as a signal transducer or transcription factor. J Clin Endocrinol Metab 2006;91(4):1526–34.

13. Vidarsdottir S, Walenkamp MJ, Pereira AM, et al. Clinical and biochemical characteristics of a male patient with a novel homozygous STAT5b mutation. J Clin Endocrinol Metab 2006;91(9):3482–5.

14. Hwa V, Camacho-Hubner C, Little BM, et al. Growth hormone insensitivity and severe short stature in siblings: a novel mutation at the exon 13-intron 13 junction of the STAT5b gene. Horm Res 2007;68(5):218–24.

15. Bernasconi A, Marino R, Ribas A, et al. Characterization of immunodeficiency in a patient with growth hormone insensitivity secondary to a novel STAT5b gene mutation. Pediatrics 2006;118(5):e1584–92.

16. Pugliese-Pires PN, Tonelli CA, Dora JM, et al. A novel STAT5B mutation causing GH insensitivity syndrome associated with hyperprolactinemia and immune dysfunction in two male siblings. Eur J Endocrinol 2010;163(2):349–55.

17. Woods KA, Camacho-Hubner C, Savage MO, et al. Intrauterine growth retardation and postnatal growth failure associated with deletion of the insulin-like growth factor I gene. N Engl J Med 1996;335:1363–7.

18. Bonapace G, Concolino D, Formicola S, et al. A novel mutation in a patient with insulin-like growth factor 1 (IGF1) deficiency. J Med Genet 2003;40(12):913–7.

19. Netchine I, Azzi S, Houang M, et al. Partial primary deficiency of insulin-like growth factor (IGF)-I activity associated with IGF1 mutation demonstrates its critical role in growth and brain development. J Clin Endocrinol Metab 2009;94(10):3913–21.

20. Walenkamp MJ, Karperien M, Pereira AM, et al. Homozygous and heterozygous expression of a novel insulin-like growth factor-I mutation. J Clin Endocrinol Metab 2005;90(5):2855–64.

21. Domene HM, Bengolea SV, Martinez AS, et al. Deficiency of the circulating insulin-like growth factor system associated with inactivation of the acid-labile subunit gene. N Engl J Med 2004;350(6):570–7.

22. David A, Rose SJ, Miraki-Moud F, et al. Acid-labile subunit deficiency and growth failure: description of two novel cases. Horm Res Paediatr 2010;73(5):328–34.
23. Domene HM, Hwa V, Argente J, et al. Human acid-labile subunit deficiency: clinical, endocrine and metabolic consequences. Horm Res 2009;72(3):129–41.
24. Domene HM, Scaglia PA, Lteif A, et al. Phenotypic effects of null and haploinsufficiency of acid-labile subunit in a family with two novel IGFALS gene mutations. J Clin Endocrinol Metab 2007;92(11):4444–50.
25. Fofanova-Gambetti OV, Hwa V, Kirsch S, et al. Three novel IGFALS gene mutations resulting in total ALS and severe circulating IGF-I/IGFBP-3 deficiency in children of different ethnic origins. Horm Res 2009;71(2):100–10.
26. Heath KE, Argente J, Barrios V, et al. Primary acid-labile subunit deficiency due to recessive IGFALS mutations results in postnatal growth deficit associated with low circulating insulin growth factor (IGF)-I, IGF binding protein-3 levels, and hyperinsulinemia. J Clin Endocrinol Metab 2008;93(5):1616–24.
27. Hwa V, Haeusler G, Pratt KL, et al. Total absence of functional acid labile subunit, resulting in severe insulin-like growth factor deficiency and moderate growth failure. J Clin Endocrinol Metab 2006;91(5):1826–31.
28. van Duyvenvoorde HA, Kempers MJ, Twickler TB, et al. Homozygous and heterozygous expression of a novel mutation of the acid-labile subunit. Eur J Endocrinol 2008;159(2):113–20.
29. Fofanova-Gambetti OV, Hwa V, Wit JM, et al. Impact of heterozygosity for acid-labile subunit (IGFALS) gene mutations on stature: results from the international acid-labile subunit consortium. J Clin Endocrinol Metab 2010;95(9):4184–91.
30. Edouard T, Grunenwald S, Gennero I, et al. Prevalence of IGF1 deficiency in prepubertal children with isolated short stature. Eur J Endocrinol 2009;161(1):43–50.
31. Ranke MB, Schweizer R, Elmlinger MW, et al. Significance of basal IGF-I, IGFBP-3 and IGFBP-2 measurements in the diagnostics of short stature in children. Horm Res 2000;54(2):60–8.
32. Van Meter Q, Midyett LK, Deeb L, et al. Prevalence of primary IGFD among untreated children with short stature in a prospective, multi-center study [abstract 715]. Proceedings of International Congress of Endocrinology. Rio de Janiero (Brazil), November, 2008.
33. Goddard AD, Covello R, Luoh SM, et al. Mutations of the growth hormone receptor in children with idiopathic short stature. N Engl J Med 1995;33:1093–8.
34. Cohen P, Germak J, Rogol AD, et al. Variable degree of growth hormone (GH) and insulin-like growth factor (IGF) sensitivity in children with idiopathic short stature compared with GH-deficient patients: evidence from an IGF-based dosing study of short children. J Clin Endocrinol Metab 2010;95(5):2089–98.
35. Eggermann T. Russell-Silver syndrome. Am J Med Genet C Semin Med Genet 2010;154C(3):355–64.
36. Gicquel C, Rossignol S, Cabrol S, et al. Epimutation of the telomeric imprinting center region on chromosome 11p15 in Silver-Russell syndrome. Nat Genet 2005;37(9):1003–7.
37. Binder G, Seidel AK, Weber K, et al. IGF-II serum levels are normal in children with Silver-Russell syndrome who frequently carry epimutations at the IGF2 locus. J Clin Endocrinol Metab 2006;91(11):4709–12.
38. Binder G, Seidel AK, Martin DD, et al. The endocrine phenotype in silver-russell syndrome is defined by the underlying epigenetic alteration. J Clin Endocrinol Metab 2008;93(4):1402–7.
39. Abuzzahab MJ, Schneider A, Goddard A, et al. IGF-I receptor mutations resulting in intrauterine and postnatal growth retardation. N Engl J Med 2003;349(23):2211–22.

40. Fang P, Schwartz ID, Johnson BD, et al. Familial short stature caused by haploinsufficiency of the insulin-like growth factor I receptor due to nonsense-mediated messenger ribonucleic acid decay. J Clin Endocrinol Metab 2009;94(5):1740–7.
41. Inagaki K, Tiulpakov A, Rubtsov P, et al. A familial IGF-1 receptor mutant leads to short stature: clinical and biochemical characterization. J Clin Endocrinol Metab 2007;92:1542–8.
42. Kawashima Y, Kanzaki S, Yang F, et al. Mutation at cleavage site of IGF receptor in a short stature child born with intrauterine growth retardation. J Clin Endocrinol Metab 2005;90:4679–87.
43. Kruis T, Klammt J, Galli-Tsinopoulou A, et al. Heterozygous mutation within a kinase-conserved motif of the insulin-like growth factor I receptor causes intrauterine and postnatal growth retardation. J Clin Endocrinol Metab 2010;95(3): 1137–42.
44. Walenkamp MJ, van der Kamp HJ, Pereira AM, et al. A variable degree of intrauterine and postnatal growth retardation in a family with a missense mutation in the insulin-like growth factor I receptor. J Clin Endocrinol Metab 2006;91(8):3062–70.
45. Wallborn T, Wuller S, Klammt J, et al. A heterozygous mutation of the insulin-like growth factor-I receptor causes retention of the nascent protein in the endoplasmic reticulum and results in intrauterine and postnatal growth retardation. J Clin Endocrinol Metab 2010;95(5):2316–24.
46. Choi JH, Kang M, Kim GH, et al. Clinical and functional characteristics of a novel heterozygous mutation of the IGF1R gene and IGF1R haploinsufficiency due to terminal 15q26.2->qter deletion in patients with intrauterine growth retardation and postnatal catch-up growth failure. J Clin Endocrinol Metab 2011;96(1): E130–4.
47. Sundararajan S, Banach W, Chernausek SD. Defective glucose homeostasis in a child with a genetically-acquired function defect in the IGF-I receptor [abstract 432]. Proceedings of the Pediatric Societies' Annual Meeting 2004.
48. Kulkarni RN, Holzenberger M, Shih DQ, et al. beta-cell-specific deletion of the Igf1 receptor leads to hyperinsulinemia and glucose intolerance but does not alter beta-cell mass. Nat Genet 2002;31(1):111–5.
49. Liu J-P, Baker J, Perkins AS, et al. Mice carrying null mutations of the genes encoding insulin-like growth factor I (Igf-1) and the type 1 IGF receptor (Igf1r). Cell 1993;75:59–72.
50. Frystyk J, Freda P, Clemmons DR. The current status of IGF-I assays–a 2009 update. Growth Horm IGF Res 2010;20(1):8–18.
51. Brabant G, von zur Muhlen A, Wuster C, et al. Serum insulin-like growth factor I reference values for an automated chemiluminescence immunoassay system: results from a multicenter study. Horm Res 2003;60(2):53–60.
52. Frystyk J. Utility of free IGF-I measurements. Pituitary 2007;10(2):181–7.
53. Yakar S, Liu JL, Stannard B, et al. Normal growth and development in the absence of hepatic insulin-like growth factor I. Proc Natl Acad Sci U S A 1999; 96(13):7324–9.
54. Yakar S, Rosen CJ, Beamer WG, et al. Circulating levels of IGF-1 directly regulate bone growth and density. J Clin Invest 2002;110(6):771–81.
55. Cianfarani S, Liguori A, Germani D. IGF-I and IGFBP-3 assessment in the management of childhood onset growth hormone deficiency. Endocr Dev 2005; 9:66–75.
56. Hauffa BP, Lehmann N, Bettendorf M, et al. Central laboratory reassessment of IGF-I, IGF-binding protein-3, and GH serum concentrations measured at local treatment centers in growth-impaired children: implications for the agreement

between outpatient screening and the results of somatotropic axis functional testing. Eur J Endocrinol 2007;157(5):597–603.

57. Kamp GA, Zwinderman AH, Van Doorn J, et al. Biochemical markers of growth hormone (GH) sensitivity in children with idiopathic short stature: individual capacity of IGF-I generation after high-dose GH treatment determines the growth response to GH. Clin Endocrinol (Oxf) 2002;57(3):315–25.

58. Dahlgren J, Kristrom B, Niklasson A, et al. Models predicting the growth response to growth hormone treatment in short children independent of GH status, birth size and gestational age. BMC Med Inform Decis Mak 2007;7:40.

59. Kristrom B, Jansson C, Rosberg S, et al. Growth response to growth hormone (GH) treatment relates to serum insulin-like growth factor I (IGF-I) and IGF-binding protein-3 in short children with various GH secretion capacities. Swedish Study Group for Growth Hormone Treatment. J Clin Endocrinol Metab 1997;82(9):2889–98.

60. Schonau E, Westermann F, Rauch F, et al. A new and accurate prediction model for growth response to growth hormone treatment in children with growth hormone deficiency. Eur J Endocrinol 2001;144(1):13–20.

61. Cohen P, Rogol AD, Deal CL, et al. Consensus statement on the diagnosis and treatment of children with idiopathic short stature: a summary of the Growth Hormone Research Society, the Lawson Wilkins Pediatric Endocrine Society, and the European Society for Paediatric Endocrinology Workshop. J Clin Endocrinol Metab 2008;93(11):4210–7.

62. Cohen P, Rogol AD, Howard CP, et al. Insulin growth factor-based dosing of growth hormone therapy in children: a randomized, controlled study. J Clin Endocrinol Metab 2007;92(7):2480–6.

63. Hankinson SE, Willett WC, Colditz GA, et al. Circulating concentrations of insulin-like growth factor-I and risk of breast cancer. Lancet 1998;351(9113):1393–6.

64. Guevara-Aguirre J, Balasubramanian P, Guevara-Aguirre M, et al. Growth hormone receptor deficiency is associated with a major reduction in pro-aging signaling, cancer, and diabetes in humans. Sci Transl Med 2011;3(70):70ra13.

65. Samani AA, Yakar S, LeRoith D, et al. The role of the IGF system in cancer growth and metastasis: overview and recent insights. Endocr Rev 2007;28(1):20–47.

66. Grahnen A, Kastrup K, Heinrich U, et al. Pharmacokinetics of recombinant human insulin-like growth factor I given subcutaneously to healthy volunteers and to patients with growth hormone receptor deficiency. Acta Paediatr Suppl 1993;82(Suppl 391):9–13 [discussion: 14].

67. Camacho-Hubner C, Rose S, Preece MA, et al. Pharmacokinetic studies of re-combinant human insulin-like growth factor I (rhIGF-I)/rhIGF-binding protein-3 complex administered to patients with growth hormone insensitivity syndrome. J Clin Endocrinol Metab 2006;91(4):1246–53.

68. Backeljauw PF, Underwood LE. Therapy for 6.5–7.5 years with recombinant insulin-like growth factor I in children with growth hormone insensitivity syndrome: a clinical research center study. J Clin Endocrinol Metab 2001;86(4):1504–10.

69. Chernausek SD, Backeljauw PF, Frane J, et al. Long-term treatment with recombi-nant insulin-like growth factor (IGF)-I in children with severe IGF-I deficiency due to growth hormone insensitivity. J Clin Endocrinol Metab 2007;92(3):902–10.

70. Guevara-Aguirre J, Rosenbloom AL, Vasconez O, et al. Two-year treatment of growth hormone (GH) receptor deficiency with recombinant insulin-like growth factor I in 22 children: comparison of two dosage levels and to GH-treated GH deficiency. J Clin Endocrinol Metab 1997;82(2):629–33.

71. Guevara-Aguirre J, Vasconez O, Martinez V, et al. A randomized, double blind, placebo-controlled trial on safety and efficacy of recombinant human insulin-like growth factor-I in children with growth hormone receptor deficiency. J Clin Endocrinol Metab 1995;80(4):1393–8.

72. Klinger B, Laron Z. Three year IGF-I treatment of children with Laron syndrome. J Pediatr Endocrinol Metab 1995;8(3):149–58.

73. Ranke MB, Savage MO, Chatelain PG, et al. Long-term treatment of growth hormone insensitivity syndrome with IGF-I. Results of the European Multicentre Study. The Working Group on Growth Hormone Insensitivity Syndromes. Horm Res 1999;51(3):128–34.

74. Laron Z, Ginsberg S, Lilos P, et al. Long-term IGF-I treatment of children with Laron syndrome increases adiposity. Growth Horm IGF Res 2006;16(1):61–4.

75. Backeljauw PF, Calikoglu AS, Kuntze J, et al. Final and near-final adult height in patients with severe primary insulin-like growth factor-I deficiency after long-term treatment with recombinant human insulin-like growth factor-I (rhIGF-I). Paper presented at: Combined Meeting of Lawson Wilkens Pediatric Endocrine Society and European Society for Pediatric Endocrinology. New York, September, 2009.

76. Ranke MB. Treatment of growth hormone insensitivity syndrome (GHIS) with insulin-like growth factor (IGF-I). In: Ross RJ, Savage MO, editors. Growth hormone resistance. London: Bailliere-Tindall; 1996. p. 401–10.

77. Camacho-Hubner C, Underwood LE, Yordam N, et al. Once daily rhIGF-1/rhIGFBP-3 treatment improves growth in children with severe primary IGF-I deficiency: results of a multicenter clinical trial. Paper presented at: Proceedings of the Endocrine Society's 88th Annual Meeting. Boston (MA), June, 2006.

78. Walker JL, Ginalska-Malinowska M, Romer TE, et al. Effects of the infusion of insulin-like growth factor I in a child with growth hormone insensitivity syndrome (Laron Dwarfism). N Engl J Med 1991;324:1483–8.

79. Kuntze J, Franklin S, Hertz J, et al. Safety of increlex treatment in the IGFD registry. Program and Abstracts of the 90th Annual Meeting of The Endocrine Society. San Francisco (CA), 2008. p. 2–564.

80. Buckway CK, Guevara-Aguirre J, Pratt KL, et al. The IGF-I generation test revisited: a marker of GH sensitivity. J Clin Endocrinol Metab 2001;86(11):5176–83.

81. Bright GM, Rogers D, Gonzalez-Mendoza L, et al. Safety and efficacy of once-daily rhIGF-I treatment in prepubertal children with primary IGF-I deficiency: results from a clinical trial. Program of the International Congress of Endocrinology. Rio de Janeiro (Brazil), November, 2008. p. 00719.

82. Midyett LK, Rogol AD, Van Meter QL, et al. Recombinant insulin-like growth factor (IGF)-I treatment in short children with low IGF-I levels: first-year results from a randomized clinical trial. J Clin Endocrinol Metab 2010;95(2):611–9.

83. Midyett LK, Reiner B, Frane JW, et al. First-year height velocity and safety results from a phase II, randomized, open-label, active-treatment controlled trial of rhGH/rhIGF-1 co-administration in short, prepubertal children with low IGF-1 and normal stimulated GH level. Paper presented at: Endocrine Society Annual Meeting. San Diego (CA), June, 2010.

84. Lango Allen H, Estrada K, Lettre G, et al. Hundreds of variants clustered in genomic loci and biological pathways affect human height. Nature 2010; 467(7317):832–8.

The Insulin-Like Growth Factors in Adipogenesis and Obesity

A. Garten, PhD, S. Schuster, W. Kiess, MD*

KEYWORDS

- Insulin-like growth factors • Growth hormone • Adipogenesis • Obesity

KEY POINTS

- Growth hormone (GH) treatment induces a reduction in adipocyte size and enhances lipolysis in patients with untreated growth hormone deficiency (GHD).
- GH acts directly via activation of the GH receptor or indirectly via insulin-like growth factor (IGF)-I.
- Insulin-like growth factor (IGF)-I is a critical mediator of preadipocyte proliferation, differentiation, and survival.
- Results from clinical studies on GH treatment in patients with GH deficiency or GH insensitivity syndrome can be used to dissect GH and IGF as well as IGF-binding protein (IGFBP) actions in vivo.

First evidence for the importance of growth hormone (GH) and insulin-like growth factor (IGF)-I in adipocyte differentiation and metabolism came from patients with untreated GH deficiency that generally are obese and have enlarged adipocytes. GH treatment induced a reduction in adipocyte size and enhanced lipolysis (reviewed in Ref.[1]). Therefore, adipose tissue was recognized as a major target of GH action (reviewed in Ref.[2]).

GH is a 191-amino-acid, single-chain polypeptide that is synthesized, stored, and secreted in various molecular forms by the somatotroph cells within the lateral wings of the anterior pituitary gland in a pulsatile manner. GH release is mainly regulated by growth hormone–releasing hormone (GHRH) and somatotropin release-inhibiting factor (somatostatin), both of which are secreted by neurosecretory nuclei within the hypothalamus. Several other factors have an impact on GH balance. Circulating GH and IGF-I decrease GH release via a negative feedback mechanism. Ghrelin, a 28-kDa polypeptide, stimulates both food intake and GH secretion. In the central nervous system, ghrelin stimulates appetite and is therefore an important link

Department of Women and Child Health, Hospital for Children and Adolescents, Center for Pediatric Research Leipzig (CPL), University Hospitals, Liebigstraße 20a, 04103 Leipzig, Germany
* Corresponding author.
E-mail address: Wieland.Kiess@medizin.uni-leipzig.de

Endocrinol Metab Clin N Am 41 (2012) 283–295
doi:10.1016/j.ecl.2012.04.011
0889-8529/12/$ – see front matter © 2012 Elsevier Inc. All rights reserved.

between the regulation of energy homeostasis and the activity of the GH/IGF-I axis (reviewed in Ref.[3]). Physiologic stimulators include exercise and deep sleep, while GH secretion is negatively influenced by free fatty acids. An overview of the regulation of GH secretion is given in **Fig. 1**.

GH circulates partially bound to growth hormone–binding protein (GHBP), which is a truncated part of the GH receptor (GHR).

GH acts directly via activation of the GHR, mainly during periods of fuel shortage (fasting, prolonged exercise). The indirect actions of GH are mediated by IGF-I. Circulating IGF-I is predominately stimulated by GH, and is mainly produced in the liver in the presence of sufficient nutrient intake and elevated portal insulin levels (reviewed in Ref.[4]). IGF-I circulates as a ternary complex bound to IGF-binding proteins (IGFBPs) and acid-labile subunit (ALS). In addition, many other tissues and cell types are able to synthesize IGF-I (reviewed in Ref.[5]).

In in vitro studies on primary preadipocytes, GH inhibited adipocyte differentiation but stimulated preadipocyte proliferation.[6,7] The mechanism by which GH inhibits the differentiation of primary preadipocytes to adipocytes is not well understood. Whereas GH treatment of preadipocytes leads to stimulation of cell proliferation via upregulation of IGF-I secretion, the inhibition of glucose uptake and lipogenesis as well as the stimulation of lipolysis by GH in mature adipocytes seem to be independent of IGF-I.[6,7] No influence of GH on the expression of the classic lipolytic enzymes such as adipocyte triglyceride lipase, hormone-sensitive lipase (HSL), or monoglyceride lipase has been shown in humans,[8] although GH has been demonstrated to increase HSL activity.[9]

In contrast to earlier studies, adipose tissue is now regarded as a major source of circulating IGF-I.[10] IGF-I is a critical mediator of preadipocyte proliferation, differentiation, and survival. Apart from systemic effects, IGF-I activates the IGF-I receptor

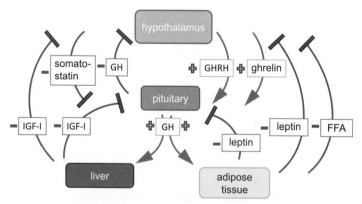

Fig. 1. An overview of the regulation of growth hormone (GH) and insulin-like growth factor I (IGF-I) secretion. Green arrows and plus-signs indicate a stimulatory effect, while red lines and minus-signs show inhibitory actions. GH is released from the pituitary upon stimulation with growth hormone–releasing hormone (GHRH) or ghrelin, which originate from the hypothalamus. There are numerous inhibitory effectors of GH release: somatostatin from the hypothalamus, leptin and free fatty acids (FFA) from adipose tissue. Negative feedback loops are elicited by GH itself or IGF-I from the liver or adipose tissue. IGF-I is released upon stimulation of hepatocytes or adipocytes by GH. (*Adapted from* Ahima RS, Saper CB, Flier JS, et al. Leptin regulation of neuroendocrine systems. Front Neuroendocrinol 2000;21:263–307; and Veldhuis JD. A tripeptidyl ensemble perspective of interactive control of growth hormone secretion. Horm Res 2003;60(Suppl 1):86–101.)

(IGF1R) in an autocrine or paracrine fashion in neighboring adipocytes, with a feedback mechanism regulating *IGF-I* mRNA expression.[11] IGF-I also activates the insulin receptor (IR) in preadipocytes. In addition, the formation of insulin/IGF-I hybrid receptors has been described.[12] IGF-I and insulin seem to act synergistically to induce adipocyte differentiation. IGF-I alone can induce CCAAT/enhancer binding protein α (C/EBPα) and adipocyte lipid binding protein (aP2) mRNA expression, but not lipid droplet accumulation associated with maturation.[13]

IGF-II is known to regulate fetal growth. Less is known about IGF-II action on adipocytes. Studies of *igf2* gene polymorphisms in pigs implicated an influence of IGF-II on fat deposition.[14] In an in vitro model of rat adipocyte progenitor cells, IGF-II stimulated adipocyte differentiation.[15]

The bioavailability of IGF-I is modulated by IGFBP-3 and other IGFBPs. The secretion of IGFBP-2, -3, and -4 is upregulated during adipocyte differentiation.[16,17] IGFBP-3 is thought to act by both binding to and sequestering IGF-I, and to exert IGF-I–independent effects. In adipocytes from visceral adipose tissue, IGFBP-3 was found to reduce insulin-stimulated 2-deoxyglucose uptake.[18] IGFBP-3 also blocks in vitro differentiation of the mouse preadipocyte cell line 3T3-L1 in an IGF-I–independent manner. By contrast, both IGF-I and IGFBP-3 stimulated glycerol-3-phosphate dehydrogenase activity during differentiation of visceral and subcutaneous preadipocytes isolated from adipose tissue of children (reviewed in Ref.[19]).

IGFBP-1 inhibits in vitro adipose differentiation by IGF-I, probably by preventing IGF-I binding to the IGF1R.[20] Systemic overexpression of IGFBP-1 or IGFBP-2 was found to protect mice from diet-induced or age-induced obesity and insulin resistance.[21,22]

EXPERIMENTAL/IN VITRO EVIDENCE
Changes in the IGF System During Adipose Differentiation In Vitro

The GH/IGF system changes during adipocyte differentiation. GHR mRNA expression is upregulated during adipogenesis of the murine adipocyte cell line 3T3-L1[23] and binding of GH to adipocyte precursors increases during differentiation.[7] The ratio of IR to IGF1R expression increases approximately 10-fold during differentiation, due to an increased IR expression. Preadipocytes express IGF1R and IR isoform A, whereas mature adipocytes express predominantly both isoform A and isoform B of the IR.[24] The increased IR expression is reflected by an increase in insulin sensitivity, with an EC_{50} for the stimulation of glucose uptake at 10^{-11} M insulin in adipocytes, compared with 10^{-9} M insulin in preadipocytes.[12]

The secretion of IGF-I and IGFBP-3 was shown to increase during adipocyte differentiation. GH was a positive regulator only in preadipocytes, whereas insulin stimulated the release of both proteins also in mature adipocytes.[17] By contrast, IGF-II and IGFBP-5 expression was shown to decrease in differentiating porcine adipocytes.[25]

Signaling Pathways of GH/IGF in Adipocytes

GH signaling
By binding to and activating its receptor, GH initiates multiple signaling pathways. On receptor activation, the GHR-associated Janus kinase 2 (JAK2) is activated, phosphorylates itself and the GHR, and can recruit several signaling molecules. In turn, this leads to the activation of signal transducers and activators of transcription (STATs), ERK1/2 or phosphatidylinositol-3 (PI3)-kinase.[26] Whereas some studies suggest PI3-kinase or protein kinase C to be essential for the activation of ERK1/2 by GH,[27,28] others show that the adapter proteins Shc and Grb2 initiate the signaling cascade leading to ERK1/2 activation.[29]

The growth-promoting action of GH is mediated by the JAK2-STAT5a/b pathway, the activity of which is terminated by the suppressor of cytokine signaling (SOCS) proteins. SOCS2 is a key regulator of GHR sensitivity, regulating cellular GHR levels through direct ubiquitination.[30]

A potential effector of GH is Sirt1, a nicotinamide adenine dinucleotide (NAD)-dependent deacetylase that is implicated in the regulation of differentiation, energy metabolism, and stress responses. In preadipocytes, Sirt1 represses adipocyte differentiation via repression of peroxisome proliferator-activated receptor γ (PPARγ). In differentiated adipocytes, upregulation of Sirt1 triggers lipolysis and decreases lipogenesis.[31,32] GH has already been shown to increase the expression of Sirt1 and activation of adenosine-monophosphate kinase in other cellular contexts.[33,34] The activity of Sirt1 is regulated by Nampt, the key enzyme in NAD biosynthesis starting from nicotinamide. GH has been shown to downregulate *Nampt* expression in 3T3-L1 adipocytes.[35]

Mammalian target of rapamycin complex 1 (mTORC1) is another metabolic regulator that has recently been shown to regulate triglyceride storage. Inhibition of mTORC1 by rapamycin induces lipolysis and increases plasma free fatty acid levels in humans.[36] It has been shown that GH acutely activates protein synthesis through signaling via mTORC1.[37] GH can modulate mTOR signaling by increasing the tyrosine phosphorylation of upstream signaling molecules insulin receptor substrate (IRS)-1, IRS-2, JAK2, and Shc.[38]

Insulin/IGF signaling

Insulin/IGF signaling is very complex, because there are 3 ligands (IGF-I, IGF-II, and insulin) binding to at least 3 receptors (IGF1R, IR isoform A, and IR isoform B) with different affinities. The formation of hybrid receptors adds even more complexity and variability to the IGF system. IGF1R has a higher affinity for IGFs, but can be activated by high insulin concentrations (eg, during differentiation of adipocyte cell culture models). Of the insulin receptor isoforms, IR B has a highly preferential affinity for insulin compared with the IGFs, and IR A, which differs from IR B only by the deletion of 12 amino acids, is predominantly a receptor for insulin and IGF-II. IR–IGF1R hybrids appear to behave more like IGF1R, with preferential affinity for IGF-I over insulin. IGF-II also has a specific receptor (IGF2R), which is structurally distinct from the IGF1R or IR. The IGF2R regulates intracellular trafficking of mannose-6-phosphate proteins such as lysosomal enzymes, and influences IGF signaling by sequestering IGF-II.[19]

To make matters even more complicated, Huang and colleagues[39] found that GH induces the formation of a complex that includes GHR, JAK2, and IGF1R in the preadipocyte cell lines 3T3-L1 and 3T3-F442A. Complex formation does not appear to be dependent on GH-induced activation of the ERK or PI3-kinase signaling pathways or on the tyrosine phosphorylation of GHR, JAK2, or IGF1R. Furthermore, GH and IGF-I act synergistically to induce ERK activation and IGF-I enhances GH-induced assembly of conformationally active GHRs.

IGF-I and insulin act through multiple signaling pathways. Several studies performed with cultivated adipocytes from various animals demonstrated that IGF-I is implicated in the regulation of adipocyte differentiation and cell cycle by activation of the PI3-kinase/AKT pathway. This activation is initiated by receptor autophosphorylation and subsequent phosphorylation of IRS-1 or IRS-2. PI3-kinase associates with IRS-1 or -2 and produces the phospholipid messenger phosphatidylinositol-3,4, 5-trisphosphate (PI-3,4,5-P3), which in turn recruits 3'-phosphoinosite-dependent protein kinase-1 (PDK1) and AKT to the cell membrane. AKT is activated by Thr308-phosphorylation through PDK1. AKT can phosphorylate several substrates relevant to insulin-like signaling. The mTORC1 is activated via AKT-mediated phosphorylation and inhibition of tuberous sclerosis complex 2. Recent work suggests that mTORC1 also plays an important role in lipid biosynthesis by promoting the cleavage and activation of sterol response element binding protein 1 (SREBP1). Cleaved SREBP1 is a transcription factor that promotes the expression of diverse genes with important roles in lipid synthesis, including fatty acid synthase (FASN), glycerol-3-phosphate acyltransferases (GPAT), ATP citrate lyase (ACLY), acetyl-CoA carboxylase (ACC), stearoyl-CoA desaturase 1 (SCD1), and glucokinase (GK).[40]

IGF-I stimulates proliferation of 3T3-L1 preadipocytes through activation of mitogen-activated protein kinase (MAPK), which is mediated through the Src family of nonreceptor tyrosine kinases.[41] Another study found that insulin stimulation of 3T3-L1 led to phosphorylation of the atypical protein kinase WNK1, which is a negative regulator of preadipocyte proliferation.[42]

A fundamental function of insulin is the maintenance of glucose homeostasis by increasing the rate of glucose uptake into myocytes and adipocytes. Both GH and IGF-I have been shown to inhibit insulin-stimulated glucose uptake. Chronic GH pretreatment of the 3T3-L1 preadipocyte cell line inhibits insulin-induced glucose uptake without affecting glucose transporter 4 (GLUT4) translocation, through the reduction of IRS-2–associated PI3-kinase activity.[43] IGF-I administration has the same effect in 3T3-L1 adipocytes. However, IGF-I was shown to stimulate the production of reactive oxygen species and thereby disturb insulin-mediated tyrosine phosphorylation of IRS-1.[44]

IGFBP-3 signaling

Apart from specific and high-affinity binding of IGFs, IGFBP-3 can modulate proliferation and cell survival in an IGF-independent manner. IGFBP-3 can translocate to the nucleus and bind to retinoid X receptor α and PPARγ, thereby inhibiting adipose differentiation.[45] By reducing GLUT4 translocation to the plasma membrane and Thr308 phosphorylation of AKT, IGFBP-3 attenuated insulin-stimulated glucose uptake.[18] In other cell types, IGFBP-3 was shown to activate PI3-kinase. This effect was inhibited by pertussis toxin, indicating the involvement of a pertussis toxin–sensitive G protein.[46]

A summary of the effects of GH, IGF-I, and IGFBP-3 on (pre)adipocytes in vitro is given in **Table 1**.

CLINICAL CONSIDERATIONS
Regulation of Adipose Mass

Adipose mass is determined by both the volume and number of adipocytes. Adipocyte number may increase through proliferation and differentiation of preadipocytes.[50] Adults with severe obesity exhibit an increased total fat cell number independent of the onset of obesity. Adipose tissue of adults contains a remarkable number of specific precursor cells that are able to differentiate into mature fat cells under appropriate conditions.[1]

Because GH induces secretion of IGF-I and IGFBP-3, it is difficult to separate the effects of GH, IGF-I, and IGFBP-3 in vivo. Much of the information on the effects of GH in vivo comes from treatment of patients with GH deficiency (GHD). By systematically reviewing blinded, randomized, placebo-controlled trials of GH treatment in adult patients with GHD, Maison and colleagues[51] found a negative effect of GH treatment on fat mass and an improvement in low-density lipoprotein (LDL) and serum cholesterol levels. Adipose tissue of adult individuals with untreated GHD was shown to contain adipocytes with a very large diameter. Of importance is that this was accompanied by increased expression of proinflammatory markers and inflammatory

Table 1
Effects of GH, IGF-I, and IGFBP-3 on (pre)adipocytes in vitro

Hormone	Effect	Adipocyte Model	Reference
GH	↑ Differentiation	Rodent cell lines (3T3-F442A)	47
	↓ Differentiation	Primary human	6
	↓ GAPDH activity		
	↓ Cellular glucose uptake, incorporation of glucose into lipids		
	↑ Lipolysis		
	↓ Differentiation	Primary rat	7
	↓ GAPDH activity		
	↓ Cellular glucose uptake		
	↓ Lipogenesis		
	↑ IGF-I synthesis		
	↑ Proliferation of precursor cells		
	↑ Lipolysis		
	↓ Insulin-stimulated glucose uptake	3T3-L1	43
IGF-I	↑ Proliferation	3T3-L1	41
	↓ Death-receptor–mediated induction of apoptosis	SGBS, primary human	48
	↑ Differentiation	Human mesenchymal stem cells (HMSCs)	49
	↑ Proliferation		
	↑ Expression of C/EBPα and aP2 mRNA	Rat mesenteric stromal vascular cells (mSVCs)	13
	↓ Insulin-stimulated glucose uptake	3T3-L1	44
IGFBP-3	↓ Insulin-stimulated glucose uptake	3T3-L1	18
	↓ Differentiation	3T3-L1	45

↓, decreasing effect; ↑, increasing effect.
Abbreviations: GAPDH, glyceraldehyde-3-phosphate dehydrogenase; SGBS, Simpson-Golabi-Behmel syndrome.

cytokines as well as impaired insulin action in obese patients with GHD, whereas lean individuals with GHD had low protein levels in several cytokines and growth factors, indicating defective adipocyte differentiation and proliferation as well as attenuated angiogenesis and neurogenesis.[52] Children with GHD were described to be generally moderately obese. At the cellular level, an increased mean adipocyte volume but a reduced number of fat cells was detected, compared with healthy children. After GH substitution, these changes were shifted toward normal.[1]

GH treatment was shown to regulate several genes involved in triglyceride hydrolysis and storage, diacylglycerol synthesis, and the expression of components of extracellular matrix and transforming growth factor β signaling pathways, as has been shown in adipose tissue biopsies from male subjects with GHD. Moreover, GH was able to decrease hydroxysteroid-(11β)-dehydrogenase 1, which activates local cortisol production. Accordingly, GH may be able to reduce the amount of locally produced cortisol in adipose tissue.[8]

Individuals with obesity that is not associated with an endocrinopathy were shown to have a lower *GHR* mRNA expression in omental as well as subcutaneous adipose tissues, compared with lean subjects. This fact might offer one explanation as to why GH treatment is not effective in patients with idiopathic obesity.[53]

Body fat mass influences basal and stimulated GH release, both of which are attenuated by increased body fat (reviewed in Ref.[54]). Obese subjects were found to have lower bioactive GH and elevated GHBP serum concentrations in comparison with lean individuals after exercise.[55] Serum levels of GHBP were also found to be increased in obese children and adolescents, and correlated with waist circumference.[56] In addition, GH serum levels were reported to be decreased by short-term overeating without a concomitant increase in body weight. This reduction was due to a decreased amplitude of the GH pulse and was accompanied by a reduction in IGFBP-1 serum levels, which resulted in increased free IGF-I serum concentrations.[57] This finding is supported by results from an earlier study showing that despite GH hyposecretion in obesity, total IGF-I and IGFBP-3 serum concentrations did not differ between obese and lean male subjects. However, free IGF-I concentrations were higher in obese subjects, probably because of decreased hepatic IGFBP-1 and IGFBP-2 production.[58]

Effects of IGF-I alone can be evaluated in patients with GH insensitivity syndrome (GHIS) resulting from mutations in the GH receptor and consequent IGF-I deficiency. These patients have metabolic disturbances that include obesity and, particularly in young individuals, spontaneous hypoglycemia caused by lack of GH effects on lipolysis and hepatic glucose production. In elderly patients, fasting hyperinsulinemia is prevalent and the risk of type 2 diabetes is increased.[59,60] IGF-I treatment of adult patients with GHIS decreased body fat mass while lean body mass increased. Measures of lipolytic activity and fat oxidation increased as well, concomitant with an increase in plasma free fatty acid and β-hydroxybutyrate concentrations and a reduced plasma insulin concentration.[61]

Visceral Versus Subcutaneous Adipose Tissue

Clinical studies have shown that in visceral adipose depots, adipocytes are less sensitive to insulin than those found in subcutaneous sites, and they appear less able to differentiate into mature adipocytes,[62] indicating that impairment of adipocyte differentiation occurs in a site-specific manner. A current hypothesis argues that in people whose fat stores are unable to differentiate optimally, excess calories are more likely to be stored in sites other than fat, such as liver, skeletal muscle, and heart, thus contributing to metabolic dysregulation with insulin resistance (reviewed in Ref.[19]). A recent study supported the finding that visceral fat deposition is associated with insulin resistance while an increase in subcutaneous fat depots is associated with a protection from insulin resistance.[63]

Significant differences exist between the growth patterns of different adipose depots. In rats fed ad libitum it was shown that the cumulative growth of the 2 intra-abdominal fat depots (mesenteric and epididymal) was due mostly to hypertrophy (increases in cell volume of 83% and 64%, respectively), whereas the growth of the other 2 depots (retroperitoneal and inguinal) was due predominantly to hyperplasia (increases in cell number of 58% and 65%, respectively).[64] This difference was found to be reflected by depot-specific expression patterns of the IGF-I and leptin genes. expression of both genes was highest in retroperitoneal and epididymal depots, followed by mesenteric and subcutaneous inguinal depots. Both leptin and IGF-I mRNAs, when expressed per 10^6 adipocytes, correlated with the adipocyte volume, suggesting that the autocrine/paracrine actions of these cytokines could modulate region-specific patterns of adipose tissue growth.[65] A more recent study reported that IGF-I–stimulated DNA synthesis was significantly lower in omental preadipocytes than in subcutaneous preadipocytes from obese subjects. IGF-I–mediated phosphorylation of the IGF1R and the ERK pathway was comparable in subcutaneous and omental cells. However, omental preadipocytes had decreased IRS-1 protein associated with increased

IRS-1-degradation. Consequently, IGF-I–stimulated phosphorylation of AKT on serine (473) but not threonine (308) was decreased in omental cells, and activation of downstream targets, including p70 S6 kinase, glycogen synthase kinase 3, and the transcription factor Forkhead box O1, was also impaired. CyclinD1 abundance was decreased in omental cells because of increased degradation. These results propose an intrinsic defect in IGF-I activation of the AKT pathway in omental preadipocytes from obese subjects that involves IRS-1 and could contribute to the distinct growth phenotype of preadipocytes in visceral fat of obese subjects.[66] In contrast to these results, Bashan and colleagues[67] demonstrated that tyrosine phosphorylation and signal transduction to AKT after insulin stimulation of omental fat was not inferior to that detected in fragments of subcutaneous fat tissue. Instead a stronger activation of stress-related kinases such as p38 MAPK and JNK was observed.

In acromegaly, a state of GH and IGF-I excess, both visceral and subcutaneous adipose tissue, but most markedly visceral adipose tissue, were shown to be decreased whereas intramuscular visceral adipose was greater. This finding suggests that increased visceral adipose in muscle could be associated with GH-induced insulin resistance.[68]

Adipose Tissue and Glucose Homeostasis

An emerging function for adipose tissue is the regulation of whole-body glucose homeostasis and insulin sensitivity. Supporting evidence came from a mouse model overexpressing GLUT4 in adipose tissue, which displayed increased glucose tolerance.[69] Tightly linked to this important role of adipose tissue is the fact that individuals with low birth weight have an increased risk of developing type 2 diabetes and other features of the metabolic syndrome later in life. A study comparing the expression of insulin/IGF-signaling molecules in adipose tissue of low-birth-weight and normal-birth-weight young males found a lower expression of genes for GLUT4 and PI3-kinase p85 and p110 subunits, as well as for IRS-1.[70] These results were supported by findings from another study involving children born small for gestational age (SGA) and control subjects born appropriate for gestational age (AGA). The content of IGF1R, IR, ERK1/2, and AKT was lower in subcutaneous adipocytes from SGA compared with that from AGA children. ERK1/2 phosphorylation after stimulation of adipocytes with insulin or IGF-I was decreased in SGA.[71]

An overview of the effects of GH and IGF-I on adipose tissue–related responses in vivo is given in **Table 2**.

Table 2
Effects of GH and IGF-I on adipose tissue–related responses in vivo

Hormone	Effect	Subjects/Animal Models	Reference
GH/IGF-I	↓ Adipocyte size ↑ Adipocyte number	Human subjects with GHD	1
GH/IGF-I	↑ Lipolysis ↑ Lipid oxidation	Human male subjects with GHD, adipose tissue biopsies	8
GH	↓ Insulin sensitivity	Liver IGF-I–deficient mice	72
GH	↑ Lipolysis ↑ Circulating free fatty acid concentrations	Humans, abdominal and femoral adipose tissue	73
GH	↑ Circulating IGF-I levels	Insulin-dependent diabetics and healthy subjects	74

↓, decreasing effect; ↑, increasing effect.

OPEN QUESTIONS

Nowadays a wealth of information is available about the differentiation process of adipocytes, the multitude of factors influencing this process, and the clinical consequences of high or low circulating GH or IGFs. Sometimes it is difficult, however, to reconcile the results of different studies, especially when the effects seen in cell lines are the opposite of effects observed in primary cells. For example, GH has been described to stimulate differentiation in the murine adipocyte cell line 3T3-F442A,[47] whereas primary preadipocytes incubated with GH did not differentiate.[6] Results from preadipocyte cell lines have to be viewed cautiously, because the immortalization process might influence the signaling pathways and therefore the cellular responses to GH or IGF stimuli. IGF-I and IGFBP-3 are known to have antiapoptotic and proapoptotic effects, respectively, in cancer cell lines,[75,76] which might confound cell responses of immortalized preadipocyte cell lines.

Another experimental strategy is the use of primary adipocyte cultures of various animals (rat, pig, mouse). In addition to the uncertainty as to whether these adipocyte cultures behave like human adipocytes, there might be differences specific to adipose depot that have to be taken into account when interpreting the results.

When using primary human material, differing study outcomes do not only occur because of technical differences (the use of isolated adipocytes, in vivo biopsies, or tissue-fragment explants) but also as a result of patient selection.[67] In addition, in vivo it is difficult to decide whether the observed effects are caused by GH directly or by increased expression of IGF-I or IGFBPs.

Taken together, the available evidence suggests that GH and IGF-I are indeed important regulators of adipocyte survival and differentiation. In addition, in obese subjects a blunted GH/IGF-I response is being observed on a regular basis. GH and/or IGF-I are nevertheless unable to influence the development of obesity in healthy subjects.

REFERENCES

1. Wabitsch M, Hauner H, Heinze E, et al. The role of growth hormone/insulin-like growth factors in adipocyte differentiation. Metabolism 1995;44:(10 Suppl 4):45–9.
2. Blüher S, Kratzsch J, Kiess W. Insulin-like growth factor I, growth hormone and insulin in white adipose tissue. Best Pract Res Clin Endocrinol Metab 2005;19: 577–87.
3. Gahete MD, Durán-Prado M, Luque RM, et al. Understanding the multifactorial control of growth hormone release by somatotropes: lessons from comparative endocrinology. Ann N Y Acad Sci 2009;1163:137–53.
4. Møller N, Jørgensen JO. Effects of growth hormone on glucose, lipid, and protein metabolism in human subjects. Endocr Rev 2009;30:152–77.
5. Kaplan SA, Cohen P. The somatomedin hypothesis 2007: 50 years later. J Clin Endocrinol Metab 2007;92:4529–35.
6. Wabitsch M, Braun S, Hauner H, et al. Mitogenic and antiadipogenic properties of human growth hormone in differentiating human adipocyte precursor cells in primary culture. Pediatr Res 1996;40:450–6.
7. Wabitsch M, Heinze E, Hauner H, et al. Biological effects of human growth hormone in rat adipocyte precursor cells and newly differentiated adipocytes in primary culture. Metabolism 1996;45:34–42.
8. Zhao JT, Cowley MJ, Lee P, et al. Identification of novel GH-regulated pathway of lipid metabolism in adipose tissue: a gene expression study in hypopituitary men. J Clin Endocrinol Metab 2011;96:E1188–96.

9. Vijayakumar A, Novosyadlyy R, Wu Y, et al. Biological effects of growth hormone on carbohydrate and lipid metabolism. Growth Horm IGF Res 2010;20:1–7.

10. Möller C, Arner P, Sonnenfeld T, et al. Quantitative comparison of insulin-like growth factor mRNA levels in human and rat tissues analysed by a solution hybridization assay. J Mol Endocrinol 1991;7:213–22.

11. Klöting N, Koch L, Wunderlich T, et al. Autocrine IGF-1 action in adipocytes controls systemic IGF-1 concentrations and growth. Diabetes 2008;57:2074–82.

12. Bäck K, Brännmark C, Strålfors P, et al. Differential effects of IGF-I, IGF-II and insulin in human preadipocytes and adipocytes—role of insulin and IGF-I receptors. Mol Cell Endocrinol 2011;339:130–5.

13. Sato T, Nagafuku M, Shimizu K, et al. Physiological levels of insulin and IGF-1 synergistically enhance the differentiation of mesenteric adipocytes. Cell Biol Int 2008;32:1397–404.

14. Nezer L, Moreau B, Brouwers W, et al. An imprinted QTL with major effect on muscle mass and fat deposition maps to the IGF2 locus in pigs. Nat Genet 1999;21:155–6.

15. Bellows CG, Jia D, Jia Y, et al. Different effects of insulin and insulin-like growth factors I and II on osteoprogenitors and adipocyte progenitors in fetal rat bone cell populations. Calcif Tissue Int 2006;79:57–65.

16. Boney CM, Moats-Staats BM, Stiles AD, et al. Expression of insulin-like growth factor-I (IGF-I) and IGF-binding proteins during adipogenesis. Endocrinology 1994;135:1863–8.

17. Wabitsch M, Heinze E, Debatin KM, et al. IGF-I and IGFBP-3-expression in cultured human preadipocytes and adipocytes. Horm Metab Res 2000;32:555–9.

18. Chan S, Twigg S, Firth S, et al. Insulin-like growth factor binding protein 3 leads to insulin resistance in adipocytes. J Clin Endocrinol Metab 2005;90:6588–95.

19. Baxter RB, Twigg SM. Actions of IGF binding proteins and related proteins in adipose tissue. Trends Endocrinol Metab 2009;20:499–505.

20. Siddals KW, Westwood M, Gibson JM, et al. IGF-binding protein-1 inhibits IGF effects on adipocyte function: implications for insulin-like actions at the adipocyte. J Endocrinol 2002;174:289–97.

21. Rajkumar K, Modric T, Murphy LJ. Impaired adipogenesis in insulin-like growth factor binding protein-1 transgenic mice. J Endocrinol 1999;162:457–65.

22. Wheatcroft SB, Kearney MT, Shah AM, et al. IGF-binding protein-2 protects against the development of obesity and insulin resistance. Diabetes 2007;56:285–94.

23. Iida K, Takahashi Y, Kaji H, et al. Diverse regulation of full-length and truncated growth hormone receptor expression in 3T3-L1 adipocytes. Mol Cell Endocrinol 2003;210:21–9.

24. Bäck K, Arnqvist HJ. Changes in insulin and IGF-I receptor expression during differentiation of human preadipocytes. Growth Horm IGF Res 2009;19:101–11.

25. Gardan D, Mourot J, Louveau I. Decreased expression of the IGF-II gene during porcine adipose cell differentiation. Mol Cell Endocrinol 2008;292:63–8.

26. Rosenfeld RG, Hwa V. New molecular mechanisms of GH resistance. Eur J Endocrinol 2004;151:S11–5.

27. Clarkson RW, Chen CM, Harrison S, et al. Early responses of trans-activating factors to growth hormone in preadipocytes: differential regulation of CCAAT enhancer-binding protein-beta (C/EBP beta) and C/EBP delta. Mol Endocrinol 1995;9:108–20.

28. Kilgour E, Gout I, Anderson NG. Requirement for phosphoinositide 3-OH kinase in growth hormone signalling to the mitogen-activated protein kinase and p70s6k pathways. Biochem J 1996;315:517–22.

29. VanderKuur JA, Butch ER, Waters SB, et al. Signalling molecules involved in coupling growth hormone receptor to MAP kinase activation. Endocrinology 1997;138:4301–7.
30. Vesterlund M, Zadjali F, Persson T, et al. The SOCS2 ubiquitin ligase complex regulates growth hormone receptor levels. PLoS One 2011;6:e25358.
31. Picard F, Kurtev M, Chung N, et al. Sirt1 promotes fat mobilization in white adipocytes by repressing PPAR-gamma. Nature 2004;429:771–6.
32. Fischer-Posovszky P, Kukulus V, Tews D, et al. Resveratrol regulates human adipocyte number and function in a Sirt1-dependent manner. Am J Clin Nutr 2010;92:5–15.
33. Qin Y, Tian YP. Exploring the molecular mechanisms underlying the potentiation of exogenous growth hormone on alcohol-induced fatty liver diseases in mice. J Transl Med 2010;8:120.
34. Cuesta S, Kireev R, Forman K, et al. Growth hormone can improve insulin resistance and differentiation in pancreas of senescence accelerated prone male mice (SAMP8). Growth Horm IGF Res 2011;21:63–8.
35. Kralisch S, Klein J, Lossner U, et al. Hormonal regulation of the novel adipocytokine visfatin in 3T3-L1 adipocytes. J Endocrinol 2005;185(3):R1–8.
36. Soliman GA, Acosta-Jaquez HA, Fingar DC. mTORC1 inhibition via rapamycin promotes triacylglycerol lipolysis and release of free fatty acids in 3T3-L1 adipocytes. Lipids 2010;45:1089–100.
37. Hayashi AA, Proud CG. The rapid activation of protein synthesis by growth hormone requires signaling through mTOR. Am J Physiol Endocrinol Metab 2007;292:E1647–55.
38. Thirone AC, Carvalho CR, Saad MJ. Growth hormone stimulates the tyrosine kinase activity of JAK2 and induces tyrosine phosphorylation of insulin receptor substrates and Shc in rat tissues. Endocrinology 1999;140:55–62.
39. Huang Y, Kim SO, Yang N, et al. Physical and functional interaction of growth hormone and insulin-like growth factor-I signaling elements. Mol Endocrinol 2004;18:1471–85.
40. Laplante M, Sabatini DM. An emerging role of mTOR in lipid biosynthesis. Curr Biol 2009;19:R1046–52.
41. Sekimoto H, Boney CM. C-terminal Src kinase (CSK) modulates insulin-like growth factor-I signaling through Src in 3T3-L1 differentiation. Endocrinology 2003;144:2546–52.
42. Jiang ZY, Zhou QL, Holik J, et al. Identification of WNK1 as a substrate of Akt/protein kinase B and a negative regulator of insulin-stimulated mitogenesis in 3T3-L1 cells. J Biol Chem 2005;280(22):21622–8.
43. Sasaki-Suzuki N, Arai K, Ogata T, et al. Growth hormone inhibition of glucose uptake in adipocytes occurs without affecting GLUT4 translocation through an insulin receptor substrate-2-phosphatidylinositol 3-kinase-dependent pathway. J Biol Chem 2009;284:6061–70.
44. Fukuoka H, Iida K, Nishizawa H, et al. IGF-I stimulates reactive oxygen species (ROS) production and inhibits insulin-dependent glucose uptake via ROS in 3T3-L1 adipocytes. Growth Horm IGF Res 2010;20:212–9.
45. Chan SS, Schedlich LJ, Twigg SM, et al. Inhibition of adipocyte differentiation by insulin-like growth factor-binding protein-3. Am J Physiol Endocrinol Metab 2009;296:E654–63.
46. Ricort JM, Binoux M. Insulin-like growth factor binding protein-3 stimulates phosphatidylinositol 3-kinase in MCF-7 breast carcinoma cells. Biochem Biophys Res Commun 2004;314:1044–9.

47. Morikawa M, Nixon T, Green H. Growth hormone and the adipose conversion of 3T3 cells. Cell 1982;29:783–9.
48. Fischer-Posovszky P, Tornqvist H, Debatin KM, et al. Inhibition of death-receptor mediated apoptosis in human adipocytes by the insulin-like growth factor I (IGF-I)/IGF-I receptor autocrine circuit. Endocrinology 2004;145:1849–59.
49. Scavo LM, Karas M, Murray M, et al. Insulin-like growth factor-I stimulates both cell growth and lipogenesis during differentiation of human mesenchymal stem cells into adipocytes. J Clin Endocrinol Metab 2004;89:3543–53.
50. Hauner H, Entenmann G, Wabitsch M, et al. Promoting effect of glucocorticoids on the differentiation of human adipocyte precursor cells cultured in a chemically defined medium. J Clin Invest 1989;84:1663–70.
51. Maison P, Griffin S, Nicoue-Beglah M, et al. Impact of growth hormone (GH) treatment on cardiovascular risk factors in GH-deficient adults: a metaanalysis of blinded, randomized, placebo-controlled trials. J Clin Endocrinol Metab 2004; 89:2192–9.
52. Ukropec J, Penesová A, Skopková M, et al. Adipokine protein expression pattern in growth hormone deficiency predisposes to the increased fat cell size and the whole body metabolic derangements. J Clin Endocrinol Metab 2008;93:2255–62.
53. Erman A, Veilleux A, Tchernof A, et al. Human growth hormone receptor (GHR) expression in obesity: I. GHR mRNA expression in omental and subcutaneous adipose tissues of obese women. Int J Obes (Lond) 2011;35:1511–9.
54. Kreitschmann-Andermahr I, Suarez P, Jennings R, et al. GH/IGF-I regulation in obesity—mechanisms and practical consequences in children and adults. Horm Res Paediatr 2010;73:153–60.
55. Thomas GA, Kraemer WJ, Kennett MJ, et al. Immunoreactive and bioactive growth hormone responses to resistance exercise in men who are lean or obese. J Appl Physiol 2011;111:465–72.
56. Kratzsch J, Dehmel B, Pulzer F, et al. Increased serum GHBP levels in obese pubertal children and adolescents: relationship to body composition, leptin and indicators of metabolic disturbances. Int J Obes Relat Metab Disord 1997;21: 1130–6.
57. Cornford AS, Barkan AL, Horowitz JF. Rapid suppression of growth hormone concentration by overeating: potential mediation by hyperinsulinemia. J Clin Endocrinol Metab 2011;96:824–30.
58. Nam SY, Lee EJ, Kim KR, et al. Effect of obesity on total and free insulin-like growth factor (IGF)-1, and their relationship to IGF-binding protein (BP)-1, IGFBP-2, IGFBP-3, insulin, and growth hormone. Int J Obes Relat Metab Disord 1997;21:355–9.
59. Laron Z, Avitzur Y, Klinger B. Carbohydrate metabolism in primary growth hormone resistance (Laron syndrome) before and during insulin-like growth factor-I treatment. Metabolism 1995;44(Suppl 4):113–8.
60. Laron Z, Ginsberg S, Lilos P, et al. Body composition in untreated adult patients with Laron syndrome (primary GH insensitivity). Clin Endocrinol (Oxf) 2006;65:114–7.
61. Mauras N, Martinez V, Rini A, et al. Recombinant human insulin-like growth factor I has significant anabolic effects in adults with growth hormone receptor deficiency: studies on protein, glucose, and lipid metabolism. J Clin Endocrinol Metab 2000;85:3036–42.
62. Tchkonia T, Tchoukalova YD, Giorgadze N, et al. Abundance of two human pre-adipocyte subtypes with distinct capacities for replication, adipogenesis, and apoptosis varies among fat depots. Am J Physiol Endocrinol Metab 2005;288: E267–77.

63. McLaughlin T, Lamendola C, Liu A, et al. Preferential fat deposition in sub-cutaneous versus visceral depots is associated with insulin sensitivity. J Clin Endocrinol Metab 2011;96:E1756–60.

64. DiGirolamo M, Fine JB, Tagra K, et al. Qualitative regional differences in adipose tissue growth and cellularity in male Wistar rats fed ad libitum. Am J Physiol 1998; 274:R1460–7.

65. Villafuerte BC, Fine JB, Bai Y, et al. Expressions of leptin and insulin-like growth factor-I are highly correlated and region-specific in adipose tissue of growing rats. Obes Res 2000;8:646–55.

66. Cleveland-Donovan K, Maile LA, Tsiaras WG, et al. IGF-I activation of the AKT pathway is impaired in visceral but not subcutaneous preadipocytes from obese subjects. Endocrinology 2010;151:3752–63.

67. Bashan N, Dorfman K, Tarnovscki T, et al. Mitogen-activated protein kinases, inhibitory-kappaB kinase, and insulin signaling in human omental versus subcu-taneous adipose tissue in obesity. Endocrinology 2007;148:2955–62.

68. Freda PU, Shen W, Heymsfield SB, et al. Lower visceral and subcutaneous but higher intermuscular adipose tissue depots in patients with growth hormone and insulin-like growth factor I excess due to acromegaly. J Clin Endocrinol Metab 2008;9:2334–43.

69. Shepherd PR, Gnudi L, Tozzo E, et al. Adipose tissue hyperplasia and enhanced glucose disposal in transgenic mice over-expressing GLUT 4 selectively in adipose tissue. J Biol Chem 1993;268:22243–6.

70. Ozanne SE, Jensen CB, Tingey JK, et al. Decreased protein levels of key insulin signaling molecules in adipose tissue from young men with a low birthweight—potential link to increased risk of diabetes? Diabetologia 2006;49:2993–9.

71. Iñiguez G, Ormazabal P, López T, et al. IGF-1R/ERK content and response to IGF-I and insulin in adipocytes from small for gestational age children. Growth Horm IGF Res 2009;19:256–61.

72. Yakar S, Setser J, Zhao H, et al. Inhibition of growth hormone action improves insulin sensitivity in liver IGF-1-deficient mice. J Clin Invest 2004;113:96–105.

73. Gravholt CH, Schmitz O, Simonsen L, et al. Effects of a physiological GH pulse on interstitial glycerol in abdominal and femoral adipose tissue. Am J Physiol 1999; 277:E848–54.

74. Wurzburger MI, Prelevic GM, Sonksen PH, et al. The effect of recombinant human growth hormone on regulation of growth hormone secretion and blood glucose in insulin-dependent diabetes. J Clin Endocrinol Metab 1993;77:267–72.

75. Varela-Nieto I, Hartl M, Gorospe I, et al. Anti-apoptotic actions of insulin-like growth factors: lessons from development and implications in neoplastic cell transformation. Curr Pharm Des 2007;13:687–703.

76. Paharkova-Vatchkova V, Lee KW. Nuclear export and mitochondrial and endo-plasmic reticulum localization of IGF-binding protein 3 regulate its apoptotic properties. Endocr Relat Cancer 2010;17:293–302.

Multifaceted Role of Insulin-Like Growth Factors and Mammalian Target of Rapamycin in Skeletal Muscle

Robert A. Frost, PhD*, Charles H. Lang, PhD

KEYWORDS

- Insulin-like growth factors • Mammalian target of rapamycin • Skeletal muscle
- Muscle mass

KEY POINTS

- Amino acids, consumed as part of a protein rich meal, signal via mTOR to increase the synthesis of muscle protein and maintain muscle mass.
- Hormones, growth factors, nutrients and exercise cooperate in maintaining muscle mass and function as we age.
- A symbiotic relationship exists between mitochondria and skeletal muscle whereby amino acids and exercise increase mitochondrial number energizing muscle contraction and promoting muscle hypertrophy.
- Follistatin overexpression increases muscle mass via an IGF-IR and mTOR mediated pathway, providing hope that pharmaceuticals based on these pathways may be beneficial in muscle pathologies.
- Chronic alcohol consumption impairs mTOR signaling in skeletal muscle an effect that can be overcome by the administration of a binary complex of IGF-I and IGFBP-3.

INSULIN-LIKE GROWTH FACTOR AND MAMMALIAN TARGET OF RAPAMYCIN IN SKELETAL MUSCLE HEALTH: THE WHYS AND THE WHEREFORES

Insulin and insulin-like growth factors (IGF-I and IGF-II) are evolutionarily conserved peptides that are expressed in organisms as evolutionarily diverse as nematodes and humans.[1] In the adult, these peptides orchestrate metabolic responses to nutrients, hormones, and stress.[2]

IGFs and their receptors are also critical for the proliferation of muscle stem cells and recovery from muscle injury.[3,4] Skeletal muscle is especially dependent on IGF

Funding Sources: Dr Lang: NIH Grants GM038032 and AA11290.
Conflict of Interest: None.
Department of Cellular and Molecular Physiology, Pennsylvania State University College of Medicine, 500 University Drive, Hershey, PA 17033, USA
* Corresponding author.
E-mail address: RFROST@PSU.EDU

Endocrinol Metab Clin N Am 41 (2012) 297–322
doi:10.1016/j.ecl.2012.04.012
0889-8529/12/$ – see front matter © 2012 Elsevier Inc. All rights reserved.

endo.theclinics.com

signaling during development, because mice null for the IGF-I receptor (IGF-IR) show severe muscle cell hypoplasia.[5,6] Specific deletion of the IGF-IR in skeletal muscle also reduces the number of myonuclei per myofiber and myofiber cross-sectional area, suggesting that IGF-IR signaling mediates both the addition of nuclei to fibers and the maintenance of myofiber size.[7] In contrast, mice null for IGF-I expression in peripheral tissues (including skeletal muscle) show body weights indistinguishable from control littermates when endocrine IGF-I is supplied from a hepatic transgene, signifying that a combination of autocrine-derived, paracrine-derived, and endocrine-derived IGFs contribute to the maintenance of muscle mass.[7–10]

A variety of pathophysiologic conditions adversely affect muscle mass and function, including glucocorticoid excess, sepsis, muscular injury and dystrophies, inactivity, alcohol, and aging. Almost all of these states have on occasion been linked to a reduction in either circulating IGF-I levels or IGF signaling, although a definitive cause and effect relationship is often lacking.[11–20] It is therefore of interest from a human health perspective to understand how IGFs affect muscle at the cellular, molecular, and organismal level to determine how and when the clinical use of IGFs or therapies that simulate their signaling pathways may be beneficial.[21–25]

Numerous laboratories have determined that nutrients, growth factors, hormones, and muscle activity all generate cellular signals that have the capacity to maintain or grow muscle mass. Although signaling through insulin receptor substrate (IRS-1 and IRS-2) and Akt are important, a key focal point at which all of these signals meet and integrate in skeletal muscle is the protein kinase known as the mammalian target of rapamycin (mTOR).[13,26,27] Because mTOR is critical for muscle function and its tissue-specific deletion results in muscular dystrophy, it seems appropriate to review the role played by IGFs and mTOR in muscle during health and disease.[28,29] This review broadly evaluates the role of IGFs and mTOR in the maintenance of muscle mass and function and how this relationship is altered in pathophysiologic conditions affecting skeletal muscle.

MUSCLE IGFs AND NUTRITION: SUBSTRATES AND SIGNALING

It has long been appreciated that optimal nutrition, including sufficient caloric and protein intake, is necessary for muscle growth during development, postnatal growth, and puberty.[30–32] The growth hormone (GH)–IGF-I axis and muscle per se are influenced by amino acids, fatty acids, and micronutrients that provide a milieu in which optimal muscle growth may occur.[33–37] Essential amino acids (EAAs) account for nearly all of the ability of a well-balanced meal to stimulate muscle protein synthesis.[38,39] Furthermore, the branched-chain amino acids (BCAA, eg, leucine, isoleucine, and valine), a subset of the EAAs, mediate this response.[40] Combined with the ability of amino acids to stimulate both insulin and GH release, these nutrients provide a strong and potentially persistent anabolic signal for skeletal muscle.[41]

BCAA not only serve as substrates for protein synthesis but also as signaling molecules that act independently of growth factor receptors, phosphoinositide 3-kinase (PI3K), and Akt to activate mTOR by facilitating its direct binding to the Ras homologue enriched in brain (Rheb).[42–45] EAA uptake is required for this effect because AA uptake inhibitors such as D-phenylalanine block mTOR activation by EAA. The small interfering RNA (siRNA)-mediated knockdown of the solute carrier SLC7A5/SLC3A2 (an EAA and glutamine cotransporter) also curtails mTOR signaling to its substrates ribosomal protein S6 kinase-1 (S6K1) and eukaryotic initiation factor 4E binding protein (4E-BP1).[46] Optimal mTOR signaling therefore occurs when the intracellular level of glutamine is sufficient for the cotransport of glutamine out of the cell followed by the ensuing movement of leucine into the cell and the activation of mTOR.[47] Leucine transport and the stimulation of mTOR are also enhanced by IGF-I, providing additive effects on the activation of mTOR in muscle cells (**Fig. 1**).[48]

Although the exact nature of the intracellular BCAA sensor in mammalian cells remains elusive, several proteins have been identified that mediate signaling between amino acids and Rheb. The key step in this process seems to be the movement of mTOR from a cytosolic location to a late endosomal or lysosomal surface. Small guanosine triphosphatases (GTPases), referred to as the Rag proteins (Rag A-D), form heterodimers that when activated by amino acids bring mTOR and Rheb together on the lysosome.[49,50] Three targeting proteins (p14, p21, and MP1, known collectively as the Ragulator) tether the Rags, mTOR, and Rheb to the lysosome.[51] Colocalization of Rags and Rheb may allow mTOR to respond to spikes in the intracellular concentration of amino acids as well as amino acids released as a consequence of lysosomal protein breakdown. This colocalization positions mTOR to commence signaling and activate translation initiation in response to fresh amino acids after a meal. Amino

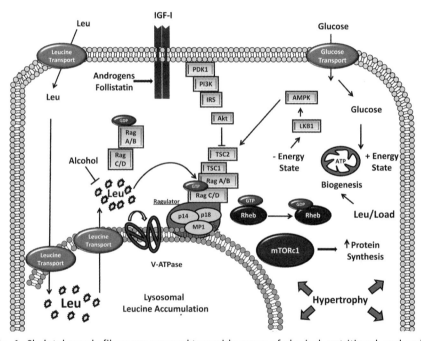

Fig. 1. Skeletal muscle fibers are exposed to a wide range of physical, nutritional, and endocrine signals. When provided on a consistent basis, the amino acid leucine and the peptide hormone IGF-I as well as physical stretch/load stimulate muscle hypertrophy. Amino acid transporters move leucine into the cell from extracellular sources and this process is enhanced by IGF-I. Leucine is transported into the lysosome, where it is also generated from the breakdown of cellular proteins by autophagy. The vacuolar ATPase in concert with 3 Ragulator proteins allow for release of leucine from the lysosome and recruitment of GTP-loaded Rag heterodimers and mTOR. Tethered to the lysosomal surface by the Ragulator, mTOR can interact with Rheb and raptor. The active raptor/mTOR complex phosphorylates mTOR substrates, such as the translation initiation factor 4E-BP1, to stimulate protein synthesis and muscle hypertrophy. IGF-I, by stimulating phosphoinositide-dependent kinase-1 (PDK1), Akt, and tuberous sclerosis protein 2 (TSC2) phosphorylation relieves the negative input of negative energy charge imposed on TSC2 and mTOR by adenosine monophosphate-activated protein kinase. Overall energy balance is improved with glucose, leucine, and exercise, all of which increase mitochondrial biogenesis and the capacity to form adenosine triphosphate.

acids signal using an inside-out mechanism, by which they must first accumulate within the lysosome followed by a rotation of the vacuolar adenosine triphosphatase (ATPase), which allows the amino acids to be released to the surface and activate the Rag proteins and mTOR (see **Fig. 1**).[52] The importance of intralysosomal accumulation of amino acids in mTOR activation was revealed by the fact that over-expression of a proton-assisted amino acid transporter (PAT-1/Slc36a1) in lysosomes prevented mTOR activation because of the ability of PAT-1 to extrude amino acids from the lysosomal lumen.[52,53] The importance of these transporters in mediating catabolism-induced defects in mTOR signaling remains unclear. Regulated transloca-tion of PAT-1 or other transporters between the plasma membrane and the lysosome may be an innate mechanism by which muscle cells regulate mTOR signaling.[54,55]

Our current understanding is that mTOR regulates both protein synthesis and autopha-gic protein degradation in muscle.[56] Nowhere is this dual role more apparent than in a premature aging model (the Klotho null mouse), in which mice show atrophy of the masseter and tongue muscles that limits food and protein intake. These mice show normal signaling upstream of mTOR in the masseter but the phosphorylation of mTOR and its downstream substrates is compromised.[57] The lack of exogenous amino acids leads to a vicious cycle of continued autophagy and muscle atrophy. Given the known interaction between Klotho and IGF-I it would be interesting to test whether the mTOR defect could be rescued by overexpression or exogenous administration of IGF-I.[58] It is likely that even although mTOR is situated on the lysosome, it does not always receive a sufficient amino acid signal to prevent autophagic cell death during prolonged periods of nutrient deprivation.[59] In this case, loss of mTOR activity on the lysosome surface may result in dephosphorylation of a transcription factor that binds to the E-box (TFEB) and the translocation of TFEB to the nucleus, where it upregulates[7] the expression of genes involved in vacuolar biogenesis, thereby perpetuating the atrophy process.[60]

Rag proteins may not be the only small GTPases to regulate the intracellular localization of mTOR. Recently, Saci and colleagues[61] showed that Rac1, a member of the Rho family, is necessary for the activation of mTOR complex (mTORc-1 and mTORc-2) by growth factors. Rac1 binds directly to mTOR via a c-terminal RKR motif, and binding is lost when these residues were mutated to alanine. Growth factors and serum stimulate the Rac1-dependent translocation of mTOR from a perinuclear local-ization to the plasma membrane.[61] Conversely, Rac1 deletion in mouse embryonic fibroblasts decreases cell size and inhibits the phosphorylation of mTOR substrates.

Additional studies suggest that BCAA also stimulate mTOR by decreasing the nega-tive input from 5'-adenosine monophosphate-activated protein kinase (AMPK).[62] During nutrient stress, AMPK phosphorylates TSC2 on S and T to increase the GTPase activating protein (GAP) activity of TSC2 toward Rheb, thereby inhibiting mTOR activity.[63] AMPK also phosphorylates Raptor on S792 to inhibit the interaction of mTOR with its substrates.[64] Nutrient stress also induces a p38 kinase/p38-regulated kinase (PRAK) pathway that phosphorylates Rheb on S130 to inhibit Rheb nucleotide binding and thus mTOR activity.[65] Thus, leucine and other BCAA, by inhibiting AMPK or PRAK, may facilitate the normal activation of Rheb and mTOR to stimulate protein accretion in skeletal muscle.

In contrast to nutrients, growth factors such as IGF-I stimulate mTOR via an IGF-IR, PI3K, Akt pathway that disrupts the TSC1 and TSC2 complex. This protein-protein complex normally represses mTOR signaling, but when TSC2 is phosphorylated on multiple serine residues (S939 and S981), TSC2 binds to 14-3-3 proteins that sequester TSC2 away from Rheb.[8]

TSC2 is a GAP for Rheb that converts Rheb from an active GTP-bound form to an inactive GDP-bound state. Therefore, the sequestration of TSC2 with 14-3-3 increases the relative amount of GTP-bound Rheb, and this activates mTOR in muscle cells.[66] The importance of TSC1 and TSC2 in the regulation of mTOR and protein synthesis is highlighted by the observation that overexpression of TSC1 in skeletal muscle leads to a more stable TSC1/2 complex, inhibition of mTOR activity, and as a result severe muscle wasting.[67] Likewise, mutation of the Akt phosphorylation sites on TSC2 to alanine prevents IGF-I from activating Rheb and inhibits mTOR activity.[66,68]

These studies emphasize that amino acids and IGF-I stimulate mTOR via separate but parallel pathways.[69] These pathways converge by stimulating both the activity of Rheb and its ability to interact with mTOR. How the binding of Rheb to mTOR activates the mTOR kinase remains controversial. Rheb stimulates phospholipase D1 (PLD1) activity and the synthesis of phosphatidic acid (PA), a known activator of mTOR.[70] Conversely, siRNA-mediated knockdown of PLD1 prevents Rheb-induced phosphorylation of mTOR substrates.

This picture is complicated by the fact that PA derived from membrane lipids may be different than PA derived from de novo glycerolipid synthesis, because the later form of PA inhibits mTORc2 activity.[71] Likewise, although PA binds directly to mTOR, it is not sufficient on its own to stimulate mTOR kinase activity in vitro, suggesting that PA needs to interact with other signaling molecules and partners and thus activates mTOR indirectly.[72] One possibility is that PA facilitates the recruitment of mTOR substrates.[72,73] This theory fits with the known ability of Rheb to enhance the binding of mTOR substrates, such as the translation initiation factor 4E-BP1 independent of the intrinsic mTOR kinase activity.[74] Recent work also suggests that PLD9-derived PA stabilizes both the mTORc1 and mTORc2 complexes, leading to greater phosphorylation of additional substrates such as Akt on S473.[75]

The parallel activation of mTOR via an amino acid induced-interaction of Rheb and mTOR and an insulin/IGF-I–induced increase in GTP-bound Rheb suggests that the two pathways allow for the fine-tuning of mTOR activity and translation initiation. This finding is especially relevant to insulin-responsive tissues such as the liver that are exposed to relatively high concentrations of amino acids after a protein-rich meal, which then triggers a rapid release of insulin into the portal circulation. Insulin or amino acids alone only minimally stimulate global hepatic protein synthesis, but in combination they robustly increase mTOR activity and protein synthesis.[76] Teleologically, it makes sense for muscle to also respond to both amino acid and growth factor stimulation. The combination of insulin and amino acids is necessary for the maximal stimulation of muscle protein synthesis observed in healthy adults, and together they enhance the anabolic effect of exercise.[77,78] Insulin and IGFs in addition to stimulating pathways upstream of mTOR also stimulate amino acid uptake and may therefore replenish intracellular levels of glutamine and leucine when these amino acids become limiting for the activation of mTOR.[48,79] In the presence of adequate amino acid availability, insulin prevents muscle protein breakdown, whereas IGF-I enhances amino acid transport and the amino acid induced increase in muscle protein synthesis.[80,81]

Amino acids, growth factors, and exercise may also function synergistically to induce muscle hypertrophy by upregulating the expression of JunB.[82–84] JunB overexpression increases the relative cross-sectional area of skeletal muscle and increases protein synthesis in C2C12 myotubes.[83] Unlike the mechanisms described earlier that alter muscle protein[10] homeostasis via Akt-dependent or mTOR-dependent pathways, JunB increases muscle size independent of mTOR activation.[83] JunB interacts with multiple transcription factors including forkhead box O3(FoxO3) and these interactions prevent the expression of genes that negatively regulate muscle mass such as the muscle-specific ubiquitin E3 ligase atrogin-1 and the activin receptor type II ligand myostatin.[83,85] Thus, muscle tissue seems to have multiple redundant, but independent, mechanisms for regulating muscle mass and its response to growth factors and feeding.

MUSCLE IGFs AND EXERCISE: MAY THE FORCE BE WITH YOU

Although IGF-I stimulates Akt and mTOR as well as protein synthesis in skeletal muscle,[86] the role of IGF-I in the context of exercise-induced hypertrophy is more tenuous.[86] For example, resistance exercise is known to increase IGF-I mRNA expression in skeletal muscle, but neither endocrine nor autocrine increases in the peptide have been reliably shown.[87–90] Recent studies in humans also imply that the total level of IGF-I peptide is unchanged in muscle microdialysis fluid during and after exercise, suggesting that no net synthesis of IGF-I occurs in exercised muscle.[91] Yet, because the amount of free IGF-I (IGF-I not bound to IGF-binding proteins [IGFBPs]) is increased in venous blood draining skeletal muscle, it seems that IGF-I could be released from IGFBPs during exercise. Thus, the overall local IGF-I bioactivity could be increased in skeletal muscle during exercise and thus stimulate hypertrophy, although the mechanism by which this may occur remains undetermined.[11,91] Although immunization of control rats with IGF-I antibody does not prevent the exercise-induced increase in protein synthesis, it does in diabetic rats.[92] These results suggest that IGF-I can compensate for insulin in hypoinsulinemic rats by enabling an anabolic response after acute resistance exercise.

Using a functional overload model in which the plantaris is forced to do the work of the excised soleus and gastrocnemius, Spangenburg and colleagues[93] showed that hypertrophy occurs equally well in control mice and mice expressing a kinase-dead form of the IGF-IR (MKR mice).

Because the MKR mice showed a decreased ability of IGF-I to stimulate Akt phosphorylation but a normal mTOR response to overload, it can be concluded that IGF-IR kinase activity is not necessary for muscle hypertrophy in this model. A similar finding has been made by Barton and colleagues,[94] in which adeno-associated virus expression of a variety of IGF-I isoforms in the tibialis failed to increase muscle mass in MKR mice. Others have also posited that the IGF-I peptide is not necessary for stretch-induced changes in mTOR signaling because conditioned media from stretched C2C12 myotubes was not sufficient to activate the phosphorylation of S6K in naive myotubes.[95] Therefore, it has been concluded that exercise-induced muscle hypertrophy is an intrinsic process independent of hormones and growth factors.[96] Yet, in a mouse model in which the tibialis anterior was electrically stimulated via the sciatic nerve, the same investigators found that electrical stimulation robustly increased S6K1 phosphorylation and this was dramatically reduced in MKR mice, suggesting the IGF-IR tyrosine kinase activity may be necessary for mTOR signaling to its substrates in this model.[97] MKR mice also show a reduced capacity to recover from muscle injury, implying that the IGF-IR is necessary for adequate myoblast fusion and differentiation during the regeneration process.[3]

Although the MKR mouse has been used to determine whether the IGF-IR is necessary for IGF-I signaling in skeletal muscle, it must be remembered that MKR mice show many compensatory changes in response to the expression of the kinase-dead receptor including hyperglycemia, insulin resistance, and decreased muscle fatty acid oxidation.[98] In addition, despite having smaller muscles, the existing muscle shows a compensatory hyperplasia and a greater number of type II glycolytic fibers, suggesting it may have a greater potential to hypertrophy independent of the IGF-IR tyrosine kinase activity.[98,99] MKR muscle also shows a basal 2-fold increase in Akt phosphorylation, a response exceeding that observed in wild-type mice overexpressing IGF-I.[94]

One interpretation of these data is that Akt and mTOR are already maximally stimulated. MKR mice also tend to be hypogonadal.[100] These and other compensatory changes may influence the final response to functional overload observed by Spangenburg and colleagues.[93] Recent work by Mavailli and colleagues[7] and Schiaffino and Mammucari[101] suggests that muscle- specific deletion of the IGF-IR might be an additional model for exploring the role of the IGF-IR in muscle hypertrophy independent of the compensatory changes observed in MKR mice.

MKR mice initially show reduced extracellular signal regulated kinase (ERK) levels in skeletal muscle compared with wild-type controls, but this is followed by a compensatory increase in ERK phosphorylation as the mice age.[99] There is now evidence that IGF-IR tyrosine kinase activity may not be necessary for ERK activation in response to IGF-I in some cell types. For example, ERK continues to be activated in cells treated with IGF-IR tyrosine kinase inhibitors and in cells expressing a kinase-dead IGF-IR.[102] These data suggest that muscle expressing the MKR mutation could still be signaling via ERK or other pathways that have not previously been appreciated as mediating the IGF-I hypertrophic response.[103] Although it is highly speculative, IGF signaling to ERK in MKR mice could activate PLD and generate PA to stimulate signaling to mTOR via an ERK pathway,[13] as recently reported by Winter and colleagues[104] in Rat2 cells. However, whether such a mechanism also occurs in hypertrophying muscle fibers remains to be determined.[104,105]

OH MY: MYOSTATIN AND FOLLISTATIN SIGNAL VIA THE IGF-IR AND mTOR

Nowhere is muscle hypertrophy more evident than in myostatin knockout mice and mice that express endogenous myostatin inhibitors such as follistatin.[106] These mice show muscle weights 2 to 3 times that of wild-type control mice. Follistatin prevents myostatin binding to the type II ActR but the mechanism by which this occurs has not been discerned. Recent work by Kalista and colleagues[107] indicates that the myostatin inhibitor follistatin causes muscle hypertrophy via IGF-IR signaling. Control mice overexpressing follistatin showed a 3-fold greater increase in muscle fiber cross-sectional area than mice expressing follistatin on the MKR background.[107] The follistatin response was also dependent on signaling pathways downstream of the IGF-IR, including mTORc1 and Akt, because the follistatin response was blunted either moderately by rapamycin or strongly by dominant-negative Akt.[107] Thus, follistatin, by increasing muscle IGFs, seems to increase both satellite cell activation and muscle hypertrophy via the classic IGF-IR/Akt/mTOR pathway.[107,108] Future work will have to determine whether follistatin, working via the IGF-IR, can also maintain both muscle fiber myonuclear domain size and muscle force.[109,110]

Recent work by Goodman and colleagues[44] reports that systemic administration of rapamycin can completely block the load-induced hypertrophy of the plantaris in a model in which the synergistic muscles (soleus and part of the gastrocnemius) are ablated. Goodman extended these findings by showing that mice expressing a muscle-specific mTOR kinase-dead transgene showed virtually no compensatory hypertrophy as evidenced by their unchanged cross-sectional area.[14]

These observations suggest that mTOR kinase activity is essential for muscle hypertrophy in this model.[111] In contrast, neither rapamycin nor the kinase-dead form of mTOR inhibited muscle hyperplasia caused by synergistic muscle ablation. This finding implies that load-induced changes in muscle mTOR activity induce mainly muscle hypertrophy but not hyperplasia.

It has been posited that because IGF peptides can also bind to IGFBPs and integrin receptors, a signal independent of IGF-IR kinase activity could be generated in the muscle of MKR mice.[112] For example, Canonici and colleagues[113] have found that the IGF-IR forms a ternary complex with E-cadherin and the α_V integrin receptor and that IGF binding initiates signaling by disrupting this complex. A similar finding was made by Saegusa and colleagues,[103] who showed direct binding of IGF-I to the $\alpha_V\beta_3$ integrin. In smooth muscle, IGF-dependent ERK signaling is dependent on direct binding of vitronectin to the β_3 receptor because disruption of binding with a β_3 antibody reduced IGF-I signaling.[114] The $\alpha_V\beta_3$ integrin receptor is present on C2C12 cells and in skeletal muscle. Therefore, it has the potential to interact with the IGF-IR and stimulate downstream signaling pathways, such as the activation of focal adhesion kinases (FAK) and the adapter protein paxillin.[115–117] FAK can transactivate IGF-IRs in which the receptor autophosphorylation sites have been mutated.[15] In addition, peptides that disrupt IGF-IR/$\alpha_V\beta_3$ interactions inhibit signaling to Akt and ERK kinases.[118,119]

Barton and colleagues[94] have reported that different IGF-I isoforms have different capacities to stimulate gene expression in skeletal muscle. IGF-I is transcribed off a single gene, but multiple mRNAs are generated by alternative splicing of exons in the gene. Muscle expresses IGF-IA and IGF-1B in rodents as well as IGF-IC in humans. Although these mRNAs produce identical IGF-I peptides, there is less homology in the E-peptides that they produce. Some have suggested that the E-peptides (ie, Ea and Eb) themselves may signal through other receptors or facilitate signaling of the IGF-I peptide.[94] Data are available indicating that the E-peptides are necessary for muscle hypertrophy because overexpression of a viral construct containing the IGF-IA or IGF-IB peptide, but not mature IGF-I, stimulated hypertrophy of the tibialis and maintained force generation in the extensor digitorum longus (EDL).[94] In addition, both the IGF-IA and IGF-IB forms were inhibited in the MKR mouse. Shavlakadze and colleagues[120] suggest that overexpression of the IGF-IA isoform in muscle is most efficacious during periods of active growth, but not in adult mice. Yet, Matheny and colleagues[121] argue that although a stable IGF-I E-propeptide exists, a final processed EB-peptide has not been identified in extracellular fluids or cell culture media. One possibility is that the E-peptides anchor the IGF-I molecule in the extracellular matrix where it is more likely to come in contact with the IGF-IR. How the E-peptide influences IGF-I signaling in skeletal muscle remains an open question and should be an area of active research.[21]

Exercise and adequate nutrition are not only important for the maintenance of muscle mass but also for the prevention of and recovery from muscle disease.[122–126] As noted earlier, a key component of the protective effects of exercise and amino acid supplementation is their ability to stimulate mTOR.[16,40,127,128] In the ensuing sections, we review how various muscle diseases affect muscle mass and function, pursue common defects, and investigate whether nutrition, exercise, and IGFs have potential therapeutic benefits.

GLUCOCORTICOIDS AND ANDROGENS: A TALE OF TWO STEROID HORMONES IN THE CONTROL OF MUSCLE MASS

The release of glucocorticoids from the adrenal cortex during stress contributes to the regulation of blood pressure, blood glucose, and the inflammatory response. Yet, glucocorticoid excess has a negative effect on muscle mass because of its ability to decrease muscle protein synthesis and increase protein degradation.[14] The synthetic glucocorticoid dexamethasone stimulates the expression of a protein regulated in development and DNA responses (REDD1) in skeletal muscle, and this protein is a putative mTOR inhibitor.[129,130] REDD1 competes with TSC2 for binding to 14-3-3 proteins such that REDD1 overexpression drives TSC2 to return Rheb to a GDP-bound form and inhibit mTOR.[131] After an 18-hour fast, corticosterone upregulates

REDD1 protein expression, which can be prevented by the glucocorticoid type II receptor antagonist RU486.[132]

REDD1 is also upregulated in several stress conditions in which mTOR and muscle protein synthesis are inhibited, including after endurance exercise, sepsis, and acute alcohol intoxication. However, a direct causal role for REDD1 in decreasing mTOR kinase activity in these conditions has not been determined.[133–135] REDD1 is also increased paradoxically by insulin and IGF-I in adipose tissue and skeletal muscle, emphasizing that the expression of REDD1 is not consistently associated with mTOR inhibition.[17,136,137] In skeletal muscle, IGF-I–induced REDD1 may act in a negative feedback loop to dampen the mitochondrial generation of reactive oxygen species (ROS) because REDD1 localizes to mitochondria, where its absence or overexpression may result in increased ROS.[138,139] REDD1 may have a similar function in glucocorticoid-induced muscle atrophy, in which ROS are also increased.[140] Although ROS are necessary for IGF-I–induced myocyte hypertrophy in C2C12 myotubes, it is not known if REDD1 is involved in this response.[141] In addition, ROS generated after treatment of C2C12 myotubes with lipopolysaccharide and interferon γ strongly inhibit mTOR activity and protein synthesis. Moreover, both parameters are restored in the presence of IGF-I and antioxidants, suggesting that a normalization of ROS levels is necessary for IGF-I–induced mTOR activity in this model.[142] Glucocorticoids can decrease muscle mass and mTOR activity by upregulating both REDD1 and the transcription Krüppel-like factor 15 (KLF15) via classic glucocorticoid receptor (GR) elements in the promoters of both genes.[143] KLF15 also binds to response elements in atrogenes, such as atrogin-1 and muscle-specific ring finger 1 (MuRF-1), and these ubiquitin ligases target the ubiquitinylation and degradation of critical structural and functional proteins within skeletal muscle, including the myosin heavy and light chains.[144–146] Glucocorticoids also increase the expression of FoxO transcription factors and FoxO1 and KLF15 cooperate to increase the promoter activity of the atrogenes in skeletal muscle.[56,143,147] Autophagy and lysosomal protein degradation pathways are also upregulated in skeletal muscle by FoxO3, resulting in a coordinated effort to mobilize amino acids for hepatic gluconeogenesis.[56,148]

Although excess glucocorticoids clearly upregulate FoxO and the translation initiation factor 4E-BP1, these proteins also maintain muscle protein homeostasis by removing protein aggregates during aging when their overexpression can increase muscle strength.[149,150] Therefore, a delicate balance of FoxO and 4E-BP1 signaling exists. The importance of FoxO and 4E-BP1 in skeletal muscle and the organism as a whole is underscored by the fact that FoxO signaling in muscle also affects metabolism in other tissues.[150] For example, overexpression of 4E-BP1 specifically in skeletal muscle, but not in other tissues of Drosophila, increases both the median and maximal life span of flies similar to that seen during caloric restriction.[150] The FoxO-dependent induction of 4E-BP1 in the fat body has also been proposed to be a metabolic brake that is activated by stress to prevent excessive fat burn during starvation.[151] Future studies need to examine whether these proteins play a similar role in vertebrate muscle.[152,153]

The mitochondrial form of the branched-chain amino transferase gene (BCATm) is also upregulated by glucocorticoids in a KLF15-dependent fashion.[143] Overexpression of KLF15 increases the activity of BCATm, resulting in enhanced oxidation of BCAA and decreased mTOR substrate phosphorylation.[143] Further, the negative effects of KLF15 can be overcome by excess BCAA. mTOR activation by BCAA do not alter the translocation of the GR into the nucleus, but do diminish GR-mediated transcriptional activity.[143] The positive effects of BCAA therefore seem to be dominant over glucocorticoids because BCAA prevent dexamethasone-induced increases in atrogenes, REDD1, and KLF15 and simultaneously maintain muscle mass, muscle cross-sectional area, and muscle strength in the gastrocnemius.[143,154,155] These data are consistent with previous reports showing that mTOR activation by upstream activators, such as IGF-I and constitutively active Akt or Rheb,[19] overcome the negative effects of dexamethasone on protein synthesis and the phosphorylation of mTOR substrates.[14,129,136,155,156]

Excess BCAA may also enhance the anti-inflammatory effects of endogenous glucocorticoids by decreasing the expression of inflammatory cytokines, as occurs in BCATm null mice.[157] Other steroid hormones, such as testosterone, may also have beneficial effects on muscle mass because of their ability to prevent glucocorticoid-induced increases in REDD1.[158,159]

The age-related decline in muscle mass and function that occurs in humans has long been believed to be caused by a coincident decline in hormones and growth factors.[160] Serum testosterone concentrations are also positively correlated with muscle mass and muscle fiber cross-sectional area in elderly people.[161] Similar to the drop in testosterone during the andropause, GH and IGF-I decline during the somatopause, and their rate of decline correlates with the decrease in muscle mass.[162] Although GH and testosterone have dramatic effects on muscle mass in young people, replacement therapies that match endogenous hormone levels have only minimal effects on muscle mass and strength during sarcopenia. In addition, exercise-induced changes in GH and testosterone do not influence muscle mass.[96,163] These data suggest that muscle shows resistance to these anabolic factors.[164,165] The mechanism behind sarcopenia is therefore multifactorial and consistent with testosterone deficiency and the development of insulin resistance. In addition, leucine resistance develops in castrated rats.[166,167] Despite these factors, the intrinsic ability of muscle to respond to exercise is largely unchanged during sarcopenia, suggesting that a multimodal approach that has exercise as its focal point but includes nutrients and hormones, when necessary, would be most efficacious at preventing muscle loss or restoring muscle mass in the perisarcopenic period.[168]

Studies from rodents have revealed that not all muscles are equally sensitive to androgens because of their differential expression of the androgen receptor (AR).[169] In addition, skeletal muscle is capable of converting dehydroepiandrosterone to testosterone but further conversion of testosterone to dihydrotestosterone may not be necessary for its anabolic effects.[170,171]

This finding is promising because testosterone-induced hyperplasia of the prostate can be blocked by 5-α reductase inhibitors, whereas the anabolic effects of testosterone are not. These data suggest that the benefits of androgens for maintaining muscle mass may be garnered without their inherent cancer risk in males.[172] Androgens seem necessary for the development of muscle mass in male but not female mice because genomic knockout of the AR decreases muscle mass and force production in a gender-dependent manner.[173] The decrease in muscle mass in AR knockout mice is uniform across several muscles, including the gastrocnemius, soleus, tibialis anterior, and the EDL, but not the heart.[173] AR knockout was associated with a decrease in maximal force generation in fast-twitch muscle (EDL) and enhanced fatigue resistance in slow-twitch muscle (soleus). These data are consistent with changes in gene expression in which androgens increase the expression of type II glycolytic fibers, which produce more force but are highly fatigable. AR null mice show no change in serum or limb muscle IGF-I or IGF-IR mRNA but show a decrease in amino acid and micronutrient transporter mRNAs (Slc38a4/SNAT4), which could influence the cotransport of glutamine and leucine consistent with the leucine resistance observed in castrated rats.[167]

Selective ablation of the AR in skeletal myofibers decreases muscle mass in the perineal muscles, which contain a high concentration of the AR, but not in the limb muscles, in which the lack of AR signaling does not decrease mass but still affects muscle structural proteins and force production.[174] AR knockout postnatally in the perineal muscles also decreased IGF-IEa mRNA, and this was associated with a decrease in muscle mass.[174] In contrast, castration of muscle-specific AR null mice decreased both muscle IGF-IEa mRNA and muscle mass, suggesting that androgens maintain muscle mass by a myofiber-specific and AR-independent mechanism. The AR, in supporting fibroblasts and satellite cells, may therefore determine autocrine IGF-I levels and muscle mass. In agreement with this theory is the finding that androgens stimulate the proliferation of human skeletal muscle cells in vitro and this is blocked by both IGF-I neutralizing antibodies and siRNA-mediated knockdown of the IGF-IR.[100] Signal transducers and activators of transcription (STAT) 5a/b, two transcription factors necessary for the maintenance of muscle mass, also maintain the expression of the AR, which is transcriptionally induced by GH. Muscle-specific knockout of STAT5a/b leads to a muscle fiber type switch from type II to type I fibers.[175] Inhibition of IGF-IR signaling in the MKR mouse also attenuates testosterone-induced gains in the mass of the perineal muscles by 60%.[100] Thus, IGF-IR signaling plays a critical role in the response of muscle to androgens.

Ibebunjo and colleagues[176] have recently discovered a potential link between the andropause and decreased muscle activity and muscle mass. These investigators found that castration decreased voluntary running speed and endurance, both of which were restored on treatment with testosterone. Testosterone increased the expression of several genes, including IGF-I, the IGF-IR, and solute carriers, but the increase in these markers occurred equally well in sedentary and exercised rats, suggesting that these genes are permissive only for the observed behavior. Although testosterone replacement was not associated with dramatic changes in muscle mass, it was associated with a transition to type IIa muscle fibers. Because the transition to type IIa fibers was greater in the mice that ran than in the sedentary animals, testosterone per se does not mediate the transition to type II fibers but is obligatory to promote the activity that drives the transition.[176]

One scheme for staving off sarcopenia may be the consumption of adequate protein during middle age. D'Antona and colleagues[177] found that mice fed a diet supplemented with BCAA showed an increase in average lifespan and enhanced mitochondrial biogenesis in skeletal muscle. The greatest mitochondrial mass was achieved in mice that received both BCAA and exercise, and the beneficial effects of BCAA on mitochondrial biogenesis could be blocked by rapamycin.[177] Many of the beneficial effects of caloric restriction on life span can be mimicked by intermittent feeding protocols in which there is little or no reduction in total caloric intake. In *Caenorhabditis elegans*, the beneficial effects of intermittent feeding require Rheb to be transiently turned on and off and for mTOR to be activated to downregulate the expression of an IGF-like peptide and increase the loco motor activity of the worms.[178]

These data suggest that hormones, growth factors, nutrients, and exercise cooperate in maintaining muscle mass and function and provide the impetus to overcome sarcopenia. Recent data suggest that this effect may occur via a centrally mediated mechanism.[176,179] AR knockout in the nervous system generates male mice that show growth retardation, a decrease in male-typical behavior, and reduced serum levels of IGF-I.[180] Although overall activity is not affected by AR knockout in the nervous system of young adult mice (2–5 months), it would be interesting to determine whether these mice are more prone to decreased activity and sarcopenia with aging (>18 months).[180] AR null mice also lack the normal feedback control regulating glucocorticoid production such that plasma adrenocorticotropic hormone and corticosterone levels are chronically increased.[181] Thus, the testosterone deficit seen with aging may be a prerequisite to a glucocorticoid-induced decrease in muscle protein. Conversely, animal studies are promising because they suggest that testosterone and tissue-selective AR modulators can reverse dexamethasone-induced atrophy of the perineal muscles and repress genes involved in glucocorticoid-induced wasting, including REDD1 and FOXO1.[158,159,182] There seem to be significant cooperative effects between amino acids, exercise, the IGF system, and androgens in the maintenance of muscle mass.

IMMOBILIZED MUSCLE: A CAST OF CHARACTERS INVOLVED IN MUSCLE ATROPHY

Immobilization of the leg muscles induces muscle atrophy and is highly relevant to clinical conditions in which patients endure long-standing bed rest.[183] During prolonged bed rest, there is a differential rate of atrophy between muscle groups, with the antigravity muscles and the plantar flexor muscles (medial gastrocnemius and soleus) showing the greatest atrophy.

The knee extensors, the hip extensors and abductors, and the muscles of the foot and ankle, such as the tibialis posterior, are also greatly affected, consistent with the use of these muscles not only for locomotion but also for supporting load.[183] In contrast, other muscles such as the toe extensors (anterior tibial muscles) and flexors (flexor digitorum longus) show little or no atrophy.[183] These observations suggest that resistance exercise protocols targeting the affected muscles could prevent damage to joints and diminish the risk of injury during the recovery phase. Immobilization is believed to make skeletal muscle resistant to the positive effects of anabolic amino acids and protein, suggesting that nutrition alone is insufficient to mount an anabolic response during bed rest.[184] Supplementation of BCAA during bed rest does not affect either muscle protein synthesis or the release of 3-methylhistidine from muscle (a marker of muscle protein breakdown) but does increase the free amino acid pool during the early recovery phase.[185] These observations suggest that a combination of amino acids and exercise might enhance muscle recovery. Recent studies indicate that provision of amino acids and exercise during bed rest increased muscle volume and strength and decreased the deposition of intramuscular fat compared with amino acid supplementation alone.[186] In a follow-up study examining potential mechanisms by which the combination of amino acids and resistance exercise restored muscle mass after bed rest, the investigators found that only the combination of exercise and amino acids increased IGF-I expression and simultaneously antagonized the increase in atrogenes.[187] Ectopic expression of IGF-I within the gastrocnemius prevented muscle atrophy by 50% in a mouse model of 7 days of hind-limb suspension.[188] IGF-I expression from the gastrocnemius also tended to increase the bone mineral content in the lumbar bones by dual-energy radiograph absorptiometry, suggesting a beneficial effect of either paracrine IGF-I or the maintenance of muscle function on bone.[188]

Recent studies suggest that FoxO and nuclear factor κB (NF-κB) transcription factors drive muscle atrophy in elderly individuals who assume a sedentary lifestyle and in rodent models of muscle immobilization.[56,189–191] Overexpression of constitutively active FoxO or NF-κB stimulates the atrophy program in mice.[192] Other data suggest that ROS, and in particular hydrogen peroxide, drive changes in muscle mass. Dodd and colleagues[193–195] have shown that overexpression of catalase partially attenuates NF-κB/FoxO signaling and the loss of muscle mass during hind-limb immobilization is consistent with the ability of some antioxidants to abate immobilization-induced muscle loss and muscle fatigue. The application of intermittent heat during the reloading period also enhanced antioxidant defenses and the recovery of muscle mass and mTOR activity.[196–198]

Although IGF-I mRNA and protein levels are not altered by immobilization, numerous genes involved in IGF signaling are downregulated in human muscle during voluntary casting.[199,200] Therefore investigators have examined whether overexpression of IGF-I can prevent immobilization-induced skeletal muscle loss. IGF-I does not inhibit the loss of muscle mass during the atrophy phase but it does enhance muscle weight gain and cross-sectional area during a 3-week reloading period.[200,201] This response suggests that casted muscle is IGF-I resistant and that muscle contraction is necessary for IGF-I to have its full biologic effect during recovery. Although IGF-I treatment is normally associated with an increase in protein synthesis in control mice, the IGF-I–induced increase in muscle mass during recovery from casting seems to be independent of changes in muscle protein synthesis and may be related to the ability of IGF-I to stimulate the proliferation and regeneration of muscle stem cells.[200] Casting in humans also decreases the expression of genes, such as SLC16A1, involved in the transport of monocarboxylates such as lactate, pyruvate, and branched-chain oxo acids derived from leucine.[199] SLC16A1, also known as MCT1, is a bidirectional transporter located on the plasma membrane of muscle cells. Genetic defects in SLC16A1 may result in a deficiency in lactate transport out of the cell, intracellular acidification, and subsequent muscle degeneration.[202] The resulting muscle acidification may also inhibit the subsequent transport of glutamine via acidosis-induced inhibition of the glutamine pump SNAT2 which is obligatory for the transport of BCAA such as leucine, activation of mTOR signaling, and protein synthesis.[203]

Growth factors may be able to overcome intracellular acidification and stimulate protein synthesis by their ability to activate the Na+/H+ antiport system and increase the pH of the intracellular compartment.[204,205]

ALCOHOL INDUCES LEUCINE AND IGF-I RESISTANCE IN SKELETAL MUSCLE

Alcoholics experience a myopathy that selectively affects type II fibers (gastrocnemius > soleus) and seems to result from a decrease in muscle protein synthesis and damage to muscle proteins.[206] Similar decrements in muscle protein synthesis are seen in animal models of both acute alcohol intoxication and chronic alcohol abuse.[207] Alcohol decreases skeletal muscle IGF-I content and makes muscle both IGF-I and insulin resistant at the level of mTOR activity.[208,209]

Although skeletal muscle is IGF-I resistant after the acute administration of alcohol, rats fed an alcohol-containing diet for 16 weeks show improved muscle protein synthesis when administered IGF-I as part of a binary complex with IGFBP-3.[210] These data suggest that the binary complex may maintain the local concentration of IGF-I in skeletal muscle for a sustained period and allow for better recovery of the muscle than a single injection of recombinant IGF-I, which is rapidly cleared from the circulation. The binary complex may also be more efficient at restoring plasma amino acids needed to transduce the IGF signal, such as glutamine and alanine.[210]

Alcohol also impairs the normal mTOR response to leucine in as little as 2.5 hours after an oral gavage of alcohol.[211] Although acute alcohol intoxication has a similar effect on mTOR activity in male and female rats, female rats seem to better tolerate the long-term effects of alcohol on muscle. Female, but not male rats, show an increase in markers of muscle protein remodeling such as atrogin-1 and MuRF-1, suggesting that female rats may be more efficient at synthesizing new protein and clearing damaged protein than males when placed on a long-term alcohol-containing diet.[212] Alcohol also accelerates muscle loss caused by unilateral hind-limb immobilization (casting a single leg), and alcohol impairs the recovery of muscle mass for at least 5 days after cast removal.[213] After unilateral hind-limb immobilization in rats, alcohol accentuates the expression of atrogin-1 and MuRF-1 and muscle recovery is improved by the proteasome inhibitor bortezomib (Velcade). These results indicate that a fairly dominant proteasome-mediated muscle proteolysis element exists in the casting model of disuse atrophy and that this can be accentuated by alcohol.

Although the mechanism by which alcohol induces leucine and IGF-I resistance has not been completely elucidated, recent data suggest that mice that have abnormally high plasma leucine levels may be protected from alcohol-induced IGF-I resistance. Mice with a whole-body knockout of the mitochondrial form of the BCAA-metabolizing enzyme BCATm show plasma leucine levels 15-fold higher than wild-type mice.[157,214] BCAA levels this high do not inhibit the effects of alcohol on muscle protein synthesis per se but they do sensitize skeletal muscle to IGF-I, allowing IGF-I to restore muscle protein synthesis to levels observed in control rats given IGF-I.[157] Excess BCAA may therefore protect the muscle from alcohol-induced changes in IGF-I sensitivity. High doses of leucine have also been shown to ameliorate the negative effects of AMPK signaling on muscle protein synthesis and to increase mitochondrial mass in muscle cells.[62,215,216]

Studies by Hong-Brown and colleagues[217] in C2C12 myoblasts suggest that alcohol differentially affects mTORc1 and mTORc2. Alcohol decreases mTORc1 activity and increases the abundance of mTORc2 components and the phosphorylation of mTORc2 substrates such as Akt on S473. These findings suggest that, in myoblasts, alcohol does not directly alter the intrinsic activity of mTOR. These investigators have also shown that alcohol disrupts leucine signaling to mTORc1 in myoblasts by suppressing the interaction of Rag A and C with mTOR.[218] A constitutively active combination of Rag A and C but not A alone overcomes the negative effect of alcohol and maintains the phosphorylation of mTOR substrates such as S6K1 and 4E-BP1.[218] This finding implies that alcohol disrupts mTOR signaling at a step either before or directly at the sensing of leucine by the Rag proteins (see **Fig. 1**).

SUMMARY

The plasticity of skeletal muscle is shown by its capacity to double or even triple in size. Overall, muscle volume may be restricted by genetic limits but muscle quantity is primarily regulated by its own use and disuse. Muscle hypertrophy is also influenced by the availability of nutrients and the presence of endocrine and autocrine hormones such as IGF-I. A concerted anabolic signal is generated by leucine, which facilitates the translocation of the kinase mTOR to the surface of the lysosome, where it is activated by Rheb, and by IGF-I, which relieves the inherent inhibition of mTOR by TSC2. mTOR is also positively regulated by short-term changes in the energy state of individual muscle fibers after a meal and secondarily by prolonged exposure to leucine, glucose, and contractile load, all of which may influence the long-term energy state by increasing mitochondrial biogenesis. mTOR, when activated, phosphorylates substrates such as the translation initiation factor 4E-BP1 to stimulate muscle protein synthesis and muscle hypertrophy. IGF-I also stimulates the self-renewal of muscle satellite cells to replace myonuclei and rebuild muscle after injury. Exercise, nutrients, and growth factors have evolved together to optimally energize mTOR and overcome the negative impact of catabolic hormones, inflammatory mediators, and muscle damage. Hence, a combination of these mTOR modifiers used in tandem may be efficacious in preventing or ameliorating reductions in muscle mass occurring in select pathologic conditions.

REFERENCES

1. Porter Abate J, Blackwell TK. Life is short, if sweet. Cell Metab 2009;10:338.
2. Spanier B, Rubio-Aliaga I, Hu H, et al. Altered signalling from germline to intestine pushes daf-2;pept-1 *Caenorhabditis elegans* into extreme longevity. Aging Cell 2010;9:636.
3. Heron-Milhavet L, Mamaeva D, LeRoith D, et al. Impaired muscle regeneration and myoblast differentiation in mice with a muscle-specific KO of IGF-IR. J Cell Physiol 2010;225:1.
4. Ten Broek RW, Grefte S, Von den Hoff JW. Regulatory factors and cell populations involved in skeletal muscle regeneration. J Cell Physiol 2010;224:7.
5. Liu JP, Baker J, Perkins AS, et al. Mice carrying null mutations of the genes encoding insulin-like growth factor I (Igf-1) and type 1 IGF receptor (Igf1r). Cell 1993;75:59.
6. Liu JL, LeRoith D. Insulin-like growth factor I is essential for postnatal growth in response to growth hormone. Endocrinology 1999;140:5178.
7. Mavalli MD, DiGirolamo DJ, Fan Y, et al. Distinct growth hormone receptor signaling modes regulate skeletal muscle development and insulin sensitivity in mice. J Clin Invest 2010;120:4007.
8. Clemmons DR. Role of IGF-I in skeletal muscle mass maintenance. Trends Endocrinol Metab 2009;20:349.
9. Stratikopoulos E, Szabolcs M, Dragatsis I, et al. The hormonal action of IGF1 in postnatal mouse growth. Proc Natl Acad Sci U S A 2008;105:19378.
10. Wu Y, Sun H, Yakar S, et al. Elevated levels of insulin-like growth factor (IGF)-I in serum rescue the severe growth retardation of IGF-I null mice. Endocrinology 2009;150:4395.
11. Han B, Zhu MJ, Ma C, et al. Rat hindlimb unloading down-regulates insulin like growth factor-1 signaling and AMP-activated protein kinase, and leads to severe atrophy of the soleus muscle. Appl Physiol Nutr Metab 2007;32:1115.
12. Gehrig SM, Ryall JG, Schertzer JD, et al. Insulin-like growth factor-I analogue protects muscles of dystrophic mdx mice from contraction-mediated damage. Exp Physiol 2008;93:1190.
13. Frost RA, Lang CH. Protein kinase B/Akt: a nexus of growth factor and cytokine signaling in determining muscle mass. J Appl Physiol 2007;103:378.
14. Schakman O, Gilson H, Kalista S, et al. Mechanisms of muscle atrophy induced by glucocorticoids. Horm Res 2009;72(Suppl 1):36.
15. Inder WJ, Jang C, Obeyesekere VR, et al. Dexamethasone administration inhibits skeletal muscle expression of the androgen receptor and IGF-1–implications for steroid-induced myopathy. Clin Endocrinol (Oxf) 2010;73:126.
16. Muscaritoli M, Bossola M, Aversa Z, et al. Prevention and treatment of cancer cachexia: new insights into an old problem. Eur J Cancer 2006;42:31.
17. Crown AL, Cottle K, Lightman SL, et al. What is the role of the insulin-like growth factor system in the pathophysiology of cancer cachexia, and how is it regulated? Clin Endocrinol (Oxf) 2002;56:723.
18. Frost RA, Lang CH. Regulation of insulin-like growth factor-I in skeletal muscle and muscle cells. Minerva Endocrinol 2003;28:53.
19. Schertzer JD, Lynch GS. Comparative evaluation of IGF-I gene transfer and IGF-I protein administration for enhancing skeletal muscle regeneration after injury. Gene Ther 2006;13:1657.
20. Demonbreun AR, Fahrenbach JP, Deveaux K, et al. Impaired muscle growth and response to insulin-like growth factor 1 in dysferlin-mediated muscular dystrophy. Hum Mol Genet 2011;20:779.

21. Vinciguerra M, Musaro A, Rosenthal N. Regulation of muscle atrophy in aging and disease. Adv Exp Med Biol 2010;694:211.
22. Schertzer JD, Gehrig SM, Ryall JG, et al. Modulation of insulin-like growth factor (IGF)-I and IGF-binding protein interactions enhances skeletal muscle regeneration and ameliorates the dystrophic pathology in mdx mice. Am J Pathol 2007; 171:1180.
23. Zdanowicz MM, Teichberg S. Effects of insulin-like growth factor-1/binding protein-3 complex on muscle atrophy in rats. Exp Biol Med (Maywood) 2003; 228:891.
24. Herndon DN, Ramzy PI, DebRoy MA, et al. Muscle protein catabolism after severe burn: effects of IGF-1/IGFBP-3 treatment. Ann Surg 1999;229:713.
25. Xu Y, Fang Y, Chen J, et al. Activation of mTOR signaling by novel fluoromethylene phosphonate analogues of phosphatidic acid. Bioorg Med Chem Lett 2004;14:1461.
26. Long YC, Cheng Z, Copps KD, et al. Insulin receptor substrates Irs1 and Irs2 coordinate skeletal muscle growth and metabolism via the Akt and AMPK pathways. Mol Cell Biol 2011;31:430.
27. McCarthy JJ, Esser KA. Anabolic and catabolic pathways regulating skeletal muscle mass. Curr Opin Clin Nutr Metab Care 2010;13:230.
28. Risson V, Mazelin L, Roceri M, et al. Muscle inactivation of mTOR causes metabolic and dystrophin defects leading to severe myopathy. J Cell Biol 2009;187:859.
29. Bentzinger CF, Romanino K, Cloetta D, et al. Skeletal muscle-specific ablation of raptor, but not of rictor, causes metabolic changes and results in muscle dystrophy. Cell Metab 2008;8:411.
30. Setia S, Sridhar MG. Changes in GH/IGF-1 axis in intrauterine growth retardation: consequences of fetal programming? Horm Metab Res 2009;41:791.
31. Kappeler L, De Magalhaes Filho C, Leneuve P, et al. Early postnatal nutrition determines somatotropic function in mice. Endocrinology 2009;150:314.
32. Christoforidis A, Maniadaki I, Stanhope R. Growth hormone/insulin-like growth factor-1 axis during puberty. Pediatr Endocrinol Rev 2005;3:5.
33. Moller N, Vendelbo MH, Kampmann U, et al. Growth hormone and protein metabolism. Clin Nutr 2009;28:597.
34. Dreyer HC, Drummond MJ, Pennings B, et al. Leucine-enriched essential amino acid and carbohydrate ingestion following resistance exercise enhances mTOR signaling and protein synthesis in human muscle. Am J Physiol Endocrinol Metab 2008;294:E392.
35. Smith GI, Atherton P, Reeds DN, et al. Dietary omega-3 fatty acid supplementation increases the rate of muscle protein synthesis in older adults: a randomized controlled trial. Am J Clin Nutr 2011;93:402.
36. Heron-Milhavet L, Haluzik M, Yakar S, et al. Muscle-specific overexpression of CD36 reverses the insulin resistance and diabetes of MKR mice. Endocrinology 2004;145:4667.
37. Gingras AA, White PJ, Chouinard PY, et al. Long-chain omega-3 fatty acids regulate bovine whole-body protein metabolism by promoting muscle insulin signalling to the Akt-mTOR-S6K1 pathway and insulin sensitivity. J Physiol 2007;579:269.
38. Rennie MJ. Exercise- and nutrient-controlled mechanisms involved in maintenance of the musculoskeletal mass. Biochem Soc Trans 2007;35:1302.
39. Wolfe RR. Skeletal muscle protein metabolism and resistance exercise. J Nutr 2006;136:525S.

40. Anthony JC, Yoshizawa F, Anthony TG, et al. Leucine stimulates translation initiation in skeletal muscle of postabsorptive rats via a rapamycin-sensitive pathway. J Nutr 2000;130:2413.
41. de Oliveira CA, Latorraca MQ, de Mello MA, et al. Mechanisms of insulin secretion in malnutrition: modulation by amino acids in rodent models. Amino Acids 2011;40:1027.
42. Apro W, Blomstrand E. Influence of supplementation with branched-chain amino acids in combination with resistance exercise on p70S6 kinase phosphorylation in resting and exercising human skeletal muscle. Acta Physiol (Oxf) 2010;200: 237.
43. Tzatsos A, Kandror KV. Nutrients suppress phosphatidylinositol 3-kinase/Akt signaling via raptor-dependent mTOR-mediated insulin receptor substrate 1 phosphorylation. Mol Cell Biol 2006;26:63.
44. Goodman CA, Miu MH, Frey JW, et al. A phosphatidylinositol 3-kinase/protein kinase B-independent activation of mammalian target of rapamycin signaling is sufficient to induce skeletal muscle hypertrophy. Mol Biol Cell 2010;21:3258.
45. Long X, Ortiz-Vega S, Lin Y, et al. Rheb binding to mammalian target of rapamycin (mTOR) is regulated by amino acid sufficiency. J Biol Chem 2005;280: 23433.
46. Nicklin P, Bergman P, Zhang B, et al. Bidirectional transport of amino acids regulates mTOR and autophagy. Cell 2009;136:521.
47. Suryawan A, Davis TA. Regulation of protein synthesis by amino acids in muscle of neonates. Front Biosci 2011;16:1445.
48. McDowell HE, Christie GR, Stenhouse G, et al. Leucine activates system A amino acid transport in L6 rat skeletal muscle cells. Am J Physiol 1995;269:C1287.
49. Avruch J, Long X, Ortiz-Vega S, et al. Amino acid regulation of TOR complex 1. Am J Physiol Endocrinol Metab 2009;296:E592.
50. Sancak Y, Peterson TR, Shaul YD, et al. The Rag GTPases bind raptor and mediate amino acid signaling to mTORC1. Science 2008;320:1496.
51. Sancak Y, Bar-Peled L, Zoncu R, et al. Ragulator-Rag complex targets mTORC1 to the lysosomal surface and is necessary for its activation by amino acids. Cell 2010;141:290.
52. Zoncu R, Bar-Peled L, Efeyan A, et al. mTORC1 senses lysosomal amino acids through an insideout mechanism that requires the vacuolar H(+)-ATPase. Science 2011;334:678.
53. Sagne C, Agulhon C, Ravassard P, et al. Identification and characterization of a lysosomal transporter for small neutral amino acids. Proc Natl Acad Sci U S A 2001;98:7206.
54. Goberdhan DC. Intracellular amino acid sensing and mTORC1-regulated growth: new ways to block an old target? Curr Opin Investig Drugs 2010;11:1360.
55. Heublein S, Kazi S, Ogmundsdottir MH, et al. Proton-assisted amino-acid transporters are conserved regulators of proliferation and amino-acid-dependent mTORC1 activation. Oncogene 2010;29:4068.
56. Zhao J, Brault JJ, Schild A, et al. FoxO3 coordinately activates protein degradation by the autophagic/lysosomal and proteasomal pathways in atrophying muscle cells. Cell Metab 2007;6:472.
57. Iida RH, Kanko S, Suga T, et al. Autophagic-lysosomal pathway functions in the masseter and tongue muscles in the klotho mouse, a mouse model for aging. Mol Cell Biochem 2011;348:89.
58. Bartke A. Long-lived Klotho mice: new insights into the roles of IGF-1 and insulin in aging. Trends Endocrinol Metab 2006;17:33.

59. Yu L, McPhee CK, Zheng L, et al. Termination of autophagy and reformation of lysosomes regulated by mTOR. Nature 2010;465:942.

60. Settembre C, Zoncu R, Medina DL, et al. A lysosome-to-nucleus signalling mechanism senses and regulates the lysosome via mTOR and TFEB. EMBO J 2012;31:1095.

61. Saci A, Cantley LC, Carpenter CL. Rac1 regulates the activity of mTORC1 and mTORC2 and controls cellular size. Mol Cell 2011;42:50.

62. Saha AK, Xu XJ, Lawson E, et al. Downregulation of AMPK accompanies leucine- and glucose-induced increases in protein synthesis and insulin resistance in rat skeletal muscle. Diabetes 2010;59:2426.

63. Inoki K, Ouyang H, Zhu T, et al. TSC2 integrates Wnt and energy signals via a coordinated phosphorylation by AMPK and GSK3 to regulate cell growth. Cell 2006;126:955.

64. Avruch J, Lin Y, Long X, et al. Recent advances in the regulation of the TOR pathway by insulin and nutrients. Curr Opin Clin Nutr Metab Care 2005;8:67.

65. Zheng M, Wang YH, Wu XN, et al. Inactivation of Rheb by PRAK-mediated phosphorylation is essential for energy-depletion-induced suppression of mTORC1. Nat Cell Biol 2011;13:263.

66. Miyazaki M, McCarthy JJ, Esser KA. Insulin like growth factor-1-induced phosphorylation and altered distribution of tuberous sclerosis complex (TSC)1/TSC2 in C2C12 myotubes. FEBS J 2010;277:2180.

67. Wan M, Wu X, Guan KL, et al. Muscle atrophy in transgenic mice expressing a human TSC1 transgene. FEBS Lett 2006;580:5621.

68. Avruch J, Hara K, Lin Y, et al. Insulin and amino-acid regulation of mTOR signaling and kinase activity through the Rheb GTPase. Oncogene 2006;25:6361.

69. Wang X, Proud CG. mTORC1 signaling: what we still don't know. J Mol Cell Biol 2011;3(4):206–20.

70. Sun Y, Fang Y, Yoon MS, et al. Phospholipase D1 is an effector of Rheb in the mTOR pathway. Proc Natl Acad Sci U S A 2008;105:8286.

71. Zhang C, Wendel AA, Keogh MR, et al. Glycerolipid signals alter mTOR complex 2 (mTORC2) to diminish insulin signaling. Proc Natl Acad Sci U S A 2012;109:1667.

72. Sengupta S, Peterson TR, Sabatini DM. Regulation of the mTOR complex 1 pathway by nutrients, growth factors, and stress. Mol Cell 2010;40:310.

73. Fang Y, Vilella-Bach M, Bachmann R, et al. Phosphatidic acid-mediated mitogenic activation of mTOR signaling. Science 2001;294:1942.

74. Sato T, Nakashima A, Guo L, et al. Specific activation of mTORC1 by Rheb G-protein in vitro involves enhanced recruitment of its substrate protein. J Biol Chem 2009; 284:12783.

75. Toschi A, Lee E, Xu L, et al. Regulation of mTORC1 and mTORC2 complex assembly by phosphatidic acid: competition with rapamycin. Mol Cell Biol 2009;29:1411.

76. Dennis MD, Baum JI, Kimball SR, et al. Mechanisms involved in the coordinate regulation of the mammalian target of rapamycin complex 1 (mTORC1) by insulin and amino acids. J Biol Chem 2011;286(10):8287–96.

77. Drummond MJ, Bell JA, Fujita S, et al. Amino acids are necessary for the insulin-induced activation of mTOR/S6K1 signaling and protein synthesis in healthy and insulin resistant human skeletal muscle. Clin Nutr 2008;27:447.

78. Tipton KD, Rasmussen BB, Miller SL, et al. Timing of amino acid-carbohydrate ingestion alters anabolic response of muscle to resistance exercise. Am J Physiol Endocrinol Metab 2001;281:E197.

79. Wasa M, Wang HS, Tazuke Y, et al. Insulin-like growth factor-I stimulates amino acid transport in a glutamine-deprived human neuroblastoma cell line. Biochim Biophys Acta 2001;1525:118.

80. Fryburg DA, Jahn LA, Hill SA, et al. Insulin and insulin-like growth factor-I enhance human skeletal muscle protein anabolism during hyperaminoacidemia by different mechanisms. J Clin Invest 1995;96:1722.

81. Henriksen EJ, Louters LL, Stump CS, et al. Effects of prior exercise on the action of insulin-like growth factor I in skeletal muscle. Am J Physiol 1992;263:E340.

82. Coletta DK, Balas B, Chavez AO, et al. Effect of acute physiological hyperinsulinemia on gene expression in human skeletal muscle in vivo. Am J Physiol Endocrinol Metab 2008;294:E910.

83. Raffaello A, Milan G, Masiero E, et al. JunB transcription factor maintains skeletal muscle mass and promotes hypertrophy. J Cell Biol 2010;191:101.

84. Trenerry MK, Carey KA, Ward AC, et al. STAT3 signaling is activated in human skeletal muscle following acute resistance exercise. J Appl Physiol 2007;102:1483.

85. Allen DL, Unterman TG. Regulation of myostatin expression and myoblast differentiation by FoxO and SMAD transcription factors. Am J Physiol Cell Physiol 2007;292:C188.

86. Bark TH, McNurlan MA, Lang CH, et al. Increased protein synthesis after acute IGF-I or insulin infusion is localized to muscle in mice. Am J Physiol 1998;275: E118.

87. Stokes KA, Sykes D, Gilbert KL, et al. Brief, high intensity exercise alters serum ghrelin and growth hormone concentrations but not IGF-I, IGF-II or IGF-I bioactivity. Growth Horm IGF Res 2010;20:289.

88. Nindl BC, Pierce JR. Insulin-like growth factor I as a biomarker of health, fitness, and training status. Med Sci Sports Exerc 2010;42:39.

89. Heinemeier KM, Olesen JL, Schjerling P, et al. Short-term strength training and the expression of myostatin and IGF-I isoforms in rat muscle and tendon: differential effects of specific contraction types. J Appl Physiol 2007;102:573.

90. Vendelbo MH, Jorgensen JO, Pedersen SB, et al. Exercise and fasting activate growth hormone-dependent myocellular signal transducer and activator of transcription-5b phosphorylation and insulin-like growth factor-I messenger ribonucleic acid expression in humans. J Clin Endocrinol Metab 2010;95:E64.

91. Berg U, Gustafsson T, Sundberg CJ, et al. Interstitial IGF-I in exercising skeletal muscle in women. Eur J Endocrinol 2007;157:427.

92. Fedele MJ, Lang CH, Farrell PA. Immunization against IGF-I prevents increases in protein synthesis in diabetic rats after resistance exercise. Am J Physiol Endocrinol Metab 2001;280:E877.

93. Spangenburg EE, Le Roith D, Ward CW, et al. A functional insulin-like growth factor receptor is not necessary for load-induced skeletal muscle hypertrophy. J Physiol 2008;586:283.

94. Barton ER, DeMeo J, Lei H. The insulin-like growth factor (IGF)-I E-peptides are required for isoform-specific gene expression and muscle hypertrophy after local IGF-I production. J Appl Physiol 2010;108:1069.

95. Hornberger TA, Armstrong DD, Koh TJ, et al. Intracellular signaling specificity in response to uniaxial vs. multiaxial stretch: implications for mechanotransduction. Am J Physiol Cell Physiol 2005;288:C185.

96. West DW, Burd NA, Staples AW, et al. Human exercise-mediated skeletal muscle hypertrophy is an intrinsic process. Int J Biochem Cell Biol 2010;42:1371.

97. Witkowski S, Lovering RM, Spangenburg EE. High-frequency electrically stimulated skeletal muscle contractions increase p70s6k phosphorylation

independent of known IGF-I sensitive signaling pathways. FEBS Lett 2010; 584:2891.

98. Vaitheesvaran B, LeRoith D, Kurland IJ. MKR mice have increased dynamic glucose disposal despite metabolic inflexibility, and hepatic and peripheral insulin insensitivity. Diabetologia 2010;53:2224.

99. Fernandez AM, Dupont J, Farrar RP, et al. Muscle-specific inactivation of the IGF-I receptor induces compensatory hyperplasia in skeletal muscle. J Clin Invest 2002;109:347.

100. Serra C, Bhasin S, Tangherlini F, et al. The role of GH and IGF-I in mediating anabolic effects of testosterone on androgen-responsive muscle. Endocrinology 2011;152:193.

101. Schiaffino S, Mammucari C. Regulation of skeletal muscle growth by the IGF1-Akt/PKB pathway: insights from genetic models. Skelet Muscle 2011;1:4.

102. Perrault R, Wright B, Storie B, et al. Tyrosine kinase-independent activation of extracellular-regulated kinase (ERK) 1/2 by the insulin-like growth factor-1 receptor. Cell Signal 2011;23(4):739–46.

103. Saegusa J, Yamaji S, Ieguchi K, et al. The direct binding of insulin-like growth factor-1 (IGF-1) to integrin alphavbeta3 is involved in IGF-1 signaling. J Biol Chem 2009;284:24106.

104. Winter JN, Fox TE, Kester M, et al. Phosphatidic acid mediates activation of mTORC1 through the ERK signaling pathway. Am J Physiol Cell Physiol 2010; 299:C335.

105. Sarbassov DD, Jones LG, Peterson CA. Extracellular signal-regulated kinase-1 and -2 respond differently to mitogenic and differentiative signaling pathways in myoblasts. Mol Endocrinol 1997;11:2038.

106. Lee SJ, McPherron AC. Regulation of myostatin activity and muscle growth. Proc Natl Acad Sci U S A 2001;98:9306.

107. Kalista S, Schakman O, Gilson H, et al. The type 1 insulin-like growth factor receptor (IGF-IR) pathway is mandatory for the follistatin-induced skeletal muscle hypertrophy. Endocrinology 2012;153:241.

108. Gilson H, Schakman O, Kalista S, et al. Follistatin induces muscle hypertrophy through satellite cell proliferation and inhibition of both myostatin and activin. Am J Physiol Endocrinol Metab 2009;297:E157.

109. Qaisar R, Renaud G, Morine K, et al. Is functional hypertrophy and specific force coupled with the addition of myonuclei at the single muscle fiber level? FASEB J 2012;26:1077.

110. Kota J, Handy CR, Haidet AM, et al. Follistatin gene delivery enhances muscle growth and strength in nonhuman primates. Sci Transl Med 2009;1:6ra15.

111. Goodman CA, Mayhew DL, Hornberger TA. Recent progress toward understanding the molecular mechanisms that regulate skeletal muscle mass. Cell Signal 2011;23:1896.

112. Stewart CE, Pell JM. Point: Counterpoint: IGF is/is not the major physiological regulator of muscle mass. Point: IGF is the major physiological regulator of muscle mass. J Appl Physiol 2010;108:1820.

113. Canonici A, Steelant W, Rigot V, et al. Insulin-like growth factor-I receptor, E-cadherin and alpha v integrin form a dynamic complex under the control of alpha-catenin. Int J Cancer 2008;122:572.

114. Maile LA, Busby WH, Sitko K, et al. Insulin-like growth factor-I signaling in smooth muscle cells is regulated by ligand binding to the 177CYDMKTTC184 sequence of the beta3-subunit of alphaVbeta3. Mol Endocrinol 2006;20:405.

115. Svendsen OS, Liden A, Nedrebo T, et al. Integrin alphavbeta3 acts downstream of insulin in normalization of interstitial fluid pressure in sepsis and in cell-mediated collagen gel contraction. Am J Physiol Heart Circ Physiol 2008;295:H555.

116. Sinanan AC, Machell JR, Wynne-Hughes GT, et al. Alpha v beta 3 and alpha v beta 5 integrins and their role in muscle precursor cell adhesion. Biol Cell 2008; 100:465.

117. Furundzija V, Fritzsche J, Kaufmann J, et al. IGF-1 increases macrophage motility via PKC/p38- dependent alphavbeta3-integrin inside-out signaling. Biochem Biophys Res Commun 2010;394:786.

118. Andersson S, D'Arcy P, Larsson O, et al. Focal adhesion kinase (FAK) activates and stabilizes IGF-1 receptor. Biochem Biophys Res Commun 2009;387:36.

119. Zheng D, Kurenova E, Ucar D, et al. Targeting of the protein interaction site between FAK and IGF-1R. Biochem Biophys Res Commun 2009;388:301.

120. Shavlakadze T, Chai J, Maley K, et al. A growth stimulus is needed for IGF-1 to induce skeletal muscle hypertrophy in vivo. J Cell Sci 2010;123:960.

121. Matheny RW Jr, Nindl BC, Adamo ML. Minireview: Mechano-growth factor: a putative product of IGF-I gene expression involved in tissue repair and regeneration. Endocrinology 2010;151:865.

122. Tsatsoulis A, Fountoulakis S. The protective role of exercise on stress system dysregulation and comorbidities. Ann N Y Acad Sci 2006;1083:196.

123. Braith RW, Magyari PM, Pierce GL, et al. Effect of resistance exercise on skeletal muscle myopathy in heart transplant recipients. Am J Cardiol 2005;95:1192.

124. Morley JE, Argiles JM, Evans WJ, et al. Nutritional recommendations for the management of sarcopenia. J Am Med Dir Assoc 2010;11:391.

125. Ahola-Erkkila S, Carroll CJ, Peltola-Mjosund K, et al. Ketogenic diet slows down mitochondrial myopathy progression in mice. Hum Mol Genet 2010;19:1974.

126. Muscaritoli M, Costelli P, Aversa Z, et al. New strategies to overcome cancer cachexia: from molecular mechanisms to the 'Parallel Pathway'. Asia Pac J Clin Nutr 2008;17(Suppl 1):387.

127. Hornberger TA, Sukhija KB, Chien S. Regulation of mTOR by mechanically induced signaling events in skeletal muscle. Cell Cycle 2006;5:1391.

128. Sakuma K, Yamaguchi A. Molecular mechanisms in aging and current strategies to counteract sarcopenia. Curr Aging Sci 2010;3:90.

129. Wang H, Kubica N, Ellisen LW, et al. Dexamethasone represses signaling through the mammalian target of rapamycin in muscle cells by enhancing expression of REDD1. J Biol Chem 2006;281:39128.

130. Corradetti MN, Inoki K, Guan KL. The stress-inducted proteins RTP801 and RTP801L are negative regulators of the mammalian target of rapamycin pathway. J Biol Chem 2005;280:9769.

131. DeYoung MP, Horak P, Sofer A, et al. Hypoxia regulates TSC1/2-mTOR signaling and tumor suppression through REDD1-mediated 14-3-3 shuttling. Genes Dev 2008;22:239.

132. McGhee NK, Jefferson LS, Kimball SR. Elevated corticosterone associated with food deprivation upregulates expression in rat skeletal muscle of the mTORC1 repressor, REDD1. J Nutr 2009;139:828.

133. Lang CH, Frost RA, Vary TC. Acute alcohol intoxication increases REDD1 in skeletal muscle. Alcohol Clin Exp Res 2008;32:796.

134. Murakami T, Hasegawa K, Yoshinaga M. Rapid induction of REDD1 expression by endurance exercise in rat skeletal muscle. Biochem Biophys Res Commun 2011;405:615.

135. Kumari R, Willing LB, Jefferson LS, et al. REDD1 (regulated in development and DNA damage response 1) expression in skeletal muscle as a surrogate biomarker of the efficiency of glucocorticoid receptor blockade. Biochem Biophys Res Commun 2011;412:644.

136. Frost RA, Huber D, Pruznak A, et al. Regulation of REDD1 by insulin-like growth factor-I in skeletal muscle and myotubes. J Cell Biochem 2009;108:1192.

137. Regazzetti C, Bost F, Le Marchand-Brustel Y, et al. Insulin induces REDD1 expression through hypoxia-inducible factor 1 activation in adipocytes. J Biol Chem 2010;285:5157.

138. Horak P, Crawford AR, Vadysirisack DD, et al. Negative feedback control of HIF-1 through REDD1-regulated ROS suppresses tumorigenesis. Proc Natl Acad Sci U S A 2010;107:4675.

139. Ellisen LW, Ramsayer KD, Johannessen CM, et al. REDD1, a developmentally regulated transcriptional target of p63 and p53, links p63 to regulation of reactive oxygen species. Mol Cell 2002;10:995.

140. Orzechowski A, Ostaszewski P, Wilczak J, et al. Rats with a glucocorticoid-induced catabolic state show symptoms of oxidative stress and spleen atrophy: the effects of age and recovery. J Vet Med A Physiol Pathol Clin Med 2002;49:256.

141. Handayaningsih AE, Iguchi G, Fukuoka H, et al. Reactive oxygen species play an essential role in IGF-I signaling and IGF-I-induced myocyte hypertrophy in C2C12 myocytes. Endocrinology 2011;152(3):912–21.

142. Frost RA, Pereyra E, Lang CH. Ethyl pyruvate preserves IGF-I sensitivity toward mTOR substrates and protein synthesis in C2C12 myotubes. Endocrinology 2011;152:151.

143. Shimizu N, Yoshikawa N, Ito N, et al. Crosstalk between glucocorticoid receptor and nutritional sensor mTOR in skeletal muscle. Cell Metab 2011;13:170.

144. Fielitz J, Kim MS, Shelton JM, et al. Myosin accumulation and striated muscle myopathy result from the loss of muscle RING finger 1 and 3. J Clin Invest 2007;117:2486.

145. Clarke BA, Drujan D, Willis MS, et al. The E3 ligase MuRF1 degrades myosin heavy chain protein in dexamethasone-treated skeletal muscle. Cell Metab 2007;6:376.

146. Cohen S, Brault JJ, Gygi SP, et al. During muscle atrophy, thick, but not thin, filament components are degraded by MuRF1-dependent ubiquitylation. J Cell Biol 2009;185:1083.

147. Waddell DS, Baehr LM, van den Brandt J, et al. The glucocorticoid receptor and FOXO1 synergistically activate the skeletal muscle atrophy-associated MuRF1 gene. Am J Physiol Endocrinol Metab 2008;295:E785.

148. Liu Y, Dentin R, Chen D, et al. A fasting inducible switch modulates gluconeogenesis via activator/coactivator exchange. Nature 2008;456:269.

149. Zhao J, Brault JJ, Schild A, et al. Coordinate activation of autophagy and the proteasome pathway by FoxO transcription factor. Autophagy 2008;4:378.

150. Demontis F, Perrimon N. FOXO/4E-BP signaling in *Drosophila* muscles regulates organism-wide proteostasis during aging. Cell 2010;143:813.

151. Teleman AA, Chen YW, Cohen SM. 4E-BP functions as a metabolic brake used under stress conditions but not during normal growth. Genes Dev 2005;19:1844.

152. Chiba T, Kamei Y, Shimizu T, et al. Overexpression of FOXO1 in skeletal muscle does not alter longevity in mice. Mech Ageing Dev 2009;130:420.

153. Zhang D, Contu R, Latronico MV, et al. MTORC1 regulates cardiac function and myocyte survival through 4E-BP1 inhibition in mice. J Clin Invest 2010;120:2805.

154. Goodman CA, Mabrey DM, Frey JW, et al. Novel insights into the regulation of skeletal muscle protein synthesis as revealed by a new nonradioactive in vivo technique. FASEB J 2011;25:1028.

155. Shah OJ, Anthony JC, Kimball SR, et al. Glucocorticoids oppose translational control by leucine in skeletal muscle. Am J Physiol Endocrinol Metab 2000; 279:E1185.

156. Schakman O, Gilson H, de Coninck V, et al. Insulin-like growth factor-I gene transfer by electroporation prevents skeletal muscle atrophy in glucocorticoid-treated rats. Endocrinology 2005;146:1789.

157. Lang CH, Lynch CJ, Vary TC. BCATm deficiency ameliorates endotoxin-induced decrease in muscle protein synthesis and improves survival in septic mice. Am J Physiol Regul Integr Comp Physiol 2010;299:R935.

158. Wu Y, Zhao W, Zhao J, et al. REDD1 is a major target of testosterone action in preventing dexamethasone-induced muscle loss. Endocrinology 2010;151:1050.

159. Qin W, Pan J, Wu Y, et al. Protection against dexamethasone-induced muscle atrophy is related to modulation by testosterone of FOXO1 and PGC-1alpha. Biochem Biophys Res Commun 2010;403:473.

160. Snyder PJ, Peachey H, Hannoush P, et al. Effect of testosterone treatment on body composition and muscle strength in men over 65 years of age. J Clin Endocrinol Metab 1999;84:2647.

161. Verdijk LB, Snijders T, Beelen M, et al. Characteristics of muscle fiber type are predictive of skeletal muscle mass and strength in elderly men. J Am Geriatr Soc 2010;58:2069.

162. Perrini S, Laviola L, Carreira MC, et al. The GH/IGF1 axis and signaling pathways in the muscle and bone: mechanisms underlying age-related skeletal muscle wasting and osteoporosis. J Endocrinol 2010;205:201.

163. West DW, Phillips SM. Anabolic processes in human skeletal muscle: restoring the identities of growth hormone and testosterone. Phys Sportsmed 2010;38:97.

164. Thomas DR. Sarcopenia. Clin Geriatr Med 2010;26:331.

165. Bhasin S, Woodhouse L, Casaburi R, et al. Older men are as responsive as young men to the anabolic effects of graded doses of testosterone on the skeletal muscle. J Clin Endocrinol Metab 2005;90:678.

166. Zitzmann M. Testosterone deficiency, insulin resistance and the metabolic syndrome. Nat Rev Endocrinol 2009;5:673.

167. Jiao Q, Pruznak AM, Huber D, et al. Castration differentially alters basal and leucine-stimulated tissue protein synthesis in skeletal muscle and adipose tissue. Am J Physiol Endocrinol Metab 2009;297(5):E1222–32.

168. Pennings B, Koopman R, Beelen M, et al. Exercising before protein intake allows for greater use of dietary protein-derived amino acids for de novo muscle protein synthesis in both young and elderly men. Am J Clin Nutr 2011;93:322.

169. Johansen JA, Breedlove SM, Jordan CL. Androgen receptor expression in the levator ani muscle of male mice. J Neuroendocrinol 2007;19:823.

170. Sato K, Iemitsu M, Aizawa K, et al. Testosterone and DHEA activate the glucose metabolism-related signaling pathway in skeletal muscle. Am J Physiol Endocrinol Metab 2008;294:E961.

171. Aizawa K, Iemitsu M, Maeda S, et al. Acute exercise activates local bioactive androgen metabolism in skeletal muscle. Steroids 2010;75:219.

172. Borst SE, Lee JH, Conover CF. Inhibition of 5alpha-reductase blocks prostate effects of testosterone without blocking anabolic effects. Am J Physiol Endocrinol Metab 2005;288:E222.

173. MacLean HE, Chiu WS, Notini AJ, et al. Impaired skeletal muscle development and function in male, but not female, genomic androgen receptor knockout mice. FASEB J 2008;22:2676.
174. Chambon C, Duteil D, Vignaud A, et al. Myocytic androgen receptor controls the strength but not the mass of limb muscles. Proc Natl Acad Sci U S A 2010;107: 14327.
175. Klover P, Chen W, Zhu BM, et al. Skeletal muscle growth and fiber composition in mice are regulated through the transcription factors STAT5a/b: linking growth hormone to the androgen receptor. FASEB J 2009;23:3140.
176. Ibebunjo C, Eash JK, Li C, et al. Voluntary running, skeletal muscle gene expression, and signaling inversely regulated by orchidectomy and testosterone replacement. Am J Physiol Endocrinol Metab 2011;300:E327.
177. D'Antona G, Ragni M, Cardile A, et al. Branched-chain amino acid supplementation promotes survival and supports cardiac and skeletal muscle mitochondrial biogenesis in middle-aged mice. Cell Metab 2010;12:362.
178. Honjoh S, Yamamoto T, Uno M, et al. Signalling through RHEB-1 mediates intermittent fasting-induced longevity in C. elegans. Nature 2009;457:726.
179. Szulc P, Duboeuf F, Marchand F, et al. Hormonal and lifestyle determinants of appendicular skeletal muscle mass in men: the MINOS study. Am J Clin Nutr 2004;80:496.
180. Raskin K, de Gendt K, Duittoz A, et al. Conditional inactivation of androgen receptor gene in the nervous system: effects on male behavioral and neuroendocrine responses. J Neurosci 2009;29:4461.
181. Miyamoto J, Matsumoto T, Shiina H, et al. The pituitary function of androgen receptor constitutes a glucocorticoid production circuit. Mol Cell Biol 2007;27: 4807.
182. Jones A, Hwang DJ, Narayanan R, et al. Effects of a novel selective androgen receptor modulator on dexamethasone-induced and hypogonadism-induced muscle atrophy. Endocrinology 2010;151:3706.
183. Belavy DL, Miokovic T, Armbrecht G, et al. Differential atrophy of the lower-limb musculature during prolonged bed-rest. Eur J Appl Physiol 2009;107:489.
184. Murton AJ, Greenhaff PL. Muscle atrophy in immobilization and senescence in humans. Curr Opin Neurol 2009;22:500.
185. Stein TP, Donaldson MR, Leskiw MJ, et al. Branched-chain amino acid supplementation during bed rest: effect on recovery. J Appl Physiol 2003;94:1345.
186. Brooks N, Cloutier GJ, Cadena SM, et al. Resistance training and timed essential amino acids protect against the loss of muscle mass and strength during 28 days of bed rest and energy deficit. J Appl Physiol 2008;105:241.
187. Brooks NE, Cadena SM, Vannier E, et al. Effects of resistance exercise combined with essential amino acid supplementation and energy deficit on markers of skeletal muscle atrophy and regeneration during bed rest and active recovery. Muscle Nerve 2010;42:927.
188. Alzghoul MB, Gerrard D, Watkins BA, et al. Ectopic expression of IGF-I and Shh by skeletal muscle inhibits disuse-mediated skeletal muscle atrophy and bone osteopenia in vivo. FASEB J 2004;18:221.
189. Cai D, Frantz JD, Tawa NE Jr, et al. IKKbeta/NF-kappaB activation causes severe muscle wasting in mice. Cell 2004;119:285.
190. Sandri M, Sandri C, Gilbert A, et al. Foxo transcription factors induce the atrophy-related ubiquitin ligase atrogin-1 and cause skeletal muscle atrophy. Cell 2004;117:399.

191. Buford TW, Cooke MB, Manini TM, et al. Effects of age and sedentary lifestyle on skeletal muscle NF-kappaB signaling in men. J Gerontol A Biol Sci Med Sci 2010;65:532.
192. Reed SA, Senf SM, Cornwell EW, et al. Inhibition of IkappaB kinase alpha (IKKα) or IKKbeta (IKKβ) plus forkhead box O (Foxo) abolishes skeletal muscle atrophy. Biochem Biophys Res Commun 2011;405:491.
193. Dodd SL, Gagnon BJ, Senf SM, et al. Ros-mediated activation of NF-kappaB and Foxo during muscle disuse. Muscle Nerve 2010;41:110.
194. Reid MB. Free radicals and muscle fatigue: of ROS, canaries, and the IOC. Free Radic Biol Med 2008;44:169.
195. Arbogast S, Smith J, Matuszczak Y, et al. Bowman-Birk inhibitor concentrate prevents atrophy, weakness, and oxidative stress in soleus muscle of hindlimb-unloaded mice. J Appl Physiol 2007;102:956.
196. Selsby JT, Rother S, Tsuda S, et al. Intermittent hyperthermia enhances skeletal muscle regrowth and attenuates oxidative damage following reloading. J Appl Physiol 2007;102:1702.
197. Selsby JT, Dodd SL. Heat treatment reduces oxidative stress and protects muscle mass during immobilization. Am J Physiol Regul Integr Comp Physiol 2005;289:R134.
198. Kakigi R, Naito H, Ogura Y, et al. Heat stress enhances mTOR signaling after resistance exercise in human skeletal muscle. J Physiol Sci 2011;61:131.
199. Chen YW, Gregory CM, Scarborough MT, et al. Transcriptional pathways associated with skeletal muscle disuse atrophy in humans. Physiol Genomics 2007; 31:510.
200. Stevens-Lapsley JE, Ye F, Liu M, et al. Impact of viral-mediated IGF-I gene transfer on skeletal muscle following cast immobilization. Am J Physiol Endocrinol Metab 2010;299:E730.
201. Criswell DS, Booth FW, DeMayo F, et al. Overexpression of IGF-I in skeletal muscle of transgenic mice does not prevent unloading-induced atrophy. Am J Physiol 1998;275:E373.
202. Merezhinskaya N, Fishbein WN, Davis JI, et al. Mutations in MCT1 cDNA in patients with symptomatic deficiency in lactate transport. Muscle Nerve 2000;23:90.
203. Evans K, Nasim Z, Brown J, et al. Acidosis-sensing glutamine pump SNAT2 determines amino acid levels and mammalian target of rapamycin signalling to protein synthesis in L6 muscle cells. J Am Soc Nephrol 2007;18:1426.
204. Chambard JC, Pouyssegur J. Intracellular pH controls growth factor-induced ribosomal protein S6 phosphorylation and protein synthesis in the G0–G1 transition of fibroblasts. Exp Cell Res 1986;164:282.
205. Woods DJ, Soden J, Tomlinson S, et al. Transmembrane Na+/H+ exchange in the rat thyroid cell strain FRTL-5: a possible role in insulin-like growth factor-I-mediated proliferation. J Mol Endocrinol 1990;4:177.
206. Fernandez-Sola J, Preedy VR, Lang CH, et al. Molecular and cellular events in alcohol-induced muscle disease. Alcohol Clin Exp Res 2007;31:1953.
207. Lang CH, Kimball SR, Frost RA, et al. Alcohol myopathy: impairment of protein synthesis and translation initiation. Int J Biochem Cell Biol 2001;33:457.
208. Kumar V, Frost RA, Lang CH. Alcohol impairs insulin and IGF-I stimulation of S6K1 but not 4E-BP1 in skeletal muscle. Am J Physiol Endocrinol Metab 2002;283:E917.
209. Lang CH, Fan J, Lipton BP, et al. Modulation of the insulin-like growth factor system by chronic alcohol feeding. Alcohol Clin Exp Res 1998;22:823.

210. Lang CH, Frost RA, Svanberg E, et al. IGF-I/IGFBP-3 ameliorates alterations in protein synthesis, eIF4E availability, and myostatin in alcohol-fed rats. Am J Physiol Endocrinol Metab 2004;286:E916.
211. Lang CH, Frost RA, Deshpande N, et al. Alcohol impairs leucine-mediated phosphorylation of 4EBP1, S6K1, eIF4G, and mTOR in skeletal muscle. Am J Physiol Endocrinol Metab 2003;285:E1205.
212. Lang CH, Frost RA, Vary TC. Skeletal muscle protein synthesis and degradation exhibit sexual dimorphism after chronic alcohol consumption but not acute intoxication. Am J Physiol Endocrinol Metab 2007;292:E1497.
213. Vargas R, Lang CH. Alcohol accelerates loss of muscle and impairs recovery of muscle mass resulting from disuse atrophy. Alcohol Clin Exp Res 2008;32:128.
214. Lang CH, Lynch CJ, Vary TC. Alcohol-induced IGF-I resistance is ameliorated in mice deficient for mitochondrial branched-chain aminotransferase. J Nutr 2010; 140:932.
215. Sun X, Zemel MB. Leucine modulation of mitochondrial mass and oxygen consumption in skeletal muscle cells and adipocytes. Nutr Metab (Lond) 2009;6:26.
216. Du M, Shen QW, Zhu MJ, et al. Leucine stimulates mammalian target of rapamycin signaling in C2C12 myoblasts in part through inhibition of adenosine monophosphate-activated protein kinase. J Anim Sci 2007;85:919.
217. Hong-Brown LQ, Brown CR, Navaratnarajah M, et al. Alcohol-induced modulation of rictor and mTORC2 activity in C2C12 myoblasts. Alcohol Clin Exp Res 1445;35.
218. Hong-Brown LQ, Brown CR, Kazi AA, et al. Rag GTPases and AMPK/TSC2/Rheb mediate the differential regulation of mTORC1 signaling in response to alcohol and leucine. Am J Physiol Cell Physiol 2012. [Epub ahead of print].

The Insulin-Like Growth Factor System in Bone
Basic and Clinical Implications

Masanobu Kawai, MD, PhD[a], Clifford J. Rosen, MD[b],*

KEYWORDS

- Insulin-like growth factors • Skeletal growth • Bone homeostasis
- Insulin-like growth factor binding protein

KEY POINTS

- The insulin-like growth factor (IGF) regulatory system is critical for skeletal growth and maintenance.
- An integrated interplay of circulating and local IGF-I determines the intricate balance of skeletal homeostasis.
- IGF binding protein regulates skeletal homeostasis in part through the modulation of IGF accessibility to the receptor and its turnover.
- IGF binding protein may confer a novel regulation through its unique domains independent of IGF binding.

INTRODUCTION

The insulin-like growth factor (IGF) regulatory system consists of IGFs (IGF-I and IGF-II), IGF receptor, and regulatory proteins including IGF-binding proteins (IGFBP-1 to IGFBP-6) and the acid-labile subunit (ALS).[1] The biological function of this system is diverse, whereby IGFs function as potent mitogens and, in some circumstances, differentiation factors. IGFs are bound in binary (to IGFBPs) or ternary complexes (IGF-ALS-IGFBP-3 or -IGFBP-5), with little free IGF-I or IGF-II in either the circulation or the extracellular fluid. IGF bioavailability is regulated by the interaction of these molecules at the receptor level; hence, changes in any component of the system can have profound effects on the biological activity of the ligands. The IGFBPs have a particularly important role in regulating IGF-I access to its receptor because their binding affinity exceeds that of the IGF receptors. What makes the IGF system unique

[a] Department of Bone and Mineral Research, Osaka Medical Center and Research Institute for Maternal and Child Health, Izumi, Osaka, Japan 594-1101; [b] Center for Translational Research, Maine Medical Center Research Institute, Scarborough, ME 04074, USA
* Corresponding author.
E-mail address: ROSENC@mmc.org

Endocrinol Metab Clin N Am 41 (2012) 323–333
doi:10.1016/j.ecl.2012.04.013
0889-8529/12/$ – see front matter

is that the IGFBPs are regulated in a cell-specific manner at the pericellular microenvironment, such that small changes in their concentrations could have a profound effect on mitogenic activity of IGF-I.[2–4] In the skeleton, IGF-I and IGF-II are extremely abundant, and are stored in their inactive form bound to several IGFBPs within the matrix. Release of the IGFs in their active form during bone modeling and remodeling is a critical aspect of skeletal homeostasis. In addition to the ubiquitous expression of the IGFs, these growth factors circulate in high concentrations and, because of the rich blood supply of the cortical and trabecular skeleton, allow exposure of bone cells to these peptides.

The main source of circulating IGF-I in mammals is the liver, and its role as an endocrine mediator of growth hormone has been established for half a century. Although nearly 80% of the circulating IGF-I comes from hepatic sources, IGF-I synthesized from the local tissues including bone may contribute to the total circulating pool as well. The expression diversity of IGF-I and the IGFBPs in a tissue-specific manner coupled with a large circulating pool adds several levels of complexity to our understanding of the role of the IGF-I/IGFBP system. However, there is little doubt that IGF-I signaling is requisite for proper skeletal accrual. This review discusses the roles of the IGF system in the regulation of skeletal homeostasis.

IGF-I REGULATORY SYSTEM AND BONE

The IGF regulatory system includes IGF-I, IGF-I receptor (IGF1R), regulatory proteins including IGFBP-1 to -6, and the ALS.[5] All of these components except ALS are expressed in relatively high concentrations within bone. IGF-I is a single-chain polypeptide and consists of 70 amino acid residues. The distribution of IGF-I in serum and skeletal environment is an important component of IGF-I action, and is determined by the relative saturation by IGFBPs. In a manner analogous to other tissues, this family of proteins can act as agonists for IGF-I or can block the actions of IGF-I by preventing access to the IGF1R in bone. The redundancy exerted by the IGFBPs in the IGF regulatory system provides an additional level of regulation, and can be used to deliver IGF-I in an endocrine fashion.

IGF-I exerts its action by binding to the IGF-I receptor, which induces receptor autophosphorylation in the intracellular kinase domain. On receptor activation several protein substrates, including insulin receptor substrate 1 (IRS-1) and Src homolog and collagen protein (SHC), are activated, and transduce multiple signaling pathways, including the PI3K/PDK-1/Akt pathway and Ras/Raf-1/MAPK 9mitogen-activated protein kinase) pathway. IRS-1 interacts with phosphatidylinositol-3-kinase (PI3K), and activation of PI3K catalyzes a phosphorylation of phosphatidylinositol-4,5-diphosphate (PIP2) to phosphatidylinositol-3,4,5-trisphosaphate (PIP3). The Increased PIP3 level activates phosphoinositide-dependent kinase 1 (PDK-1) and Akt. The Ras/Raf-1/MAPK pathway is activated through the SHC-Grb2-SOC complex, which is critical for cell proliferation. Activation of the PI3K/PDK-1/Akt pathway has been shown to be important in skeletal acquisition in vitro and in vivo.[6,7] For example, Akt1 and Akt2 double knock-out mice show severely delayed skeletal development.[7] The precise mechanisms underlying the effect of the PI3K/Akt pathway on skeleton need to be clarified; however, it is known that cell survival[8] and cell migration induced by this pathway are important. Migration of mesenchymal stem cells and/or osteoblasts is an important component in skeletal development, bone remodeling, and fracture healing. For example, during bone remodeling initial resorption by osteoclasts leads to elaboration of matrix proteins and calcium. IGF components are also released during acidification of the resorption surface, and it is thought that IGF-I may be critical for attracting osteoblast precursors to the endosteal surfaces. Whether the IGFs may also enhance osteoblast differentiation, thereby promoting bone formation, remains to be demonstrated. Previous studies have shown that dominant-negative Akt suppressed Runx2-induced osteoblastic cell migration and PI3K inhibitor suppressed IGF-I-induced cell migration of MC3T3-E1 cells.[9,10] As such, beyond its role as a mitogen, IGF-I may function as a chemotactic factor, particularly in the skeleton.

ANIMAL STUDIES

Recent advances in molecular biology and development of genetically modified mice have expanded our understanding of the role of IGF-I in the skeleton. The first evidence of the involvement of IGF-I in bone biology using a genetically engineered mouse model comes from the study in which mice lacking the *Igfl* gene were generated.[11] More than 80% of these mice died perinatally, but survivors reached adulthood and showed postnatal growth retardation. Subsequently, IGF-I heterozygous mice on CD-1 background were analyzed and demonstrated a reduction in cortical bone mineral density associated with decreased serum IGF-I levels, suggesting that IGF-I is a determinant of bone mass in postnatal life.[12] Bikle and colleagues[13] also reported a unique skeletal phenotype of IGF-I null mice. These mice exhibited a 24% reduction in the size of cortical bone and shortened femur length compared with controls, whereas trabecular bone density and connectivity were increased.[14] This mixed phenotype of these mice may be at least in part explained by their impaired osteoclastogenesis, because cocultures of osteoblasts from IGF-I null mice and osteoclast precursors from wild-type mice, as well as osteoblasts from wild-type mice and osteoclast precursors from IGF-I null mice showed reduced numbers of osteoclasts. In addition, expression of receptor activator of nuclear factor κB ligand (RANKL) was impaired in IGF-I null osteoblasts isolated from the bone marrow, and expression of RANKL, RANK, and macrophage colony-stimulating factor in long bones were all reduced in IGF-I null mice.

IGF-I transgenic mice under the control of metallothionein promoter resulted in increased body weight and disproportionate overgrowth of some organs with elevated serum IGF-I levels, but skeletal size and morphology was normal.[15] IGF1R-deficient mice showed organ hypoplasia, delayed skeletal calcification, severe growth retardation, and invariably died postnatally as a result of respiratory dysfunction. The fact that cross-breeding of IGF-I null mice and IGF1R null mice exhibit a phenotype, which is indistinguishable from the one noted in IGF1R null mice, indicates that IGF-I mediates its action exclusively through the IGF1R.[11]

To overcome the long-standing struggle to identify the role of locally produced IGF-I, IGF-I transgenic mice under the osteocalcin promoter were generated.[16] Serum IGF-I levels and body growth were not altered in these mice, but they showed increased bone mineral density and trabecular bone volume, though cortical bone volume was not altered. The change was accompanied by increased bone formation. Of note is that osteoblast number was not altered. Thus, the anabolic effect of locally produced IGF-I by osteoblasts is exerted by enhancing osteoblast function, not by recruiting osteoblasts from osteogenic precursor cells. In line with these observations, mice lacking IGF1R in an osteoblast-specific manner were of normal body size and weight, but demonstrated reduced trabecular bone volume, connectivity, and trabecular number, as well as increased trabecular spacing.[17]

In addition to the locally produced IGF-I, critical roles of circulating IGF-I in skeletal homeostasis have been clarified using genetically engineered mouse models. Yaker and colleagues[18,19] generated a liver-specific IGF-I deficient mouse (LID mouse) under the control of albumin promoter and clarified the role of IGF-I produced by liver on the skeleton. LID mice showed relatively normal development despite the reduction in serum IGF-I levels by 75%; surprisingly, femur length and body weight decreased by only 6%, but cortical bone volume was reduced by 26% and trabecular bone volume was preserved. Periosteal circumference and cross-sectional area were also markedly reduced.[20] To gain more insights regarding the role of circulating IGF-I in bone mass, the ALS was deleted in another mouse model (ALSKO mouse). As expected, serum IGF-I levels in ALSKO mice were reduced by 65% and cortical bone volume was reduced. Double knock-out liver IGF-I and ALS mice demonstrated a marked decrease in serum IGF-I of 85% to 90%, despite normal expression of skeletal IGF-I. The skeletal phenotype of these mice included reduced cortical bone volume and significant growth retardation with disordered growth plates. Taken together, these data suggest that circulating IGF-I is important for longitudinal growth, and the modeling of bone, particularly periosteal expansion. To better understand the role of circulating IGF-I, 2 independent groups generated transgenic mice expressing IGF-I in liver on an IGF-I null background. Stratikopoulos and colleagues[21] produced a mouse model in which IGF-I cDNA is regulated under a native promoter/enhancer of IGF-I gene only in liver on an *Igf1* null background, and revealed that endocrine IGF-I contributed approximately 30% of the adult mouse body size. Similarly, Elis and colleagues[22] generated *Igf1* transgenic mice under transthyretin promoter on an *Igf1* null background (KO-HIT [hepatic IGF-I transgenic mice]). KO-HIT mice showed an approximately 3-fold increase in serum IGF-I levels. The body weight of KO-HIT mice was comparable with that of controls up to 16 weeks, but these mice showed shorter femorae at 4 weeks of age and exhibited catch-up growth by 8 weeks of age. These data suggested that locally expressed IGF-I is important in the regulation of body length during first the 4 weeks of life, but circulating IGF-I can compensate for the loss of local IGF-I after 4 weeks of age. In respect of the skeletal phenotype, KO-HIT mice had shorter femorae and smaller bone size at 4 weeks of age, but then showed a marked increase in these parameters. Thus, circulating IGF-I can compensate for the loss of locally produced IGF-I in a developmentally stage-specific manner.

Analyses of the role of signaling molecules that lie downstream of IGF1R activation have provided another level of evidence to support the importance of IGF-I in skeletal homeostasis. For example, insulin receptor substrates (IRSs) are the best defined IGF1R substrates and consist of 4 members. Several studies have demonstrated that IRS-1 is involved in bone acquisition.[23] IRS-1 null mice show severe osteopenia with low bone turnover. IRS-1–deficient osteoblasts from these mice revealed that IRS-1 deficiency reduces cell proliferation and differentiation in response to IGF-I and cannot support osteoclastogenesis, leading to low-turnover osteopenia. PTEN (phosphatase and tensin homolog deleted on chromosome 10) is a lipid phosphatase and opposes IGF-I signaling by dephosphorylating PIP3 to PIP2. Mice deficient in PTEN only in osteoblasts were created by use of the human osteocalcin promoter. These mice showed progressively increasing bone mineral density throughout life. The PI3K pathway was activated constitutively in these mice, and the osteoblasts were protected from apoptosis.[24] These findings indicate the importance of PTEN and the PI3K system in bone acquisition.

ROLE OF THE IGFBPs IN THE SKELETON

IGF-I bioactivity is modulated by the IGFBPs (IGFBP-1 to -6), and their role in skeletal acquisition has been analyzed using genetically altered mice. The function of IGFBPs with respect to IGF-I signaling depends on the relative molar ratio between IGFBPs and IGF-I, but IGFBPs are primarily considered to work as inhibitors for IGF-I, as is true for IGFBP-2, which has been shown to block IGF-I binding to its receptor. Hence, IGFBP-2 has been regarded as a negative regulator for IGF-I–induced bone acquisition. For example, in vitro analysis revealed that IGFBP-2 inhibited IGF-I–stimulated bone cell proliferation, collagen synthesis, and bone formation. In vivo, overexpression of *Igfbp2* has been demonstrated to reduce bone mass and inhibit growth hormone (GH)-stimulated linear growth in GH transgenic mice, possibly by antagonizing the GH/IGF-I axis.[25] Of note, the effect of IGFBP-2 on bone accrual is also evidenced by human studies in which serum IGFBP-2 levels were inversely associated with bone mass.[26–28] Amin and colleagues[26] reported that IGFBP-2 levels increased with age and that serum IGFBP-2 levels showed negative association with bone mineral density in both men and women. van den Beld and colleagues[27] showed that higher serum IGFBP-2 levels were associated with a higher degree of disability and a lower physical performance, muscle strength, and bone mineral density of proximal femur. However, growing evidence demonstrates that the effect of IGFBP-2 on bone mass is context specific, such that IGFBP-2 has an anabolic effect on skeleton. For example, Khosla and colleagues[29,30] reported that IGFBP-2 stimulated bone formation in association with IGF-II in patients with hepatitis C–associated osteosclerosis. *Igfbp2*$^{-/-}$ mice have been shown to exhibit a gender-specific and compartment-specific skeletal phenotype; *Igfbp2*$^{-/-}$ females had increased cortical thickness with a greater periosteal circumference, whereas *Igfbp2*$^{-/-}$ males had reduced cortical bone size. Trabecular bone volume was reduced by 20% in *Igfbp2*$^{-/-}$ males whereas trabecular bone was not affected in female *Igfbp2*$^{-/-}$ mice. PTEN expression was enhanced in osteoblasts isolated from bone marrow of *Igfbp2*$^{-/-}$ mice compared with controls. Because PTEN regulates IGF-I signaling in a negative direction, IGF-I signaling may be impaired in *Igfbp2*$^{-/-}$ mice. Recently, the authors have identified a unique heparin-binding domain (HBD) in IGFBP-2 which, at least in part, mediates the anabolic effect of IGFBP-2. Administration of the HBD of IGFBP-2 in *Igfbp2*$^{-/-}$ mice partially rescued the osteopenic phenotype of these mice. The molecular mechanisms of the HBD of IGFBP-2 needs to be determined, but the HBD is implicated in downregulating PTEN expression and activates IGF-I signaling pathway in osteoblasts, indicating that the effect of the HBD on bone acquisition is in part mediated by the reduction of PTEN expression in osteoblastic cells.

IGFBP-3 is the predominant IGFBP, and forms a tertiary complex with IGF-I and ALS. Similar to other IGFBPs, IGFBP-3 can have an antagonistic effect on IGF-I signaling. Skeletal phenotypes of *Igfbp3* transgenic mice demonstrated decreased cortical and trabecular bone mineral density.[31] However, there is some evidence to suggest that IGFBP-3 can have a positive effect on bone formation in some situations. For example, IGFBP-3 has been shown to bind to the type I collagen molecule, thereby playing a role in storing IGFs within the skeletal matrix.

IGFBP-4 is one of the most abundant IGFBPs synthesized by bone cells, and has been shown to be inhibitory for IGF-I signaling in vitro. Targeted overexpression of *Igfbp4* in bone using the human osteocalcin promoter results in postnatal growth retardation, altered bone turnover, and low bone mass.[32] *Igfbp4*$^{-/-}$ mice also have modest growth retardation at birth and reduced bone mineral density, suggesting that it may play an important role as a storage protein in bone.[33] IGFBP-5 can bind extracellular matrices through a conserved HBD. Its role in bone formation has been considered both within the realm of its role as a storage protein and as a potential agonist for IGF-I, although a receptor for IGFBP-5 has not been identified. Transgenic

Igfbp5 mice under the control of osteocalcin promoter showed decreased bone volume with low bone formation.[34] Taken together, these lines of evidence demonstrate that physiologic levels of IGFBPs have an anabolic effect on skeleton, at least in part through targeting IGF-I to the skeletal microenvironment.

ROLE OF IGF-I IN THE SKELETON
Human Studies

It is well established that serum IGF-I levels are positively associated with bone mass.[5] For example, serum IGF-I levels peak at puberty when the bone acquisition is maximized, and decline with aging accompanied by the aging-related bone loss. This positive correlation is also relevant in neonates.[35] Clinical studies of patients with disturbances in the GH–IGF-I axis have provided significant evidence of the importance of IGF-I in maintaining the bone mass. Children and adults with GH deficiency, whose serum levels of IGF-I are low, have low areal bone mineral density (aBMD), and bone mass recovers after GH replacement therapy associated with significant increments in serum IGF-I.[36–38] In patients with a GH-receptor deficiency (primary IGF-I deficiency, Laron syndrome), bone mass has long been suggested to be low, but this tenet might not be true because there is increasing evidence that when volumetric bone mineral density is measured there are no changes in bone mass, probably due to the small bone area and short stature of these patients.[39,40] A similar trend is also observed in patients with severe IGF-I deficiency caused by homozygous mutation in the *Igf1* gene[41–44] and patients with mutation in the *Igf1 receptor* gene.[45–47] These findings are informative, but conclusions may be tenuous, owing to several covariates and small subject numbers.

Cohort studies in adult populations have also provided clinical evidence of the positive relationship between IGF-I and bone mass, but this might be context specific because there is evidence that serum IGF-I levels are not associated with bone mass in men.[48] Langlois and colleagues[48] investigated the relationship between serum IGF-I and bone mineral density from the Framingham Heart Study, and reported that IGF-I levels were positively correlated with aBMD at all sites of the hip, radius, and lumbar spine in women, whereas IGF-I was not significantly associated with bone mineral density in men. Bauer and colleagues[49] examined the relationship of IGF-I and IGFBP-3 to hip fractures in 9704 women from the Study of Osteoporotic Fractures. In that study, women in the lowest quartile for serum IGF-I had a 60% greater risk of hip or spine fracture, whereas IGFBP-3 did not show any correlation. Garnero and colleagues[50] also demonstrated that serum IGF-I levels in older individuals were related to hip fracture risk. These studies suggest there is a positive correlation between serum IGF-I concentrations and bone mineral density. However, it is unclear how IGF-I is involved in the pathogenesis of osteoporosis, because serum IGF-I levels are strongly influenced by catabolic states, undernutrition, surgery, and advanced age, all of which are risk factors for fractures.

Linkage analysis in humans has also implicated the possible role of *Igf1* gene as contributing to the bone mass.[51,52] For example, CA-repeat promoter polymorphisms in the *Igf1* gene have been shown to be associated with bone mass.[53–55] However, the importance of CA-repeat polymorphisms needs to be clarified because some studies could not find any association between bone mineral density and this polymorphism in premenopausal Caucasian and African American women[56] and in premenopausal Chinese women.[57] These data suggest that IGF-I polymorphisms may be associated with bone mass, but there is significant genetic heterogeneity.

Clinical Studies with IGFs and IGFBPs

Recombinant human IGF-I (rhIGF-I) has been used with success to treat GH resistance and IGF-I deficiency syndromes in children, although clinical use is not widespread, in part because of metabolic adverse effects including hypoglycemia and hypophosphatemia.[58] On the other hand, administration of rhIGF-I to enhance bone formation and improve bone mass has been met with major limitations. The first long-term study was initially done nearly 20 years ago.[59] However, clinical trial studies of rhIGF-I in osteoporotic patients have been limited. In a trial of 16 healthy elderly women (71.9 ± 1.3 years of age), a high dose of rhIGF-I (60 μg/kg/d) or a low dose of rhIGF-I (15 μg/kg/d) was administered for 28 days, and bone resorption and formation markers were analyzed.[60] The high-dose rhIGF-I increased both bone resorption and bone formation markers, but low-dose rhIGF-I did not affect bone resorption markers. Subsequent work proved that IGF-I was a potent stimulus for osteoclast differentiation,[61] suggesting that IGF-I was a "coupler" of bone remodeling; that is, a stimulus for both resorption and formation. In addition, there were concerns from that first study about clinically significant hypoglycemia. Boonen and colleagues[62] reported that the administration of a complex, IGF-I coupled to IGFBP-3, resulted in reduced bone loss from the femur in elderly patients with hip fractures, as well as some improvement in functional outcomes. However, no further studies were subsequently conducted using this complex in skeletal disorders (**Fig. 1**).

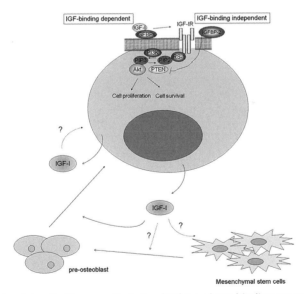

Fig. 1. The role of insulin-like growth factor (IGF)-I and IGF-binding proteins (IGFBPs) in osteoblast differentiation. IGFBPs regulate the accessibility of IGF-I to its receptor through a manner dependent on IGF-I binding. In addition, IGFBPs can exert the unique function in a manner independent of IGF-I binding. For example, IGFBP-2 suppresses PTEN expression in osteoblastic cells through its unique heparin-binding domain, resulting in enhanced IGF-I/Akt signaling. IGF-I produced from osteoblasts plays a critical role in osteoblast maturation and migration, but its role in the proliferation and/or differentiation of mesenchymal stem cells remains to be elucidated. IR, insulin receptor; IRS-1, insulin receptor substrate 1; PI3K, phosphatidylinositol-3-kinase; PIP2, phosphatidylinositol-4,5-diphosphate; PIP3, phosphatidylinositol-3,4,5-trisphosphate; PTEN, phosphatase and tensin homolog.

SUMMARY

There is no doubt that the IGF regulatory system (both locally and systemically) is critical for skeletal growth and maintenance. This fact is reinforced by studies showing that rhIGF-I has been used with success in a limited number of growth disorders. With respect to adults, serum levels of IGF-I have been strongly associated with osteoporosis, as have several IGFBPs. However, trials using recombinant IGF peptides or complexes to treat age-related bone disease have been limited by lack of strong anabolic activity, and significant off-target actions such as hypoglycemia and the potential for malignant transformation. Notwithstanding, ongoing animal studies using genetic models have provided fresh insight into the role of these growth factors in skeletal homeostasis.

REFERENCES

1. Rosen CJ, Donahue LR, Hunter SJ. Insulin-like growth factors and bone: the osteoporosis connection. Proc Soc Exp Biol Med 1994;206:83–102.
2. Hwa V, Oh Y, Rosenfeld RG. The insulin-like growth factor-binding protein (IGFBP) superfamily. Endocr Rev 1999;20:761–87.
3. Jones JI, Clemmons DR. Insulin-like growth factors and their binding proteins: biological actions. Endocr Rev 1995;16:3–34.
4. Firth SM, Baxter RC. Cellular actions of the insulin-like growth factor binding proteins. Endocr Rev 2002;23:824–54.
5. Niu T, Rosen CJ. The insulin-like growth factor-I gene and osteoporosis: a critical appraisal. Gene 2005;361:38–56.
6. Ghosh-Choudhury N, Abboud SL, Nishimura R, et al. Requirement of BMP-2-induced phosphatidylinositol 3-kinase and Akt serine/threonine kinase in osteoblast differentiation and Smad-dependent BMP-2 gene transcription. J Biol Chem 2002;277:33361–8.
7. Peng XD, Xu PZ, Chen ML, et al. Dwarfism, impaired skin development, skeletal muscle atrophy, delayed bone development, and impeded adipogenesis in mice lacking Akt1 and Akt2. Genes Dev 2003;17:1352–65.
8. Grey A, Chen Q, Xu X, et al. Parallel phosphatidylinositol-3 kinase and p42/44 mitogen-activated protein kinase signaling pathways subserve the mitogenic and antiapoptotic actions of insulin-like growth factor I in osteoblastic cells. Endocrinology 2003;144:4886–93.
9. Nakasaki M, Yoshioka K, Miyamoto Y, et al. IGF-I secreted by osteoblasts acts as a potent chemotactic factor for osteoblasts. Bone 2008;43: 869–79.
10. Fujita T, Azuma Y, Fukuyama R, et al. Runx2 induces osteoblast and chondrocyte differentiation and enhances their migration by coupling with PI3K-Akt signaling. J Cell Biol 2004;166:85–95.
11. Liu JP, Baker J, Perkins AS, et al. Mice carrying null mutations of the genes encoding insulin-like growth factor I (Igf-1) and type 1 IGF receptor (Igf1r). Cell 1993;75:59–72.
12. He J, Rosen CJ, Adams DJ, et al. Postnatal growth and bone mass in mice with IGF-I haploinsufficiency. Bone 2006;38:826–35.
13. Bikle D, Majumdar S, Laib A, et al. The skeletal structure of insulin-like growth factor I-deficient mice. J Bone Miner Res 2001;16:2320–9.
14. Wang Y, Nishida S, Elalieh HZ, et al. Role of IGF-I signaling in regulating osteoclastogenesis. J Bone Miner Res 2006;21:1350–8.

15. Mathews LS, Hammer RE, Behringer RR, et al. Growth enhancement of transgenic mice expressing human insulin-like growth factor I. Endocrinology 1988; 123:2827–33.
16. Zhao G, Monier-Faugere MC, Langub MC, et al. Targeted overexpression of insulin-like growth factor I to osteoblasts of transgenic mice: increased trabecular bone volume without increased osteoblast proliferation. Endocrinology 2000;141: 2674–82.
17. Zhang M, Xuan S, Bouxsein ML, et al. Osteoblast-specific knockout of the insulin-like growth factor (IGF) receptor gene reveals an essential role of IGF signaling in bone matrix mineralization. J Biol Chem 2002;277:44005–12.
18. Yakar S, Liu JL, Stannard B, et al. Normal growth and development in the absence of hepatic insulin-like growth factor I. Proc Natl Acad Sci U S A 1999; 96:7324–9.
19. Yakar S, Rosen CJ, Beamer WG, et al. Circulating levels of IGF-1 directly regulate bone growth and density. J Clin Invest 2002;110:771–81.
20. Bouxsein ML, Rosen CJ, Turner CH, et al. Generation of a new congenic mouse strain to test the relationships among serum insulin-like growth factor I, bone mineral density, and skeletal morphology in vivo. J Bone Miner Res 2002;17:570–9.
21. Stratikopoulos E, Szabolcs M, Dragatsis I, et al. The hormonal action of IGF1 in postnatal mouse growth. Proc Natl Acad Sci U S A 2008;105:19378–83.
22. Elis S, Courtland HW, Wu Y, et al. Elevated serum levels of IGF-1 are sufficient to establish normal body size and skeletal properties, even in the absence of tissue IGF-1. J Bone Miner Res 2010;25(6):1257–66.
23. Ogata N, Chikazu D, Kubota N, et al. Insulin receptor substrate-1 in osteoblast is indispensable for maintaining bone turnover. J Clin Invest 2000;105:935–43.
24. Liu X, Bruxvoort KJ, Zylstra CR, et al. Lifelong accumulation of bone in mice lacking Pten in osteoblasts. Proc Natl Acad Sci U S A 2007;104:2259–64.
25. Hoeflich A, Nedbal S, Blum WF, et al. Growth inhibition in giant growth hormone transgenic mice by overexpression of insulin-like growth factor-binding protein-2. Endocrinology 2001;142:1889–98.
26. Amin S, Riggs BL, Atkinson EJ, et al. A potentially deleterious role of IGFBP-2 on bone density in aging men and women. J Bone Miner Res 2004;19:1075–83.
27. van den Beld AW, Blum WF, Pols HA, et al. Serum insulin-like growth factor binding protein-2 levels as an indicator of functional ability in elderly men. Eur J Endocrinol 2003;148:627–34.
28. Nakaoka D, Sugimoto T, Kaji H, et al. Determinants of bone mineral density and spinal fracture risk in postmenopausal Japanese women. Osteoporos Int 2001; 12:548–54.
29. Conover CA, Johnstone EW, Turner RT, et al. Subcutaneous administration of insulin-like growth factor (IGF)-II/IGF binding protein-2 complex stimulates bone formation and prevents loss of bone mineral density in a rat model of disuse osteoporosis. Growth Horm IGF Res 2002;12:178–83.
30. Khosla S, Hassoun AA, Baker BK, et al. Insulin-like growth factor system abnormalities in hepatitis C-associated osteosclerosis. Potential insights into increasing bone mass in adults. J Clin Invest 1998;101:2165–73.
31. Silha JV, Mishra S, Rosen CJ, et al. Perturbations in bone formation and resorption in insulin-like growth factor binding protein-3 transgenic mice. J Bone Miner Res 2003;18:1834–41.
32. Zhang M, Faugere MC, Malluche H, et al. Paracrine overexpression of IGFBP-4 in osteoblasts of transgenic mice decreases bone turnover and causes global growth retardation. J Bone Miner Res 2003;18:836–43.

33. Ning Y, Schuller AG, Conover CA, et al. Insulin-like growth factor (IGF) binding protein-4 is both a positive and negative regulator of IGF activity in vivo. Mol Endocrinol 2008;22:1213–25.
34. Devlin RD, Du Z, Buccilli V, et al. Transgenic mice overexpressing insulin-like growth factor binding protein-5 display transiently decreased osteoblastic function and osteopenia. Endocrinology 2002;143:3955–62.
35. Javaid MK, Godfrey KM, Taylor P, et al. Umbilical venous IGF-1 concentration, neonatal bone mass, and body composition. J Bone Miner Res 2004;19:56–63.
36. Holmes SJ, Economou G, Whitehouse RW, et al. Reduced bone mineral density in patients with adult onset growth hormone deficiency. J Clin Endocrinol Metab 1994;78:669–74.
37. Saggese G, Baroncelli GI, Bertelloni S, et al. Effects of long-term treatment with growth hormone on bone and mineral metabolism in children with growth hormone deficiency. J Pediatr 1993;122:37–45.
38. Rosen T, Hansson T, Granhed H, et al. Reduced bone mineral content in adult patients with growth hormone deficiency. Acta Endocrinol (Copenh) 1993;129:201–6.
39. Bachrach LK, Marcus R, Ott SM, et al. Bone mineral, histomorphometry, and body composition in adults with growth hormone receptor deficiency. J Bone Miner Res 1998;13:415–21.
40. Benbassat CA, Eshed V, Kamjin M, et al. Are adult patients with Laron syndrome osteopenic? A comparison between dual-energy X-ray absorptiometry and volumetric bone densities. J Clin Endocrinol Metab 2003;88:4586–9.
41. Woods KA, Camacho-Hubner C, Bergman RN, et al. Effects of insulin-like growth factor I (IGF-I) therapy on body composition and insulin resistance in IGF-I gene deletion. J Clin Endocrinol Metab 2000;85:1407–11.
42. Woods KA, Camacho-Hubner C, Savage MO, et al. Intrauterine growth retardation and postnatal growth failure associated with deletion of the insulin-like growth factor I gene. N Engl J Med 1996;335:1363–7.
43. Walenkamp MJ, Karperien M, Pereira AM, et al. Homozygous and heterozygous expression of a novel insulin-like growth factor-I mutation. J Clin Endocrinol Metab 2005;90:2855–64.
44. Bonapace G, Concolino D, Formicola S, et al. A novel mutation in a patient with insulin-like growth factor 1 (IGF1) deficiency. J Med Genet 2003;40:913–7.
45. Raile K, Klammt J, Schneider A, et al. Clinical and functional characteristics of the human Arg59Ter insulin-like growth factor I receptor (IGF1R) mutation: implications for a gene dosage effect of the human IGF1R. J Clin Endocrinol Metab 2006;91:2264–71.
46. Kawashima Y, Kanzaki S, Yang F, et al. Mutation at cleavage site of insulin-like growth factor receptor in a short-stature child born with intrauterine growth retardation. J Clin Endocrinol Metab 2005;90:4679–87.
47. Abuzzahab MJ, Schneider A, Goddard A, et al. IGF-I receptor mutations resulting in intrauterine and postnatal growth retardation. N Engl J Med 2003;349:2211–22.
48. Langlois JA, Rosen CJ, Visser M, et al. Association between insulin-like growth factor I and bone mineral density in older women and men: the Framingham Heart Study. J Clin Endocrinol Metab 1998;83:4257–62.
49. Bauer DC, Rosen C, Cauley J, et al; the SOF Research Group. Low serum IGF-1 but not IGFBP-3 predicts hip and spine fracture: the study of osteoporotic fracture. Bone 1998;23:5(Suppl 1):S561.
50. Garnero P, Sornay-Rendu E, Delmas PD. Low serum IGF-1 and occurrence of osteoporotic fractures in postmenopausal women. Lancet 2000;355:898–9.

51. Deng HW, Xu FH, Huang QY, et al. A whole-genome linkage scan suggests several genomic regions potentially containing quantitative trait Loci for osteoporosis. J Clin Endocrinol Metab 2002;87:5151–9.
52. Karasik D, Myers RH, Cupples LA, et al. Genome screen for quantitative trait loci contributing to normal variation in bone mineral density: the Framingham Study. J Bone Miner Res 2002;17:1718–27.
53. Kim JG, Roh KR, Lee JY. The relationship among serum insulin-like growth factor-I, insulin-like growth factor-I gene polymorphism, and bone mineral density in postmenopausal women in Korea. Am J Obstet Gynecol 2002;186:345–50.
54. Rivadeneira F, Houwing-Duistermaat JJ, Vaessen N, et al. Association between an insulin-like growth factor I gene promoter polymorphism and bone mineral density in the elderly: the Rotterdam Study. J Clin Endocrinol Metab 2003;88: 3878–84.
55. Rivadeneira F, Houwing-Duistermaat JJ, Beck TJ, et al. The influence of an insulin-like growth factor I gene promoter polymorphism on hip bone geometry and the risk of nonvertebral fracture in the elderly: the Rotterdam Study. J Bone Miner Res 2004;19:1280–90.
56. Takacs I, Koller DL, Peacock M, et al. Sibling pair linkage and association studies between bone mineral density and the insulin-like growth factor I gene locus. J Clin Endocrinol Metab 1999;84:4467–71.
57. Jiang DK, Shen H, Li MX, et al. No major effect of the insulin-like growth factor I gene on bone mineral density in premenopausal Chinese women. Bone 2005;36: 694–9.
58. Laron Z. Insulin-like growth factor-I treatment of children with Laron syndrome (primary growth hormone insensitivity). Pediatr Endocrinol Rev 2008;5:766–71.
59. Ebeling PR, Jones JD, O'Fallon WM, et al. Short-term effects of recombinant human insulin-like growth factor I on bone turnover in normal women. J Clin Endocrinol Metab 1993;77:1384–7.
60. Ghiron LJ, Thompson JL, Holloway L, et al. Effects of recombinant insulin-like growth factor-I and growth hormone on bone turnover in elderly women. J Bone Miner Res 1995;10:1844–52.
61. Rubin J, Ackert-Bicknell CL, Zhu L, et al. IGF-I regulates osteoprotegerin (OPG) and receptor activator of nuclear factor-kappaB ligand in vitro and OPG in vivo. J Clin Endocrinol Metab 2002;87:4273–9.
62. Boonen S, Rosen C, Bouillon R, et al. Musculoskeletal effects of the recombinant human IGF-I/IGF binding protein-3 complex in osteoporotic patients with proximal femoral fracture: a double-blind, placebo-controlled pilot study. J Clin Endocrinol Metab 2002;87:1593–9.

The Insulin-Like Growth Factor System in Cancer

S. John Weroha, MD, PhD[a], Paul Haluska, MD, PhD[b],*

KEYWORDS

- Insulin-like growth factor • Cancer risk stratification • Growth hormone
- Signal transduction

KEY POINTS

- IGF signaling is a key mediator of tumorigenesis, cancer proliferation and survival.
- The insulin receptor, particularly the A isoform, is also an IGF signaling receptor that may function as a hybrid receptor with IGF-1R or as a homoreceptor.
- Targeting IGF signaling is promising in the treatment of many types of malignancies, though determining markers of sensitivity has been challenging.
- "Crosstalk" signaling between other receptors, including EGFR and HER2, may limit the effectiveness of targeting IGF-1R.
- Clinical investigations with agents targeting IGF signaling are ongoing.

THE INSULIN-LIKE GROWTH FACTOR SYSTEM AND CANCER RISK

Insulin-like growth factor (IGF) plays an important role in tissue growth and development. As such, several studies have demonstrated the association between circulating levels of IGF-1 and -2 and cancer risk. In patients with acromegaly, an endocrine disorder characterized by a hypersecretion of growth hormone (GH) and consequently higher endogenous IGF, several studies have shown a 2-fold increased risk of gastrointestinal cancers.[1–4] Other studies have shown a modest association between higher circulating IGF-1 and -2 levels and an increased risk for prostate, breast, colorectal, and ovarian cancer.[5–11] However, several other studies do not show a similar increase in cancer risk.[12–19] Exogenous recombinant GH has been proposed as a potential cancer-promoting agent, but no convincing link between cancer risk and its use in children or adults has been identified.[20,21] The role of IGF

Disclosure of potential conflicts of interest: P.H. receives research funds from BMS, Roche, ImClone, GSK, Pfizer, Merck, and MedImmune, and is an unpaid consultant for BMS, Roche, Merck, and MedImmune.

This work was supported by the United States National Institutes of Health Grant CA136393, Mayo Clinic SPORE in Ovarian Cancer, CA116201 Mayo Clinic Breast SPORE and CA090628 K12.

[a] Department of Oncology, Mayo Clinic College of Medicine, 200 First Street Southwest, Rochester, MN 55905, USA; [b] Division of Medical Oncology, Department of Oncology, Mayo Clinic College of Medicine, 200 First Street Southwest, Rochester, MN 55905, USA

* Corresponding author.

E-mail address: haluska.paul@mayo.edu

Endocrinol Metab Clin N Am 41 (2012) 335–350

doi:10.1016/j.ecl.2012.04.014

0889-8529/12/$ – see front matter © 2012 Elsevier Inc. All rights reserved.

in cancer risk is multifactorial and, taken together, the preponderance of data suggests a slight increased risk of some cancers because of higher activity of the IGF system. Conversely, patients with congenital deficiencies in IGF-1 have a protective effect against developing cancer.[22]

THE IGF SYSTEM IN CELLULAR PROLIFERATION AND SURVIVAL

The life cycle of a normal human cell is tightly regulated by intracellular and extracellular signals, working in concert to appropriately control cellular proliferation, senescence, and apoptosis. When the sum of growth stimulatory and inhibitory signals favors proliferation, the cell enters mitosis. For example, circulating IGF-1 and IGF-2 bind to the IGF-1 receptor (IGF-1R) and trigger a signal transduction cascade that leads to increased proliferation and enhanced survival of IGF-responsive cells (**Fig. 1**). Such signaling is central to the processes of oncogenesis. The mitogenic activity of the IGF-1R is mediated through the Ras and AKT pathways, and results in the upregulation of cyclin D1 and its binding partner CDK4, leading to the phosphorylation of retinoblastoma protein, release of E2F transcription factor, and expression of downstream target genes such as cyclin E.[23,24] Moreover, IGF-1R activation downregulates the cell-cycle suppressors p27[kip1], p57[kip2], and PTEN,[25,26] indicating that multiple pathways are involved.

In addition to promoting cellular proliferation, the IGF system is a potent prosurvival stimulus. Apoptosis is the essential process of programmed cell death by which normal embryonic tissue architecture is formed and adult tissues are maintained following cellular senescence, injury, and hyperplasia. In adults, apoptosis is responsible for the elimination of senescent mammary epithelial cells during postmenopausal breast tissue involution,[27] cardiac remodeling seen in ischemic cardiomyopathy,[28] and the removal of excess lobular epithelial cells following periodic breast hyperplasia associated with menstruation.[27] However, cancer cells can often evade the normal apoptosis mechanisms and thus evade programmed cell death. The AKT pathway plays a critical role in apoptosis by inhibiting proapoptotic proteins such as BAD[29] and FKHR,[30] and activating antiapoptotic factors such as nuclear factor κB[31] and MDM2.[32] The importance of AKT in cancer-related IGF signaling is further exemplified by its role in invasion and metastasis.[33] Taken together, the IGF-1R provides a growth advantage to IGF-responsive cells by the promotion of cellular proliferation and enhanced survival.

THE INSULIN RECEPTOR AND HYBRID RECEPTORS

The insulin receptor (IR) is a tetrameric receptor consisting of 2 extracellular α and 2 intracellular β subunits, with significant overall homology to the IGF-1R and 84% homology at tyrosine kinase domains.[34] The identification of 2 isoforms generated from the alternative splicing (IR-A) of the full-length transcript (IR-B) results in a 12-amino difference between the 2 isoforms[35] and differential expression during mammalian development. IR-B is the classic form of the IR, which is primarily expressed in liver, muscle, and adipose tissues. It only binds insulin at physiologic concentrations, with predominantly metabolic effects.[36,37] On the other hand, IR-A is expressed during fetal development and in cancer cells with the ability to bind insulin as well as IGF-2, resulting in metabolic and mitogenic effects, respectively.[36] Breast and ovarian tumor cells have higher IR expression relative to normal epithelial cells,[38,39] and patients with very high IR expression have worse disease-free survival.[40]

The significant sequence homology has important implications for IGF-1R function in general, and oncogenesis in particular. The discovery that some cancers, such as thyroid, breast, and colon cancer, exhibit a higher relative abundance of IR-A compared with normal cells provided insight into the intimate association between

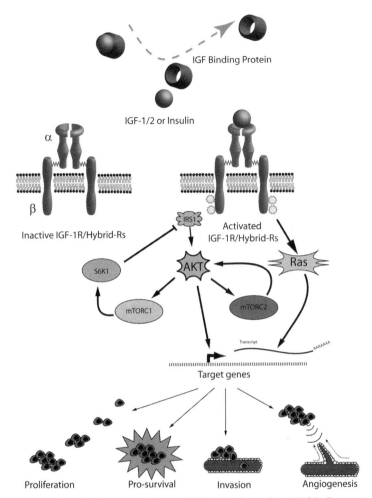

Fig. 1. Circulating insulin-like growth factor (IGF)-1/-2 is bound to IGF-binding proteins and released at the IGF receptor 1 (IGF-1R), which is composed of an α and β tetrameric receptor. This process leads to the activation of Ras and AKT with subsequent upregulation of genes involved in cell proliferation, survival, invasion, and angiogenesis. AKT is also an upstream regulator of mammalian target of rapamycin complex 1 (mTORC1) and a downstream effector of mTORC2. Both mTOR complexes play an important role in positive and negative feedback on the IGF/AKT signaling pathway. Hybrid-Rs, hybrid receptors; IRS1, insulin receptor substrate 1; S6K1, p70 S6 kinase.

the insulin and IGF systems.[36,41,42] Indeed, the homology between IR and IGF-1R permit the formation hybrid receptors (Hybrid-Rs), comprising one α/β monomer of IR and one of IGF-1R, with the hybrid receptor ligand specificity determined by the IR isoform.[43] For example, heterodimerization of IGF-1R with IR-A or IR-B gives rise to Hybrid-RA or Hybrid-RB, respectively. Both receptor hybrids have affinity for IGF-1 and IGF-2 (and to a lesser extent, insulin for Hybrid-RA) to activate downstream targets leading to cellular proliferation.[44,45]

The precise role of Hybrid-Rs in oncogenesis is under active investigation. Hybrid-Rs may increase the functional pool of receptors capable of activating the IGF system and provide further growth advantages to a subset of cells overexpressing IGF-1R,

IR-A, or both. Hybrid-Rs also have therapeutic implications, because novel therapies targeted against the IGF-1R may have lower efficacy in cancers signaling through IR-A or Hybrid-RA receptors, especially those with a high Hybrid-R:IGF-1R ratio.[46] Furthermore, hyperinsulinemic states may directly stimulate IR-A or Hybrid-RA expression and increase the bioavailability of IGF-1.[14,47] The role of Hybrid-Rs and IR isoforms in breast and other cancers is an active area of investigation.

SIGNAL TRANSDUCTION CROSS-TALK

Signaling cross-talk is characterized by the influence of one receptor/signaling system on a separate receptor/signaling system. There is growing evidence that such cross-talk in cancer cells has important implications in the efficacy of novel therapeutics. One such cross-talk pathway occurs between IGF-1R and the erbB family of receptors, which include erbB1 (epidermal growth factor receptor [EGFR]) and erbB2 (human epidermal growth factor receptor 2 [HER2]/neu) (**Fig. 2**). Treatment of breast and

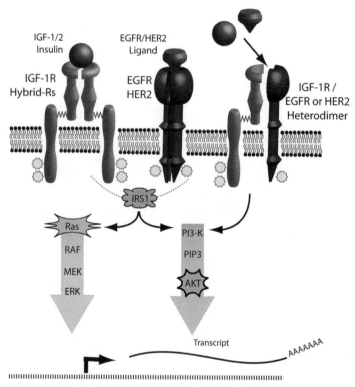

Fig. 2. IGF-1R and EGFR/HER2 cross-talk occurs by way of 2 main mechanisms. Because both pathways share a common signal transduction mediator, IRS1, resistance to inhibition of one receptor pathway can result from activation of IRS1 by the alternative receptor pathway. In addition, the formation of IGF-1R and EGFR/HER2 heterodimers increases the functional pool of receptors capable of binding IGF or EGFR/HER2 ligands, thus conferring resistance to single-agent targeted therapy. EGFR, epidermal growth factor receptor; HER2, human epidermal growth factor receptor 2; Hybrid-Rs, hybrid receptors; IGF, insulin-like growth factor; IGF-1R, IGF receptor 1; IRS1, insulin receptor substrate 1; PI3K, phosphatidylinositol-3-kinase.

ovarian cancer cells with the duel IGF-1R/IR tyrosine kinase inhibitor (TKI) BMS-536924 caused a reciprocal upregulation of the erbB family of receptors, which conferred resistance to IGF-1R inhibition.[48] Conversely, treatment of EGFR-dependent, tamoxifen-resistant breast cancer cells with the EGFR-selective TKI gefitinib led to activated IGF-1R signaling and subsequent resistance to EGFR inhibition.[49] Similarly, trastuzumab, a monoclonal antibody that binds HER2, is used to treat HER2-positive breast cancer, but resistance is problematic[50] and in vitro studies with SKBR3 breast cancer cells implicate activated IGF-1R in this process,[51] which is reversed by inhibition of IGF-1R.[52] One mechanism of resistance to IGF-1R or erbB targeted therapy occurs by the heterodimerization of IGF-1R with erbB receptors,[52,53] which provides an alternative signaling pathway to activate downstream mediators of cell proliferation and survival (see **Fig. 2**). Another example of cross-talk involves the estrogen receptor (ER), which is an important therapeutic target in adjuvant treatment of breast cancer. The IGF-1R may contribute to tamoxifen resistance by 2 possible mechanisms: (1) IGF-mediated activation of AKT and subsequent estrogen-independent activation of ER,[54] or (2) a direct interaction between ER and IGF-1R.[55] An emerging body of evidence supports an additional layer of cross-talk involving mammalian target of rapamycin (mTOR), a downstream effector of AKT with effects on cell proliferation, survival, and angiogenesis. The interaction of mTOR with either Raptor or Rictor results in the formation of functionally distinct mTOR complex 1 (mTORC1) or 2 (mTORC2), respectively. Activation of mTORC1 leads to S6K1-mediated destabilization of insulin receptor substrate 1 (IRS1) and subsequent inhibition of IR and IGF-1R signaling,[56] providing a negative feedback loop to downregulate AKT (see **Fig. 1**). Conversely, activation of mTORC2 leads to the upregulation of AKT by the specific phosphorylation of serine 473.[57] This IGF-1R/AKT/mTOR signaling cross-talk has important therapeutic implications because rapalogs such as sirolimus, temsirolimus, everolimus, and ridaforolimus preferentially inhibit mTORC1 and can promote AKT activation by increased mTORC2 activation in addition to a loss of feedback inhibition.[58]

The aforementioned examples of reciprocal cross-talk underscore the complexity of the IGF system in cancer and the need for multipathway targeting. Indeed, concomitant treatment of ovarian cancer cells with BMS-536924 and BMS-599626, a pan-HER inhibitor, demonstrated synergistic antiproliferative activity.[48] Dual therapy is currently being investigated in clinical trials with IMC-A12 (anti–IGF-IR antibody) and cetuximab (anti-EGFR antibody) in patients with head and neck cancer, and IMC-A12 and lapatinib (a TKI against HER2) in patients with breast cancer.[59] Although a recent clinical trial investigating IMC-A12 and cetuximab in patients with colorectal cancer did not show a benefit with IGF-1R inhibition,[60] study patients were resistant to prior anti-EGFR therapy, and staining for activated AKT, a marker of EGFR and IGF-1R signaling, did not correlate with outcome. With respect to mTOR/IGF-1R dual targeted therapy, early results from a phase I clinical trial evaluating ridaforolimus (small-molecule inhibitor of mTOR) and the IGF-1R antibody dalotozumab demonstrate clinical benefit in 16.1% of patients with advanced cancer and 21.7% of patients with breast cancer.[61] These data suggest that multiple pathways are interconnected, and support the argument for customized cancer therapy based on pathway activation rather than histologic diagnosis alone.

IGF-BINDING PROTEINS

There are 6 IGF-binding proteins (IGFBPs) with high affinity for IGF-1 and IGF-2. Serum concentrations of IGF are affected primarily by IGFBP3, which is the most abundant binding protein with the highest affinity for IGF-1 and IGF-2.[62] Although

IGFBPs are synthesized primarily in the liver, many normal and malignant tissues such as lung, breast, and ovarian cancers express IGFBPs.[63–65] These molecules are thought to influence malignancy by several mechanisms. First, they regulate bioavailability and half-life of IGF-1/-2 in the circulation, and provide a mechanism for transport to target organs. Second, IGFBPs modulate the activity of IGF through important interactions with extracellular proteases that degrade IGFBPs, resulting in the release of ligand and subsequent activation of IGF-1R. These proteolytic fragments, particularly of IGFBP-5 and -3, may also have ligand-independent biological activity.[66,67]

The involvement of IGFBPs in cancer varies by the type of malignancy. For example, IGFBP-2, -3, and -5 are associated with glioblastoma more commonly than with other brain tumors, and IGFBP-3 in particular is associated with shorter overall survival.[68] In breast cancer cells, IGFBP-5 is associated with metastasis[69] and poor prognosis.[70] However, the specific mechanisms by which IGFBPs affect tumor progression are complex, and published data are sometimes discrepant. For instance, despite the aforementioned association between IGFBP-5 and metastasis, forced overexpression of IGFBP-5 in breast cancer cell lines actually inhibits cell growth.[71] Further studies have determined that the subcellular localization of IGFBP-5 influences its biological effect. Indeed, cytoplasmic IGFBP-5 promotes cell proliferation and motility[72] whereas nuclear IGFBP-5 does not.[71] Ligand-independent activity for IGFBP-5[73] is thought to involve the AKT pathway, with effects on ovarian cancer angiogenesis.[74] IGFBP-2 has also demonstrated ligand-independent activity, mediated by interactions with cell-surface integrins.[75,76] Another binding protein with ligand-independent activity is IGFBP-4, which physically interacts with Frz8, a Wnt receptor, in cardiomyocytes and inhibits activation by Wnt3A ligand.[77] This discovery adds to the complexity of the IGF system and previously mentioned pathway cross-talk. However, the impact of IGFBP-4 on Wnt signaling in cancer biology remains to be characterized.

SPECIFIC CANCERS
Breast

Breast cancer is the most common malignancy in American women and is the second most common cause of death attributable to cancer.[78] The IGF system has a presence in most solid and hematologic malignancies, including breast cancer. The extent of IGF-1R expression in breast cancer varies by methodology but may approach 90% of tumors.[79] This high expression presents a potentially greater opportunity for targeted therapy than does HER2, which is present in 20% to 25% of all breast cancers. Although the prognostic value of IGF-1R expression is debatable,[80,81] in vitro studies have demonstrated that IGF-1 contributes to breast cancer growth by promoting cell proliferation and chemotherapy resistance.[82,83] The role of IGF-1, IGF-1R, IGFBPs, Hybrid-Rs, and IGF signaling cross-talk in breast cancer are discussed above. Targeting these cross-talk pathways in breast cancer remains an active area of clinical investigation.

Sarcomas

Genetic and cytogenetic aberrations are predominate oncogenic forces in sarcoma development, and this may have downstream consequences for the IGF system. For example, Ewing sarcoma (ES) is characterized by a t(11;22) translocation producing the EWSR1-FLI1 fusion protein, which acts as an aberrant transcription factor, leading to the upregulation of downstream targets such as c-myc,[84] cyclin D1,[85] and platelet-derived growth factor (PDGF)-C.[86] IGF-1R expression is a prerequisite to EWSR1-FLI1–mediated transformation,[87] required for ES cell survival,[88] and attenuates the efficacy of cytotoxic chemotherapy.[89] Inhibition of the IGF-1R with NVP-AEW541, a small-molecule inhibitor, induces cell-cycle arrest and apoptosis in vitro and reduces in vivo growth of ES cells.[90] A phase I single-agent clinical trial with a fully human IGF-1R monoclonal antibody inhibitor, figitumumab (CP-751,871) demonstrated clinical benefit (objective response or stable disease) in 50% (n = 16) of ES patients.[91] In a follow-up phase II trial with 125 ES patients with recurrent or refractory disease, objective responses were observed in 14.4%.[92] A smaller phase II trial with 35 ES or desmoplastic small round-cell tumor patients demonstrated an objective response rate of 6% with single-agent AMG 479.[93] The modest clinical responses despite strong preclinical data support the contention that patients should be selected based on a tumor phenotype rather than on histologic classification. Moreover, the activation of parallel but interconnected signal transduction pathways in ES suggested a potential role for multipathway targeting of IGF-1R and mTOR.[94–96]

Less is known about the IGF system in other sarcomas, but interesting observations have been made that have not yet been described for carcinomas. For instance, alveolar rhabdomyosarcoma is a pediatric sarcoma characterized by a t(2;13) translocation that results in a Pax3-FKHR fusion gene. The Pax3-FKHR fusion protein can transactivate the *IGFR1* gene,[97] leading to an overexpression of IGF-1R with growth and survival advantages that are abrogated by IGF-1R knockdown.[98] In gastrointestinal stromal cell tumors (GIST), *KIT*/PDGF receptor (*PDGFR*)-α wild-type tumors are less responsive to imatinib therapy and pose a therapeutic challenge.[99] This subset of GIST exhibits *IGF1R* gene amplification and overexpression that drives cell growth and survival, suggesting a possible role for IGF targeting.[100]

Gliomas

Gliomas are malignant central nervous tumors that include ependymomas, astrocytomas, oligodendrogliomas, and mixed gliomas. Glioblastoma multiforme (GBM) is the most common and aggressive subtype of astrocytoma. The primary treatment is surgical resection followed by chemotherapy and radiation therapy. However, prognosis remains poor and recurrence is common. Cumulative data indicate an important role for the IGF system in glioblastoma progression. For example, C6 glioblastoma cells exhibit growth inhibition when IGF-1R is downregulated in vivo and in vitro,[101] and inhibition of IGF-1R by picropodophyllin (a small-molecule TKI) inhibits cell growth by reduced AKT activation.[102] The prosurvival influence of IGF-1R has been linked to increased expression of Bcl-2.[103] GBM is known for its ability to invade the surrounding brain parenchyma as well as to stimulate angiogenesis. The IGF system is implicated in this process as perivascular tumor cells express higher levels of IGF-1R,[104] which is known to modulate production of vascular endothelial growth factor.[105] In addition, treatment of glioblastoma cells with IGF-1 increases cellular migration.[106] Taken together with the observation that tumor cells within the margins of infiltration express higher levels of IGF-1R,[104] the IGF system is intimately linked to glioblastoma tumor invasion. Although radiation therapy is effective in prolonging survival of patients, local recurrences may actually be promoted by radiation therapy through activation of EGFR, IGF-1R, and PDGFR,[107,108] while inhibition of these pathways increases radiosensitivity.[108] An additional example of signal transduction cross-talk has been reported in GBM, as IGF-1R upregulation can induce resistance to EGFR inhibition.[109] Thus, targeting IGF signaling in gliomas may be a promising anticancer strategy.

Lung Cancer

Lung cancer is the second most common malignancy afflicting American patients. Although platinum-based chemotherapy may provide modest benefit for advanced disease, lung cancer remained the most common cause of cancer deaths in 2010.[78] The IGF system has been implicated in essentially all phases of lung cancer oncogenesis. For instance, high-grade bronchial dysplasia produces greater paracrine and autocrine IGF than benign bronchial epithelial cells,[110] suggesting the IGF system has an early role in lung cancer development. In addition, non–small cell lung cancer (NSCLC) cells, particularly the squamous cell subtype, is associated with increased *IGF1R* gene copy number and mRNA/protein expression,[111] providing a growth and survival advantage to malignant cells and resistance to chemotherapy.[112] Inhibition of IGF-1R with figitumumab (an anti–IGF-IR antibody) leads to downregulated receptor expression, inhibition of tumor growth,[113] and radiosensitization of cancer cells.[114] Promising preclinical data and results from a phase I clinical trial with figitumumab in advanced cancers[115] led to a phase II trial with combination therapy in NSCLC.[116] The objective response rate was 54% for all NSCLC subtypes, but reached an impressive 78% in patients with the squamous-cell subtype. Although the subsequent phase III trial with figitumumab as first-line treatment in NSCLC cancer was greatly anticipated, it was stopped early when interim analysis failed to show a benefit in the figitumumab arm.[117]

Ovarian

Ovarian cancer is the fifth most common cause of death attributable to cancer in women.[78] Epidemiologic data has linked IGF-1R to high tumor grade and stage, and is associated with poor survival.[118] Although localized disease is associated with a 93% 5-year survival rate, 79% of patients are stage III or IV at the time of initial diagnosis.[78] After debulking surgery and 6 cycles of platinum-based chemotherapy, 75% of patients will achieve complete remission, but three-quarters of these will relapse within 20 months on average.[119] Retreatment with a platinum-based regimen is reasonable after a 6-month platinum-free period, but resistance is common and may be attributed to increased IGF-1R expression in ovarian tumor cells.[120] Although primary ovarian tumor cell cultures do not overexpress IGF, dysregulation of IGF homeostasis by the overexpression of IGFBP-2 in ovarian cancer cells may sequester and maintain an elevated localized pool of IGF for activation of IGF-1R.[63,121] A phase II clinical trial is currently evaluating the efficacy and tolerability of front-line AMG-479, a fully human monoclonal antibody against the IGF-1R, in combination with carboplatin and paclitaxel in advanced-stage, optimally debulked epithelial ovarian, primary peritoneal, and fallopian tube cancer (TRIO-014).

SUMMARY

The IGF system has been implicated in the oncogenesis of essentially all solid and hematologic malignancies. The central involvement of IGF signaling in tumor cell proliferation, survival, invasion, and metastasis makes it an attractive therapeutic target. The IGF signaling pathway has also been directly implicated in resistance to clinically important therapies, including hormonal agents, HER receptor targeting agents, radiation, and cytotoxic chemotherapy. Indeed, several clinical trials are currently evaluating the efficacy of IGF-1R inhibition to either overcome these resistance mechanisms or directly induce antiproliferative effects on tumors dependent on IGF signaling. Current strategies include monoclonal antibodies directed at IGF-1R, TKIs with activity against IGF-1R ± IR and antiligand antibodies. The optimal strategy for targeting IGF signaling in patients with cancer is not clear. The modest benefits reported thus far underscore the need for a better understanding of IGF signaling, which would enable clinicians to identify the subset of patients with the greatest likelihood of attaining benefit from this targeted approach.

REFERENCES

1. Baris D, Gridley G, Ron E, et al. Acromegaly and cancer risk: a cohort study in Sweden and Denmark. Cancer Causes Control 2002;13(5):395–400.
2. Kauppinen-Makelin R, Sane T, Valimaki MJ, et al. Increased cancer incidence in acromegaly—a nationwide survey. Clin Endocrinol (Oxf) 2010;72(2):278–9.
3. Orme SM, McNally RJ, Cartwright RA, et al. Mortality and cancer incidence in acromegaly: a retrospective cohort study. United Kingdom Acromegaly Study Group. J Clin Endocrinol Metab 1998;83(8):2730–4.
4. Ron E, Gridley G, Hrubec Z, et al. Acromegaly and gastrointestinal cancer. Cancer 1991;68(8):1673–7.
5. Jenkins PJ, Frajese V, Jones AM, et al. Insulin-like growth factor I and the development of colorectal neoplasia in acromegaly. J Clin Endocrinol Metab 2000; 85(9):3218–21.
6. Key TJ, Appleby PN, Reeves GK, et al. Insulin-like growth factor 1 (IGF1), IGF binding protein 3 (IGFBP3), and breast cancer risk: pooled individual data analysis of 17 prospective studies. Lancet Oncol 2010;11(6):530–42.
7. Lukanova A, Lundin E, Toniolo P, et al. Circulating levels of insulin-like growth factor-I and risk of ovarian cancer. Int J Cancer 2002;101(6):549–54.
8. Renehan AG, Painter JE, O'Halloran D, et al. Circulating insulinlike growth factor II and colorectal adenomas. J Clin Endocrinol Metab 2000;85(9):3402–8.
9. Renehan AG, Zwahlen M, Minder C, et al. Insulin-like growth factor (IGF)-I, IGF binding protein-3, and cancer risk: systematic review and meta-regression analysis. Lancet 2004;363(9418):1346–53.
10. Rinaldi S, Cleveland R, Norat T, et al. Serum levels of IGF-I, IGFBP-3 and colorectal cancer risk: results from the EPIC cohort, plus a meta-analysis of prospective studies. Int J Cancer 2010;126(7):1702–15.
11. Roddam AW, Allen NE, Appleby P, et al. Insulin-like growth factors, their binding proteins, and prostate cancer risk: analysis of individual patient data from 12 prospective studies. Ann Intern Med 2008;149(7):461–71 W83–8.
12. Allen NE, Key TJ, Appleby PN, et al. Serum insulin-like growth factor (IGF)-I and IGF-binding protein-3 concentrations and prostate cancer risk: results from the European Prospective Investigation into Cancer and Nutrition. Cancer Epidemiol Biomarkers Prev 2007;16(6):1121–7.
13. Finne P, Auvinen A, Koistinen H, et al. Insulinlike growth factor I is not a useful marker of prostate cancer in men with elevated levels of prostate-specific antigen. J Clin Endocrinol Metab 2000;85(8):2744–7.
14. Lukanova A, Zeleniuch-Jacquotte A, Lundin E, et al. Prediagnostic levels of C-peptide, IGF-I, IGFBP -1, -2 and -3 and risk of endometrial cancer. Int J Cancer 2004;108(2):262–8.
15. Mikami K, Ozasa K, Nakao M, et al. Prostate cancer risk in relation to insulin-like growth factor (IGF)-I and IGF-binding protein-3: A nested case-control study in large scale cohort study in Japan. Asian Pac J Cancer Prev 2009;10(Suppl): 57–61.
16. Pham TM, Fujino Y, Kikuchi S, et al. A nested case-control study of stomach cancer and serum insulin-like growth factor (IGF)-1, IGF-2 and IGF-binding protein (IGFBP)-3. Eur J Cancer 2007;43(10):1611–6.

17. Sakauchi F, Nojima M, Mori M, et al. Serum insulin-like growth factors I and II, insulin-like growth factor binding protein-3 and risk of breast cancer in the Japan Collaborative Cohort study. Asian Pac J Cancer Prev 2009;10(Suppl):51–5.

18. Spitz MR, Barnett MJ, Goodman GE, et al. Serum insulin-like growth factor (IGF) and IGF-binding protein levels and risk of lung cancer: a case-control study nested in the beta-Carotene and Retinol Efficacy Trial Cohort. Cancer Epidemiol Biomarkers Prev 2002;11(11):1413–8.

19. Suzuki S, Kojima M, Tokudome S, et al. Insulin-like growth factor (IGF)-I, IGF-II, IGF binding protein-3, and risk of colorectal cancer: a nested case-control study in the Japan Collaborative Cohort study. Asian Pac J Cancer Prev 2009; 10(Suppl):45–9.

20. Renehan AG, Brennan BM. Acromegaly, growth hormone and cancer risk. Best Pract Res Clin Endocrinol Metab 2008;22(4):639–57.

21. Svensson J, Bengtsson BA. Safety aspects of GH replacement. Eur J Endocrinol 2009;161(Suppl 1):S65–74.

22. Shevah O, Laron Z. Patients with congenital deficiency of IGF-I seem protected from the development of malignancies: a preliminary report. Growth Horm IGF Res 2007;17(1):54–7.

23. Lavoie JN, L'Allemain G, Brunet A, et al. Cyclin D1 expression is regulated positively by the p42/p44MAPK and negatively by the p38/HOGMAPK pathway. J Biol Chem 1996;271(34):20608–16.

24. Hamelers IH, van Schaik RF, Sipkema J, et al. Insulin-like growth factor I triggers nuclear accumulation of cyclin D1 in MCF-7S breast cancer cells. J Biol Chem 2002;277(49):47645–52.

25. Mairet-Coello G, Tury A, DiCicco-Bloom E. Insulin-like growth factor-1 promotes G(1)/S cell cycle progression through bidirectional regulation of cyclins and cyclin-dependent kinase inhibitors via the phosphatidylinositol 3-kinase/Akt pathway in developing rat cerebral cortex. J Neurosci 2009;29(3):775–88.

26. Ma J, Sawai H, Matsuo Y, et al. IGF-1 mediates PTEN suppression and enhances cell invasion and proliferation via activation of the IGF-1/PI3K/Akt signaling pathway in pancreatic cancer cells. J Surg Res 2010;160(1):90–101.

27. Strange R, Metcalfe T, Thackray L, et al. Apoptosis in normal and neoplastic mammary gland development. Microsc Res Tech 2001;52(2):171–81.

28. Sun Y. Oxidative stress and cardiac repair/remodeling following infarction. Am J Med Sci 2007;334(3):197–205.

29. Datta SR, Dudek H, Tao X, et al. Akt phosphorylation of BAD couples survival signals to the cell-intrinsic death machinery. Cell 1997;91(2):231–41.

30. Brunet A, Bonni A, Zigmond MJ, et al. Akt promotes cell survival by phosphorylating and inhibiting a Forkhead transcription factor. Cell 1999;96(6):857–68.

31. Kane LP, Shapiro VS, Stokoe D, et al. Induction of NF-kappaB by the Akt/PKB kinase. Curr Biol 1999;9(11):601–4.

32. Mayo LD, Donner DB. A phosphatidylinositol 3-kinase/Akt pathway promotes translocation of Mdm2 from the cytoplasm to the nucleus. Proc Natl Acad Sci U S A 2001;98(20):11598–603.

33. Zhang D, Brodt P. Type 1 insulin-like growth factor regulates MT1-MMP synthesis and tumor invasion via PI 3-kinase/Akt signaling. Oncogene 2003;22(7):974–82.

34. Ullrich A, Gray A, Tam AW, et al. Insulin-like growth factor I receptor primary structure: comparison with insulin receptor suggests structural determinants that define functional specificity. EMBO J 1986;5(10):2503–12.

35. Moller DE, Yokota A, Caro JF, et al. Tissue-specific expression of two alternatively spliced insulin receptor mRNAs in man. Mol Endocrinol 1989;3(8):1263–9.

36. Frasca F, Pandini G, Scalia P, et al. Insulin receptor isoform A, a newly recognized, high-affinity insulin-like growth factor II receptor in fetal and cancer cells. Mol Cell Biol 1999;19(5):3278–88.

37. Kido Y, Nakae J, Accili D. Clinical review 125: the insulin receptor and its cellular targets. J Clin Endocrinol Metab 2001;86(3):972–9.

38. Papa V, Pezzino V, Costantino A, et al. Elevated insulin receptor content in human breast cancer. J Clin Invest 1990;86(5):1503–10.

39. Kalli KR, Falowo OI, Bale LK, et al. Functional insulin receptors on human epithelial ovarian carcinoma cells: implications for IGF-II mitogenic signaling. Endocrinology 2002;143(9):3259–67.

40. Mathieu MC, Clark GM, Allred DC, et al. Insulin receptor expression and clinical outcome in node-negative breast cancer. Proc Assoc Am Physicians 1997; 109(6):565–71.

41. Belfiore A, Pandini G, Vella V, et al. Insulin/IGF-I hybrid receptors play a major role in IGF-I signaling in thyroid cancer. Biochimie 1999;81(4):403–7.

42. Garrouste FL, Remacle-Bonnet MM, Lehmann MM, et al. Up-regulation of insulin/insulin-like growth factor-I hybrid receptors during differentiation of HT29-D4 human colonic carcinoma cells. Endocrinology 1997;138(5):2021–32.

43. Pandini G, Frasca F, Mineo R, et al. Insulin/insulin-like growth factor I hybrid receptors have different biological characteristics depending on the insulin receptor isoform involved. J Biol Chem 2002;277(42):39684–95.

44. Benyoucef S, Surinya KH, Hadaschik D, et al. Characterization of insulin/IGF hybrid receptors: contributions of the insulin receptor L2 and Fn1 domains and the alternatively spliced exon 11 sequence to ligand binding and receptor activation. Biochem J 2007;403(3):603–13.

45. Slaaby R, Schaffer L, Lautrup-Larsen I, et al. Hybrid receptors formed by insulin receptor (IR) and insulin-like growth factor I receptor (IGF-IR) have low insulin and high IGF-1 affinity irrespective of the IR splice variant. J Biol Chem 2006; 281(36):25869–74.

46. Pandini G, Wurch T, Akla B, et al. Functional responses and in vivo anti-tumour activity of h7C10: a humanised monoclonal antibody with neutralising activity against the insulin-like growth factor-1 (IGF-1) receptor and insulin/IGF-1 hybrid receptors. Eur J Cancer 2007;43(8):1318–27.

47. Jenab M, Riboli E, Cleveland RJ, et al. Serum C-peptide, IGFBP-1 and IGFBP-2 and risk of colon and rectal cancers in the European Prospective Investigation into Cancer and Nutrition. Int J Cancer 2007;121(2):368–76.

48. Haluska P, Carboni JM, TenEyck C, et al. HER receptor signaling confers resistance to the insulin-like growth factor-I receptor inhibitor, BMS-536924. Mol Cancer Ther 2008;7(9):2589–98.

49. Knowlden JM, Jones HE, Barrow D, et al. Insulin receptor substrate-1 involvement in epidermal growth factor receptor and insulin-like growth factor receptor signalling: implication for gefitinib ('Iressa') response and resistance. Breast Cancer Res Treat 2008;111(1):79–91.

50. Vogel CL, Cobleigh MA, Tripathy D, et al. Efficacy and safety of trastuzumab as a single agent in first-line treatment of HER2-overexpressing metastatic breast cancer. J Clin Oncol 2002;20(3):719–26.

51. Lu Y, Zi X, Zhao Y, et al. Insulin-like growth factor-I receptor signaling and resistance to trastuzumab (Herceptin). J Natl Cancer Inst 2001;93(24): 1852–7.

52. Nahta R, Yuan LX, Zhang B, et al. Insulin-like growth factor-I receptor/ human epidermal growth factor receptor 2 heterodimerization contributes

to trastuzumab resistance of breast cancer cells. Cancer Res 2005;65(23): 11118–28.

53. Morgillo F, Woo JK, Kim ES, et al. Heterodimerization of insulin-like growth factor receptor/epidermal growth factor receptor and induction of survivin expression counteract the antitumor action of erlotinib. Cancer Res 2006; 66(20):10100–11.

54. Campbell RA, Bhat-Nakshatri P, Patel NM, et al. Phosphatidylinositol 3-kinase/ AKT-mediated activation of estrogen receptor alpha: a new model for anti-estrogen resistance. J Biol Chem 2001;276(13):9817–24.

55. Massarweh S, Osborne CK, Creighton CJ, et al. Tamoxifen resistance in breast tumors is driven by growth factor receptor signaling with repression of classic estrogen receptor genomic function. Cancer Res 2008;68(3):826–33.

56. Shah OJ, Wang Z, Hunter T. Inappropriate activation of the TSC/Rheb/mTOR/ S6K cassette induces IRS1/2 depletion, insulin resistance, and cell survival deficiencies. Curr Biol 2004;14(18):1650–6.

57. Sarbassov DD, Guertin DA, Ali SM, et al. Phosphorylation and regulation of Akt/ PKB by the rictor-mTOR complex. Science 2005;307(5712):1098–101.

58. Huang J, Manning BD. A complex interplay between Akt, TSC2 and the two mTOR complexes. Biochem Soc Trans 2009;37(Pt 1):217–22.

59. Haluska P, Reinholz MM, Dueck AC, et al. N0733: phase II trial of capecitabine and lapatinib plus or minus cixutumumab in HER2-positive breast cancer. J Clin Oncol (ASCO Meeting Abstracts) 2010;28(Suppl 15):TPS129.

60. Reidy DL, Vakiani E, Fakih MG, et al. Randomized, phase II study of the insulin-like growth factor-1 receptor inhibitor IMC-A12, with or without cetuximab, in patients with cetuximab- or panitumumab-refractory metastatic colorectal cancer. J Clin Oncol 2010;28(27):4240–6.

61. Di Cosimo S, Bendell JC, Cervantes-Ruiperez A, et al. A phase I study of the oral mTOR inhibitor ridaforolimus (RIDA) in combination with the IGF-1R antibody dalotuzumab (DALO) in patients (pts) with advanced solid tumors. J Clin Oncol (ASCO Meeting Abstracts) 2010;28(Suppl 15):3008.

62. Shimasaki S, Ling N. Identification and molecular characterization of insulin-like growth factor binding proteins (IGFBP-1, -2, -3, -4, -5 and -6). Prog Growth Factor Res 1991;3(4):243–66.

63. Wang H, Rosen DG, Wang H, et al. Insulin-like growth factor-binding protein 2 and 5 are differentially regulated in ovarian cancer of different histologic types. Mod Pathol 2006;19(9):1149–56.

64. Jaques G, Noll K, Wegmann B, et al. Nuclear localization of insulin-like growth factor binding protein 3 in a lung cancer cell line. Endocrinology 1997;138(4): 1767–70.

65. Schedlich LJ, Young TF, Firth SM, et al. Insulin-like growth factor-binding protein (IGFBP)-3 and IGFBP-5 share a common nuclear transport pathway in T47D human breast carcinoma cells. J Biol Chem 1998;273(29):18347–52.

66. Laursen LS, Kjaer-Sorensen K, Andersen MH, et al. Regulation of insulin-like growth factor (IGF) bioactivity by sequential proteolytic cleavage of IGF binding protein-4 and -5. Mol Endocrinol 2007;21(5):1246–57.

67. Lalou C, Lassarre C, Binoux M. A proteolytic fragment of insulin-like growth factor (IGF) binding protein-3 that fails to bind IGFs inhibits the mitogenic effects of IGF-I and insulin. Endocrinology 1996;137(8):3206–12.

68. Santosh V, Arivazhagan A, Sreekanthreddy P, et al. Grade-specific expression of insulin-like growth factor-binding proteins-2, -3, and -5 in astrocytomas: IGFBP-3 emerges as a strong predictor of survival in patients with newly

diagnosed glioblastoma. Cancer Epidemiol Biomarkers Prev 2010;19(6): 1399–408.

69. Wang H, Arun BK, Fuller GN, et al. IGFBP2 and IGFBP5 overexpression correlates with the lymph node metastasis in T1 breast carcinomas. Breast J 2008; 14(3):261–7.

70. Mita K, Zhang Z, Ando Y, et al. Prognostic significance of insulin-like growth factor binding protein (IGFBP)-4 and IGFBP-5 expression in breast cancer. Jpn J Clin Oncol 2007;37(8):575–82.

71. Butt AJ, Dickson KA, McDougall F, et al. Insulin-like growth factor-binding protein-5 inhibits the growth of human breast cancer cells in vitro and in vivo. J Biol Chem 2003;278(32):29676–85.

72. Akkiprik M, Hu L, Sahin A, et al. The subcellular localization of IGFBP5 affects its cell growth and migration functions in breast cancer. BMC Cancer 2009;9:103.

73. Tripathi G, Salih DA, Drozd AC, et al. IGF-independent effects of insulin-like growth factor binding protein-5 (Igfbp5) in vivo. FASEB J 2009;23(8):2616–26.

74. Rho SB, Dong SM, Kang S, et al. Insulin-like growth factor-binding protein-5 (IGFBP-5) acts as a tumor suppressor by inhibiting angiogenesis. Carcinogenesis 2008;29(11):2106–11.

75. Schutt BS, Langkamp M, Rauschnabel U, et al. Integrin-mediated action of insulin-like growth factor binding protein-2 in tumor cells. J Mol Endocrinol 2004;32(3):859–68.

76. Wang GK, Hu L, Fuller GN, et al. An interaction between insulin-like growth factor-binding protein 2 (IGFBP2) and integrin alpha5 is essential for IGFBP2-induced cell mobility. J Biol Chem 2006;281(20):14085–91.

77. Zhu W, Shiojima I, Ito Y, et al. IGFBP-4 is an inhibitor of canonical Wnt signalling required for cardiogenesis. Nature 2008;454(7202):345–9.

78. Jemal A, Siegel R, Xu J, et al. Cancer statistics, 2010. CA Cancer J Clin 2010; 60(5):277–300.

79. Peyrat JP, Bonneterre J, Vennin PH, et al. Insulin-like growth factor 1 receptors (IGF1-R) and IGF1 in human breast tumors. J Steroid Biochem Mol Biol 1990; 37(6):823–7.

80. Railo MJ, von Smitten K, Pekonen F. The prognostic value of insulin-like growth factor-I in breast cancer patients. Results of a follow-up study on 126 patients. Eur J Cancer 1994;30A(3):307–11.

81. Papa V, Gliozzo B, Clark GM, et al. Insulin-like growth factor-I receptors are over-expressed and predict a low risk in human breast cancer. Cancer Res 1993; 53(16):3736–40.

82. Dunn SE, Hardman RA, Kari FW, et al. Insulin-like growth factor 1 (IGF-1) alters drug sensitivity of HBL100 human breast cancer cells by inhibition of apoptosis induced by diverse anticancer drugs. Cancer Res 1997;57(13):2687–93.

83. Gooch JL, Van Den Berg CL, Yee D. Insulin-like growth factor (IGF)-I rescues breast cancer cells from chemotherapy-induced cell death—proliferative and anti-apoptotic effects. Breast Cancer Res Treat 1999;56(1):1–10.

84. Bailly RA, Bosselut R, Zucman J, et al. DNA-binding and transcriptional activation properties of the EWS-FLI-1 fusion protein resulting from the t(11;22) translocation in Ewing sarcoma. Mol Cell Biol 1994;14(5):3230–41.

85. Matsumoto Y, Tanaka K, Nakatani F, et al. Downregulation and forced expression of EWS-Fli1 fusion gene results in changes in the expression of G(1)regulatory genes. Br J Cancer 2001;84(6):768–75.

86. Zwerner JP, May WA. PDGF-C is an EWS/FLI induced transforming growth factor in Ewing family tumors. Oncogene 2001;20(5):626–33.

87. Toretsky JA, Kalebic T, Blakesley V, et al. The insulin-like growth factor-I receptor is required for EWS/FLI-1 transformation of fibroblasts. J Biol Chem 1997; 272(49):30822–7.

88. Yee D, Favoni RE, Lebovic GS, et al. Insulin-like growth factor I expression by tumors of neuroectodermal origin with the t(11;22) chromosomal translocation. A potential autocrine growth factor. J Clin Invest 1990;86(6):1806–14.

89. Benini S, Manara MC, Baldini N, et al. Inhibition of insulin-like growth factor I receptor increases the antitumor activity of doxorubicin and vincristine against Ewing's sarcoma cells. Clin Cancer Res 2001;7(6):1790–7.

90. Scotlandi K, Manara MC, Nicoletti G, et al. Antitumor activity of the insulin-like growth factor-I receptor kinase inhibitor NVP-AEW541 in musculoskeletal tumors. Cancer Res 2005;65(9):3868–76.

91. Olmos D, Postel-Vinay S, Molife LR, et al. Safety, pharmacokinetics, and preliminary activity of the anti-IGF-1R antibody figitumumab (CP-751,871) in patients with sarcoma and Ewing's sarcoma: a phase 1 expansion cohort study. Lancet Oncol 2010;11(2):129–35.

92. Pappo AS, Patel S, Crowley J, et al. Activity of R1507, a monoclonal antibody to the insulin-like growth factor-1 receptor (IGF1R), in patients (pts) with recurrent or refractory Ewing's sarcoma family of tumors (ESFT): results of a phase II SARC study. J Clin Oncol (ASCO Meeting Abstracts) 2010;28(Suppl 15):10000.

93. Tap WD, Demetri GD, Barnette P, et al. AMG 479 in relapsed or refractory Ewing's family tumors (EFT) or desmoplastic small round cell tumors (DSRCT): phase II results. J Clin Oncol (ASCO Meeting Abstracts) 2010;28(Suppl 15):10001.

94. Krishnan K, Bruce B, Hewitt S, et al. Ezrin mediates growth and survival in Ewing's sarcoma through the AKT/mTOR, but not the MAPK, signaling pathway. Clin Exp Metastasis 2006;23(3–4):227–36.

95. Benini S, Manara MC, Cerisano V, et al. Contribution of MEK/MAPK and PI3-K signaling pathway to the malignant behavior of Ewing's sarcoma cells: therapeutic prospects. Int J Cancer 2004;108(3):358–66.

96. van de Luijtgaarden AC, Versleijen-Jonkers YM, Roeffen MH, et al. Predicting an optimal strategy for insulin-like growth factor 1 (IGF1) signaling interference in Ewing's sarcoma (ES). J Clin Oncol (ASCO Meeting Abstracts) 2010;28(Suppl 15):9538.

97. Ayalon D, Glaser T, Werner H. Transcriptional regulation of IGF-I receptor gene expression by the PAX3-FKHR oncoprotein. Growth Horm IGF Res 2001;11(5): 289–97.

98. Shapiro DN, Jones BG, Shapiro LH, et al. Antisense-mediated reduction in insulin-like growth factor-I receptor expression suppresses the malignant phenotype of a human alveolar rhabdomyosarcoma. J Clin Invest 1994;94(3): 1235–42.

99. Debiec-Rychter M, Dumez H, Judson I, et al. Use of c-KIT/PDGFRA mutational analysis to predict the clinical response to imatinib in patients with advanced gastrointestinal stromal tumours entered on phase I and II studies of the EORTC Soft Tissue and Bone Sarcoma Group. Eur J Cancer 2004;40(5):689–95.

100. Tarn C, Rink L, Merkel E, et al. Insulin-like growth factor 1 receptor is a potential therapeutic target for gastrointestinal stromal tumors. Proc Natl Acad Sci U S A 2008;105(24):8387–92.

101. Resnicoff M, Sell C, Rubini M, et al. Rat glioblastoma cells expressing an antisense RNA to the insulin-like growth factor-1 (IGF-1) receptor are nontumorigenic and induce regression of wild-type tumors. Cancer Res 1994; 54(8):2218–22.

102. Yin S, Girnita A, Stromberg T, et al. Targeting the insulin-like growth factor-1 receptor by picropodophyllin as a treatment option for glioblastoma. Neuro Oncol 2010;12(1):19–27.

103. Yin D, Tamaki N, Parent AD, et al. Insulin-like growth factor-I decreased etoposide-induced apoptosis in glioma cells by increasing bcl-2 expression and decreasing CPP32 activity. Neurol Res 2005;27(1):27–35.

104. Hirano H, Lopes MB, Laws ER Jr, et al. Insulin-like growth factor-1 content and pattern of expression correlates with histopathologic grade in diffusely infiltrating astrocytomas. Neuro Oncol 1999;1(2):109–19.

105. Gariboldi MB, Ravizza R, Monti E. The IGFR1 inhibitor NVP-AEW541 disrupts a pro-survival and pro-angiogenic IGF-STAT3-HIF1 pathway in human glioblastoma cells. Biochem Pharmacol 2010;80(4):455–62.

106. Schlenska-Lange A, Knupfer H, Lange TJ, et al. Cell proliferation and migration in glioblastoma multiforme cell lines are influenced by insulin-like growth factor I in vitro. Anticancer Res 2008;28(2A):1055–60.

107. Zhai GG, Malhotra R, Delaney M, et al. Radiation enhances the invasive potential of primary glioblastoma cells via activation of the Rho signaling pathway. J Neurooncol 2006;76(3):227–37.

108. Carapancea M, Cosaceanu D, Budiu R, et al. Dual targeting of IGF-1R and PDGFR inhibits proliferation in high-grade gliomas cells and induces radiosensitivity in JNK-1 expressing cells. J Neurooncol 2007;85(3):245–54.

109. Chakravarti A, Loeffler JS, Dyson NJ. Insulin-like growth factor receptor I mediates resistance to anti-epidermal growth factor receptor therapy in primary human glioblastoma cells through continued activation of phosphoinositide 3-kinase signaling. Cancer Res 2002;62(1):200–7.

110. Kim WY, Jin Q, Oh SH, et al. Elevated epithelial insulin-like growth factor expression is a risk factor for lung cancer development. Cancer Res 2009;69(18): 7439–48.

111. Dziadziuszko R, Merrick DT, Witta SE, et al. Insulin-like growth factor receptor 1 (IGF1R) gene copy number is associated with survival in operable non–small-cell lung cancer: a comparison between IGF1R fluorescent in situ hybridization, protein expression, and mRNA expression. J Clin Oncol 2010;28(13):2174–80.

112. Lee YJ, Imsumran A, Park MY, et al. Adenovirus expressing shRNA to IGF-1R enhances the chemosensitivity of lung cancer cell lines by blocking IGF-1 pathway. Lung Cancer 2007;55(3):279–86.

113. Cohen BD, Baker DA, Soderstrom C, et al. Combination therapy enhances the inhibition of tumor growth with the fully human anti-type 1 insulin-like growth factor receptor monoclonal antibody CP-751,871. Clin Cancer Res 2005;11(5):2063–73.

114. Iwasa T, Okamoto I, Suzuki M, et al. Inhibition of insulin-like growth factor 1 receptor by CP-751,871 radiosensitizes non-small cell lung cancer cells. Clin Cancer Res 2009;15(16):5117–25.

115. Karp DD, Pollak MN, Cohen RB, et al. Safety, pharmacokinetics, and pharmacodynamics of the insulin-like growth factor type 1 receptor inhibitor figitumumab (CP-751,871) in combination with paclitaxel and carboplatin. J Thorac Oncol 2009;4(11):1397–403.

116. Karp DD, Paz-Ares LG, Novello S, et al. Phase II study of the anti–insulin-like growth factor type 1 receptor antibody CP-751,871 in combination with paclitaxel and carboplatin in previously untreated, locally advanced, or metastatic non-small-cell lung cancer. J Clin Oncol 2009;27(15):2516–22.

117. Jassem J, Langer CJ, Karp DD, et al. Randomized, open label, phase III trial of figitumumab in combination with paclitaxel and carboplatin versus paclitaxel

and carboplatin in patients with non-small cell lung cancer (NSCLC). J Clin Oncol (ASCO Meeting Abstracts) 2010;28(Suppl 15):7500.

118. Sayer RA, Lancaster JM, Pittman J, et al. High insulin-like growth factor-2 (IGF-2) gene expression is an independent predictor of poor survival for patients with advanced stage serous epithelial ovarian cancer. Gynecol Oncol 2005;96(2): 355–61.

119. Ozols RF. Treatment goals in ovarian cancer. Int J Gynecol Cancer 2005; 15(Suppl 1):3–11.

120. Eckstein N, Servan K, Hildebrandt B, et al. Hyperactivation of the insulin-like growth factor receptor I signaling pathway is an essential event for cisplatin resistance of ovarian cancer cells. Cancer Res 2009;69(7):2996–3003.

121. Conover CA, Hartmann LC, Bradley S, et al. Biological characterization of human epithelial ovarian carcinoma cells in primary culture: the insulin-like growth factor system. Exp Cell Res 1998;238(2):439–49.

Insulin-Like Growth Factors in Normal and Diseased Kidney

Daniela Kiepe, MD*, Burkhard Tönshoff, MD, PhD

KEYWORDS

- IGF-system • Kidney disease • Pathophysiology • Treatment

KEY POINTS

- IGF-I is involved in the regulation of kidney development and growth, renal hemodynamics, and the regulation of certain tubular functions.
- Complex disturbances of the IGF system, which result in a functional IGF deficiency, play an important pathophysiological role in growth failure associated with chronic renal failure in children and in protein catabolism associated with end-stage renal disease.

INTRODUCTION

Insulin-like growth factor I (IGF-I) is a potent growth factor, exerting its actions by both endocrine and paracrine/autocrine mechanisms. The action of IGFs in the circulation and tissues is tightly regulated by a family of high-affinity IGF binding proteins (IGFBPs). Six distinct IGFBPs have been identified. Although structurally related, they have individual expression patterns and exert different functions, including stimulation or inhibition of IGF bioactivity, as well as IGF-independent actions.[1–3] The synthesis of the IGFBPs is also under control of IGF-I. IGF-I itself exerts its biologic effects by binding to the transmembrane type 1 IGF receptor, whose activation leads to the extensive tyrosyl-phosphorylation of insulin-receptor substrate-1, which acts as a docking protein for the downstream signal transduction pathways.[4,5] Two canonical pathways, the phosphatidylinositol-3 kinase (PI-3 kinase) and the p42/44 MAPK pathway, mediate the mitogenic, differentiating, and antiapoptotic response to IGF-I,[6] but the relative contributions to the diverse cellular actions of IGF-I vary according to the cell type.[7]

The expression of the components of the IGF system in the kidney is anatomically heterogeneous.[8,9] As elsewhere in the body, growth hormone (GH) is the major regulator for IGF-I expression in the kidney. Locally produced and circulating IGF-I has profound effects on renal structure and function, including modulation of tubular

The authors have nothing to disclose.

Department of Pediatrics I, University Children's Hospital Heidelberg, INF 430, D-69120 Heidelberg, Germany

* Corresponding author.

E-mail address: daniela.choukair@med.uni-heidelberg.de

Endocrinol Metab Clin N Am 41 (2012) 351–374

doi:10.1016/j.ecl.2012.04.015

0889-8529/12/$ – see front matter © 2012 Published by Elsevier Inc.

electrolyte transport, renal blood flow, glomerular hemodynamics, and stimulating kidney growth. Animal studies have demonstrated that IGF-I may play a role in renal regeneration after acute tubular necrosis.[10] A profound role for the IGF system has been suggested in the pathogenesis of kidney diseases, such as diabetic nephropathy, or the stimulation of compensatory kidney growth after unilateral nephrectomy.[11–13]

In this article, we review the physiology of the IGF system in the kidney and the changes and potential role of this system in selected renal diseases. Finally, we briefly discuss the potential therapeutic uses of recombinant human (rh) IGF-I for the treatment of acute and chronic kidney failure.

PHYSIOLOGY OF THE IGF SYSTEM IN THE KIDNEY
The IGF System in Renal Development

During human embryogenic development, the metanephros arises from the mesodermal nephrogenic cord and develops into the definitive kidney.[14] At about 8 weeks of gestation, nephron formation begins in the metanephros with small foci of condensed mesenchyme near the ureteric bud. This cell mass develops into an S-shaped body, of which the lower portion develops into the glomerulus. The upper portion of the S-shaped body gives rise to the proximal and distal convoluted segments and the loop of Henle.[15,16] At about the 11th week of gestation, metanephroic nephrons start functioning, and, postpartum, further development of the nephron occurs during the subsequent 3 to 4 weeks.[14]

Kidney development is highly regulated by specific growth factors, such as epidermal growth factor, transforming growth factors, platelet-derived growth factor, and also the insulin-like growth factors (IGFs). In fact, IGF-I is necessary for normal metanephric development,[17,18] because IGF-antisense oligonucleotide causes growth retardation of mouse nephroi organ culture, and also neutralizing antibodies to IGF-I and IGF-II inhibit the development and growth of rat metanephroi.[19–21] On the other hand, mouse metanephroi in organ culture become enlarged after exposure to IGF-I and the nephron population increases.[19] Hence, the IGF system is important for the development of the metanephros, but not for the differentiation of embryonic kidney mesenchyme into epithelium or interstitial cells.[22,23]

Rodent models illustrate the importance of the IGF-I system for kidney size. Mice with global overexpression of IGF-I exhibit renal and glomerular hypertrophy.[24–26] In IGF-I-transgenic, as well as in IGF-I-treated rodents, IGF-I stimulates renal growth to an approximately similar extent as it stimulates overall body growth.[24,27] In mice with global inactivation of the IGF-I gene that survive the postnatal period, the proportionally reduced kidney size is associated with reduced glomerular size and decreased numbers of nephrons.[28] The role of liver-derived circulating IGF-I for kidney size has been investigated in mice with liver-specific IGF-I knockout (KO).[29,30] Despite their secondary high circulating GH levels,[31] mice with liver-specific IGF-I KO had an absolute and relative decrease in kidney weight, however, with no alterations in kidney morphology, including the size, number, and distribution of renal structures. A microarray analysis of the kidneys of mice with liver-specific IGF-I KO revealed normal IGF-I mRNA levels, but a pronounced and tissue-specific decrease in renal IGF-II mRNA levels.[30] Given that mice overexpressing IGF-II have increased relative kidney weight,[32–34] and that postnatally elevated IGF-II selectively increased the kidney weight of total IGF-I KO mice,[34] it may be hypothesized that liver-derived circulating IGF-I increases renal IGF-II expression, resulting in symmetric renal growth.

During kidney development in the human fetus, IGF-II is greatly expressed at a gestational age of 8 to 14 weeks in the uninduced metanephric blastema and later on, formation of the S-shaped nephron is colocalized with IGFBP-2 and IGFBP-4.[35] In the maturing glomerulus, the glomerular epithelial cells express IGF-II mRNA together with IGFBP-2 and IGFBP-4 mRNAs. The renal mesenchyme in the cortex and medulla abundantly express IGF-II mRNA. Neonatal IGF-II transgenic mice exhibit a twofold to threefold increase in serum IGF-II and a significantly increased kidney weight.[32] These data indicate that IGF-II is important in the developing kidney. Interestingly, the renal IGF-II expression does not decrease postpartum, whereas it decreases in most other organs.[36]

The type 1 IGF receptor plays an important role during metanephric development. In mouse embryos maintained in organ culture, type 1 IGF receptor expression was at greatest density at day 13 of gestation, decreased thereafter, but was still present after birth.[37] Inhibition of the type 1 IGF receptor expression by antisense-oligodeoxynucleotide resulted in inhibition of kidney growth, reduction in nephron number, and disorganization of ureteric bud branching.[37,38] Hence, IGF-I acts through the type 1 IGF receptor during metanephros development.

The bioactivity of IGF-I during renal development is partially regulated by IGFBPs. In human fetuses at 14 to 18 weeks of gestation, particularly IGFBP-4, but also IGFBP-5 and IGFBP-6, are abundantly expressed in the kidney.[35,39,40] With induction by the ureteric duct, the aggregated metanephric blastema additionally expresses IGFBP-2 and IGFBP-4 mRNAs. The mature ureteric duct expresses IGFBP-3 mRNA, whereas the ampulla in contact with the metanephric blastema exclusively expresses IGFBP-2. On formation of the S-shape nephron, IGFBP-2 mRNA is expressed in the committed glomerular and epithelial cells, which also express IGF-II and IGFBP-4, whereas the mesenchyme of the vascular cleft expresses IGFBP-5 mRNA. In the maturing glomerulus, the glomerular epithelial cells express IGF-II mRNA together with IGFBP-2 and IGFBP-4, whereas IGFBP-5 mRNA is localized to the mesangium and supporting mesenchyme. As the proximal tubule is formed, the epithelium expresses less IGFBP-2 and more IGFBP-4. The renal mesenchyme in the cortex and medulla expresses abundant IGF-II and, to a lesser extent, IGFBP-4 and IGFBP-5. The epithelium of the collecting ducts and pelvicalyceal system exhibit abundant expression of IGFBP-3, but only low expression of IGF-I, IGFBP-1, and IGFBP-6. The specific temporal and spatial pattern of expression of IGFBP genes on the background of abundant IGF-II gene expression suggests that the IGFBP peptides, as modulators of IGF action, are expressed locally at specific points of nephrogenesis to interact with IGF-II to regulate mesenchymal induction, renal epithelial cell commitment, differentiation, and growth.[35]

Transgenic mice that constitutively overexpress rat IGFBP-1 exhibit normal kidney size.[41] Interestingly, mice transgenic for human IGFBP-1 show glomerular sclerosis and reduced nephron numbers.[42,43] Compared with the reduced body size of transgenic murine IGFBP-2 mice, kidney size was not reduced[44]; however, mice transgenic for human IGFBP-3 revealed small kidneys.[45,46] The kidney size of IGFBP-5 transgenic mice was also normal; in IGFBP-4 and IGFBP-6 transgenic mice, the kidneys were not investigated.[47,48] Only mice transgenic for IGFBP-1 and IGFBP-3 demonstrate a renal phenotype. Probably increased IGFBP-1 can contribute to kidney growth owing to mitogenic actions via binding to $\alpha_5\beta_1$-integrins. On the other hand, IGFBP-3, the most abundant IGFBP in serum, acts as an IGF inhibitor by competing with the type 1 IGF receptor for IGF binding, which likely contributes to the reduction in kidney size (**Table 1**).

Postnatal Expression and Regulation of the IGF System in the Kidney

The expression of the IGF system components in the kidney is highly organized with a specific distribution of each component among the different anatomic and functional segments of the nephron (**Fig. 1**).

Table 1
The concentration of intact IGFBPs and their respective fragments in CRF plasma, their correlation with parameters of longitudinal growth in children with CRF, their intrinsic and IGF-dependent effect on growth plate chondrocyte proliferation, and the effect of their respective overexpression on growth in transgenic animals

IGFBP	Concentration in CRF Plasma	Correlation to Growth in Clinical CRF	Kidney in Transgenic Animals	
			Size	Morphology
Intact IGFBP-1	Increased[129,149]	Negative[129]	Normal[41]	Reduced nephron size; glomerular sclerosis[41]
Intact IGFBP-2	Increased[129,149]	Negative[129,149]	Normal[44]	ND
C-terminal fragmented IGFBP-2	Increased[164]	ND	ND	ND
Intact IGFBP-3	Normal[149,165]	None[a,149,165]	Reduced[45,46]	ND
IGFBP-3[29]	Increased[166]	ND	ND	ND
Intact IGFBP-4	Increased[130,167]	Negative[130]	ND	ND
IGFBP-4[1−122]	+[168]	ND	ND	ND
IGFBP-4[136−237]	+[168]	ND	ND	ND
Intact IGFBP-5	Normal[a,130,167]	Positive[a,130,167]	Normal[48]	ND
IGFBP-5[1−169]	ND	ND	ND	ND
IGFBP-5[144−252]	+[169]	ND	ND	ND
Intact IGFBP-6	Increased[170]	None[170]	ND	ND

Abbreviations: CRF, chronic renal failure; IGFBP, insulin-like growth factor binding protein; +, fragments present; ND, not done.
[a] Immunoreactive IGFBP levels.

Data from Tönshoff B, Kiepe D, Ciarmatori S. Growth hormone/insulin-like growth factor system in children with chronic renal failure. Pediatr Nephrol 2005;20:279–89.

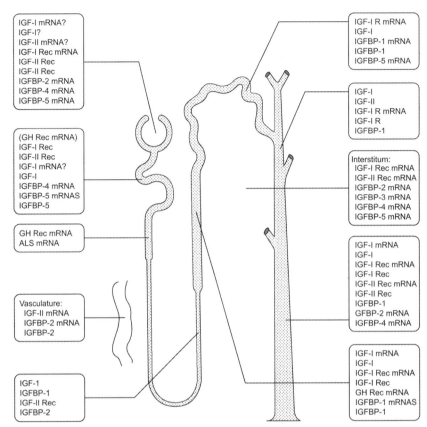

Fig. 1. Expression of GH receptors and of IGF system components in the rat nephron. The figure differentiates between protein and mRNAs. The presence of the latter suggests in situ synthesis. ?, in vitro finding, but not confirmed in in vivo studies; ALS, acid-labile subunit; Rec, receptor. (*Data from* Feld S, Hirschberg R. Growth hormone, the insulin-like growth factor system, and the kidney. Endocr Rev 1996;17:423–80.)

Because IGF-I is expressed in the kidney and the IGF-I concentration is greater in renal venous than in arterial blood, it is obvious that the kidney synthesizes this growth factor.[49] The amount of IGF-I protein extracted from the kidney is comparable to that in liver, whereas the IGF-I mRNA content of the liver is 10-fold higher compared with kidney.[50] This suggests that the major fraction of IGF-I in the kidney is derived from the circulation and is trapped in the kidney by surface receptors or by specific IGFBPs.

All components of the IGF system beside IGF-II and IGFBP-6 are expressed in the human glomerulus.[9,51–53] Also glomerular podocytes express IGF-I and the type 1 IGF receptor. Hence, IGF-I by its autocrine/paracrine mode of action likely plays an important role in podocyte migration, differentiation, and survival. The expression of type 1 IGF receptors, which is more dense in the glomerulus than in any other part of the nephron, provides the basis for the biologic effects of IGF-I on glomerular structure and function. In the proximal tubulus of rats, IGF-I is not expressed under physiologic circumstances, although it becomes transiently expressed in regenerating proximal tubules after acute injury.[54,55] Because IGF-I protein is detected along the brush border and the basolateral membrane of the proximal tubules, it is derived probably from glomerular ultrafiltration, paracrine synthesis, or peritubular circulation and has undergone receptor binding to exert its action on proximal tubule cells.[56] In rat proximal tubules, IGFBP-4 and IGFBP-5 are expressed.[8,57] In the thick ascending limb of the loop of Henle of the rat IGF-I, IGF-I receptor, and IGFBP-1 mRNA are expressed.[56,58] Distal tubular cells do not express IGF-I or IGF-II mRNA, but express the type 1 IGF receptor mRNA and IGFBP mRNA in a species-specific manner (in rat kidney, IGFBP-1 and IGFBP-5; in human kidney, IGFBP-2).[8,53,56,59] Rat collecting ducts express mRNA species for the type 1 and the type 2 IGF receptors and in addition for several IGFBPs (IGFBP-1 in rat cortical, IGFBP-2 and IGFBP-4 in rat medullary, IGFBP-2 in human cortical and medullary collecting duct).[8,9,52,53,60]

In summary, the type 1 IGF receptor is ubiquitously expressed in the kidney, whereas IGF-I expression itself is found predominantly in the loop of Henle. The strikingly heterogeneous expression of all 6 IGFBPs suggests their function of trapping IGF-I and modulating its action in the kidney. It is noteworthy that the detected IGF-I protein in the kidney derives from endogenous synthesis, but also from trapping of circulating or ultrafiltrated IGF-I by IGF receptors or specific IGFBPs.

Renal Handling of the IGFs and IGFBPs

The glomerular capillary wall and basement membrane constitutes a size-selective ultrafiltration barrier, allowing free ultrafiltration of proteins smaller than 10 kD. Larger peptides and proteins are ultrafiltrated according to their molecular size. Ultrafiltrated proteins are reabsorbed in the proximal tubules via endocytosis and undergo endocytotic uptake and lysosomal degradation in tubular cells. Only exiguous amounts of filtered proteins are excreted in the urine.[61]

Although IGF-I and IGF-II are small proteins with a respective molecular size of 7.6 kD, the amount of glomerular ultrafiltration under normal circumstances is very low, because 98% of IGFs in the circulation are bound to IGFBPs in 45-kD and 150-kD complexes. Most of the IGFs are complexed with IGFBP-3 together with an acid-labile subunit in the 150-kD ternary complex, a lesser amount of IGFs bind to IGFBP-1, IGFBP-2, IGFBP-4, and IGFBP-6 and build a 45-kD complex. Because of their larger size, these complexes are filtered through the glomerulus at much slower rates than free IGF peptides. In humans, urinary IGF-II excretion is several fold higher than that of IGF-I because of the higher IGF-II serum concentration.[62] The rate of urinary excretion is greatest in prepubertal children and tends to decline with age.[63]

Animal studies with labeled IGF-I demonstrated that renal extraction and degradation of IGF-I occur via glomerular filtration with receptor-mediated uptake of filtered IGF-I from the tubular lumen and also by uptake from peritubular capillaries through the basolateral tubular cell membrane.[64] A small amount of the internalized IGF-I may also be transported into the cell nucleus.[65] The IGFBPs that predominantly appear in the urine, although in small quantities, are IGFBP-1, IGFBP-2, and IGFBP-3, reflecting their greater abundance in serum.[62,66] In patients with glomerular diseases, the excretion of IGF/IGFBP complexes is increased[63,66,67] (see section titled "Nephrotic syndrome").

Renal Effects of the IGFs

Glomerular hemodynamics

In humans and rats, IGF-I infusion increases renal plasma flow and glomerular filtration rate (GFR) by 20% to 30% and decreases renal vascular resistance (**Fig. 2**).[68–71] In single-nephron micropuncture studies in rats, IGF-I infusion decreases the afferent and efferent arteriolar resistance, resulting in an increase of GFR, probably because of an expansion and relaxing of mesangial cells determining the surface area available for ultrafiltration.[72] Several experiments showed that IGF-I mediates its effects on glomerular hemodynamics via the type 1 IGF receptor and secondarily enhanced nitric oxide synthesis that mediates the generation of cyclic GMP.[73–76] In a number of

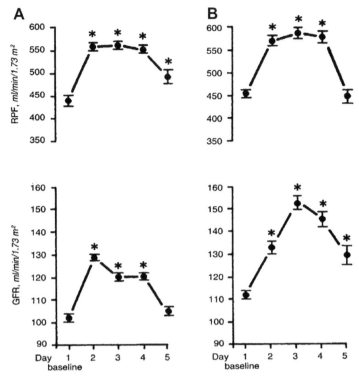

Fig. 2. IGF-I administration acutely raises renal plasma flow (RPF) and GFR in healthy human subjects without (*A*) and with (*B*) volume expansion by salt loading. Recombinant human IGF-I was administered subcutaneously on days 2 to 4. Mean ± SEM of GFR and RPF in the healthy (*A*) and saline-loaded healthy subjects (*B*); *P<.05 versus baseline. (*Reprinted from* Hirschberg R, Brunori G, Kopple JD, et al. Effects of insulin-like growth factor I on renal function in normal men. Kidney Int 1993;43:387–97; with permission.)

physiologic and pathophysiological circumstances of elevated circulating IGF-I, such as acromegalia, pregnancy, and during a high-protein diet, GFR is increased.[77] On the other hand, in chronic conditions associated with low serum IGF-I owing to isolated GH-deficiency, panhypopituitarism, GH-receptor defects (Laron dwarfism), or malnutrition, GFR is reduced.[77] In concert, these observations suggest a role of IGF-I in the maintenance of an adequate GFR.

Tubular functions
The expression of the type 1 IGF receptor in tubules is limited to the proximal, distal, and collecting tubules in both the apical and basolateral membrane providing a mechanism for IGF-I to mediate its biologic effects on tubular function. Published data have been focused on the IGF-I effect on phosphate and sodium/water reabsorption, whereas much less information is available on tubular absorption of other minerals and/or organic compounds.[78–82] Observations from patients with GH-receptor defects (Laron dwarfism) or from interventional human or animal studies indicate that IGF-I increases tubular phosphate reabsorption.[72,79,82–85] The IGF-I effect on tubular phosphate reabsorption is mediated via the type 1 IGF receptor, which is more densely expressed on the apical than on the basolateral membrane.[85] Absorption of ultrafiltrated phosphate from the tubular lumen occurs via a specific sodium-phosphate cotransporter in the

brush border membrane on proximal tubule cells. This sodium-phosphate cotrans-porter is activated independently by phosphate depletion, parathyroid hormone, and IGF-I.[86–88]

IGF-I increases sodium and water retention and this accounts for transient edema formation especially in diabetic patients treated with IGF-I.[79,89–92] In patients, short-term infusion of rhIGF-I results in a decrease of fractional sodium excretion.[80,93] Examination of the underlying mechanisms showed that sodium reabsorption is not mediated via the sodium cotransporters in the proximal tubule, but rather via the amilorid-sensitive apical sodium channel in the distal tubule.[85,94] Another mechanism accounting for sodium and water retention during IGF-I therapy is probably decreased atrial natriuretic peptide secretion and stimulated release of renin.[95]

Renal growth

Loss of renal mass is followed by compensatory renal growth, a process thought to be mediated through local growth factors, such as IGF-I. In transgenic mice models with overexpression of IGF-I, kidney and glomerular size are increased.[26,59,96–99] Increased renal mass in response to IGF-I is a result of hypertrophy of all segments of the nephron (most prominently of the proximal tubule), and also hyperplasia of glomerular and interstitial cells.[97–99]

Because IGF-I promotes renal growth, it may also be involved in compensatory kidney growth after loss of renal mass. For example, after uninephrectomy in adult rats, the IGF-I content in the remaining kidney increases early and returns to baseline after 4 days.[60,100–102] Most of the studies fail to demonstrate a concomitant increase in kidney IGF-I gene expression.[102–104] Increased type 1 IGF receptor expression and membrane-associated IGFBP-5 in the glomerulus and in proximal tubules 1 month after unilateral nephrectomy may contribute to hypertrophy of the proximal part of the nephron.[105] The expression of IGFBP-2, IGFBP-3, and IGFBP-5 are reduced in the setting of compensatory renal growth.[106]

Administration of an antagonist to the type 1 IGF receptor inhibits early compensa-tory renal growth and compensatory hyperfiltration after loss of renal mass, again underlying the important role of IGF-I in promoting compensatory renal growth.[107,108]

The response to loss of renal mass differs between immature and mature rats. First, the renal response in adult rats comprises predominantly cellular hypertrophy, whereas in weaning rats, hyperplasia prevails.[105,106] Second, in immature rats, IGF-I and type 1 IGF receptor expression is increased, especially in the ascending loop of Henle, but not in adult rats.[106,109] Third, in immature rat kidneys IGFBP-3, IGFBP-4, and IGFBP-5 mRNA expression is increased in compensatory renal growth, accompanied by an increase in plasma membrane–associated IGFBPs.[106] In summary, the intrarenal IGF system plays an important role in adaptive renal growth, especially in immature kidneys, where IGF-I accounts for the hyperplasia ongoing 1 week after unilateral nephrectomy, whereas the prevailing hypertrophy in adult kidneys appears to be independent of IGF-I.

THE IGF SYSTEM IN SELECTED RENAL DISEASES
Acute Renal Failure

Acute renal failure (ARF) results from ischemic or toxic acute kidney injury preferentially to cells of the proximal convoluted tubules and of the ascending limb of the loop of Henle, leading to cell apoptosis or necrosis.[110] During the first few days after an ischemic insult in rats, renal expression of IGF-I, the type 1 IGF receptor, and of IGFBP-2 through IGFBP-5 are downregulated.[54,55,111,112] After 2 to 3 days of recovery, regenerative cells, particularly in the proximal tubule, express transiently IGF-I mRNA, IGF-I peptide is detectable,[55,113] and the type 1 IGF receptor is upregulated.[55,112]

Because in the rat model of ARF IGF-I regulates tissue repair by increasing glomerular blood flow, stimulating tubular cell proliferation, and inhibiting apoptosis, this peptide hormone appears promising for treatment of ARF.[113] Indeed, in several rat models, rhIGF-I or des(1–3)IGF-I treatment results in accelerated recovery from ischemic ARF (**Fig. 3**).[114–117] Treatment with rhIGF-I has no effect on the expression of the type 1 IGF receptor. These promising experimental results initiated several clinical trials of IGF-I treatment in the setting of acute renal failure in humans. In a multicenter placebo-controlled study including 72 patients with severe ARF, rhIGF-I therapy did not accelerate recovery of renal function.[113] In a single-center study including 54 patients after heart surgery, prophylactic rhIGF-I treatment was associated with a smaller postoperative decline in renal function (22%) compared with placebo-treated controls (33%).[118] There were no significant differences in levels of serum creatinine at time of discharge, length of hospital stay, length of intensive care unit stay, length of intubation, or incidence of dialysis or death. The lack of effectiveness of rhIGF-I treatment in humans on recovery of ARF compared with the results in rats remains unclear and needs further investigation.

Chronic Renal Failure

Disturbances of the somatotropic hormone axis play an important pathogenic role in growth retardation in children with chronic kidney disease (CKD) and contribute to protein catabolism in adults with CKD. Multiple alterations of this hormone axis, both in the setting of clinical and experimental chronic renal failure (CRF), have been described. Random fasting serum levels of GH are normal or increased in children and adults with CRF, depending on the extent of renal failure.[119–121] The apparent discrepancy between normal or elevated GH levels and diminished longitudinal growth in CKD has led to the concept of GH insensitivity, which is caused by complex alterations in the distal components of the somatotropic hormone axis. Serum levels of IGF-I and IGF-II are normal in preterminal chronic renal failure, whereas in end-stage renal disease (ESRD) IGF-I levels are slightly decreased and IGF-II levels are slightly increased. In view of the prevailing elevated GH levels in ESRD, these serum IGF-I levels appear inadequately low. Indeed, there is both clinical and experimental

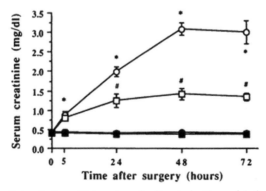

Fig. 3. Serum creatinine before (0 hour) and after induction of ischemic ARF or sham surgery. Treatment with rhIGF-I or vehicle was begun, after the measurement at 5 hours was obtained. o, ARF + vehicle; ●, sham + vehicle; □, ARF + rhIGF-I; ■, sham + rhIGF-I. * P<.05 versus sham + rhIGF-I or sham + vehicle; # P<.05 versus ARF + vehicle. (*Reprinted from* Ding H, Kopple JD, Cohen A, et al. Recombinant human insulin-like growth factor-I accelerates recovery and reduces catabolism in rats with ischemic acute renal failure. J Clin Invest 1993:91:2281–7; with permission.)

evidence for decreased hepatic production of IGF-I in CRF.[122] This hepatic insensitivity to the action of GH may be partly the consequence of reduced GH receptor expression in liver tissue and partly a consequence of disturbed GH receptor signaling.[123–125]

Although total immunoreactive IGF levels in CRF serum are normal, IGF bioactivity, measured by sulfate incorporation into porcine costal cartilage, is markedly reduced.[126,127] Similarly, the level of free IGF-I is reduced by 50% in relation to the degree of renal dysfunction.[128] This finding is one of the key abnormalities of the GH/IGF axis in children with CRF.

The discrepancy between normal total immunoreactive IGF levels and decreased IGF bioactivity has been explained by the presence of IGF inhibitors in CRF serum. Uremic serum contains low molecular weight (about 1 kDa) IGF inhibitors, the molecular structures of which have not yet been defined.[126] The prevailing inhibitory effect on IGF bioactivity in CRF serum is because of an excess of high-affinity IGFBPs. CRF serum has an IGF-binding capacity that is increased by 7-fold to 10-fold, leading to decreased IGF bioactivity of CRF serum despite normal total IGF levels.

Serum levels of intact IGFBP-1, IGFBP-2, IGFBP-4, IGFBP-6, and low molecular weight fragments of IGFBP-3 are elevated in CRF serum in relation to the degree of renal dysfunction, whereas serum levels of intact IGFBP-3 are normal. Levels of immunoreactive IGFBP-5 are not altered in CRF serum, but most IGFBP-5 is fragmented (**Fig. 4**). Decreased renal filtration and increased hepatic production of IGFBP-1 and IGFBP-2 both contribute to high levels of serum IGFBP.[129]

The underlying mechanisms of increased IGFBP serum level in CRF are multiple. The inverse correlation of IGFBP-1, IGFBP-2, IGFBP-4, and IGFBP-6 serum levels with GFR indicate a reduced elimination of IGFBPs in CRF.[130] The reason for the increased concentration of proteolytic fragments of IGFBP-3 in CRF serum is probably reduced renal filtration by the diseased kidneys. Increased proteolytic activity toward IGFBP-3 in serum, which is found in pregnancy and various catabolic states, seems not to be operative in patients with CRF.[131,132]

Experimental and clinical evidence suggests that the accumulation of high-affinity IGFBPs in CRF serum inhibit IGF action in growth plate chondrocytes by competition with the type 1 IGF receptor for IGF binding (**Figs. 5** and **6**).[133,134] These data indicate

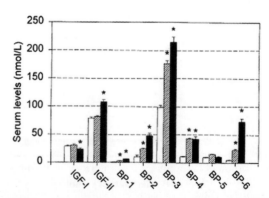

Fig. 4. Comparison of the molar serum concentrations of IGFs and IGFBPs in children with preterminal CRF (*hatched bars*) and children with ESRD (*filled bars*). The respective mean molar concentration in normal age-matched children is given in open bars for comparison. Data are means ± SEM. Statistics by analysis of variance. *$P<.05$ versus control. (*Reprinted from* Ulinski T, Mohan S, Kiepe D, et al. Serum insulin-like growth factor binding protein (IGFBP)-4 and IGFBP-5 in children with chronic renal failure: relationship to growth and glomerular filtration rate. Pediatr Nephrol 2000;14:589–97; with permission.)

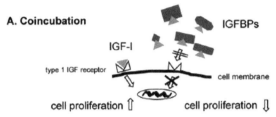

Fig. 5. Effect of IGFBP-3 in growth plate chondrocytes. Coincubation of IGFBP-3 with IGF-I inhibits cell proliferation by preventing binding of IGF-I to the type 1 IGF receptor. (*Reprinted from* Tönshoff B, Kiepe D, Ciarmatori S. Growth hormone/insulin-like growth factor system in children with chronic renal failure. Pediatr Nephrol 2005;20:279–89; with permission.)

that growth failure in CRF is mainly caused by functional IGF deficiency. Combined therapy with rhGH and rhIGF-I is therefore a logical approach.

Nephrotic Syndrome

The nephrotic syndrome is characterized by hypoalbuminemia, proteinuria, hypercholesterolemia, and/or hypertriglyceridemia. It results from various glomerular diseases, such as minimal change disease, focal-segmental glomerular sclerosis, diabetic glomerular sclerosis, various forms of glomerulonephritis, and others. As a result of damage to the glomerular filter, consisting of podocytes, the slit membrane, and the basement membrane, which serve as a size-selective ultrafiltration barrier, urinary loss of plasma

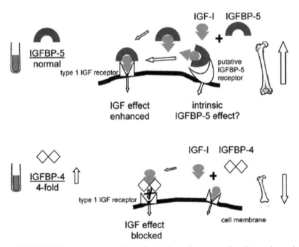

Fig. 6. IGFBP-4 and IGFBP-5 have contrasting functions in growth plate chondrocytes. IGFBP-4 levels are elevated fourfold in CRF serum and negatively correlated with longitudinal growth in children with chronic kidney disease. Both intact IGFBP-4 and the fragment IGFBP-4$^{1-122}$ have exclusive inhibitory roles in IGF-I–stimulated cells by binding IGF-I in the N-terminal domain and preventing or reducing the binding of the ligand to its signaling receptor. Serum levels of IGFBP-5 are normal and positively correlated with longitudinal growth in children with CRF. IGFBP-5 enhances IGF-I action in the growth plate, apparently by its association with the cell membrane in the C-terminal domain, thereby better presenting IGF-I to its receptor. IGFBP-5 also stimulates chondrocyte cell proliferation in the absence of exogenous IGF-I, probably by modulating endogenous IGF-I or by binding with its C-terminal domain to a specific IGFBP-5 receptor. (*Reprinted from* Tönshoff B, Kiepe D, Ciarmatori S. Growth hormone/insulin-like growth factor system in children with chronic renal failure. Pediatr Nephrol 2005;20:279–89; with permission.)

proteins and compounds bound to serum proteins occurs.[135] In patients with the nephrotic syndrome, urinary excretion of IGF-I, IGF-II, IGFBP-1, IGFBP-2, and IGFBP-3 is increased[136] and therefore serum levels of IGF-I and IGF-II are reduced by 50% and 60%, respectively.[67] In the setting of experimental nephrotic syndrome in adriamycin-treated rats, serum IGF-I levels are reduced by one-third without an increased hepatic expression of IGF-I, which could potentially compensate for the urinary IGF-I loss.[137] Serum levels of IGFBP-3 are reduced because of urinary losses and possibly because of increased protease activity toward IGFBP-3. Serum IGFBP-2 levels are increased owing to increased hepatic IGFBP-2 mRNA expression.[137] In summary, in the nephrotic syndrome, there is considerably more IGF-I bound in the 45-kD binary complex compared with the 150-kD ternary complex, as observed under physiologic conditions. Furthermore, the increased concentration of IGF-I in the ultrafiltrate in the nephrotic syndrome may stimulate the secretion of profibrotic cytokines and collagen types I and IV by proximal tubular cells and thereby contribute to progression of interstitial fibrosis and glomerular sclerosis, which is commonly found in patients with glomerular diseases.

Diabetic Nephropathy

Diabetic kidney disease is characterized by an early increase in kidney size, glomerular volume, and later by the development of mesangial proliferation, accumulation of glomerular extracellular matrix, increased urinary albumin excretion, and glomerular sclerosis, leading to diminished kidney function.[138] In experimental diabetic kidney disease, renal hypertrophy is associated with increased tissue concentration of IGF-I.[139] Further evidence that IGF-I acts as a renotropic growth factor is given by experiments with GH-deficient diabetic dwarf mice. In these animals, IGF-I serum concentration is reduced, and these diabetic dwarf mice exhibit slower and lesser initial renal and glomerular hypertrophy as well as a smaller increase in renal IGF-I compared with diabetic controls.[140] Furthermore, diabetic dwarf rats with diabetes duration of 6 months display a smaller increase in urinary albumin excretion, indicating that IGF-I may be involved in the development of diabetic kidney changes. Type 1 IGF receptor expression is significantly increased in the diabetic kidney; this overexpression in conjunction with the increased IGF-I bioavailability in diabetic nephropathy explains the increased bioactivity of IGF-I at the glomerular level.[141]

The following observations have been made regarding the renal expression of IGFBPs in the diabetic rat model. In the early phase of diabetic nephropathy, medullary IGFBP-1 mRNA is remarkably reduced, whereas cortical IGFBP-1 gene expression is markedly upregulated; this finding persists for up to 6 months (**Table 2**).[142] Interestingly, IGFBP-1 transgenic mice develop glomerulosclerosis without glomerular hypertrophy.[42,43] Probably increased IGFBP-1 can contribute to kidney growth owing to mitogenic actions via $\alpha_5\beta_1$-integrins.[77] Furthermore, in human diabetic kidneys, IGFBP-2 expression is downregulated in glomeruli suggesting a higher bioavailability of IGFs.[143]

In humans with diabetic nephropathy, the extent of urinary IGFBP-3 excretion correlates positively with albuminuria.[144] In addition, the urinary protease activity toward IGFBP-3 is increased and leads to a higher urinary concentration of the 18-kD IGFBP-3 fragment. It has been hypothesized that the increased urinary proteolytic cleavage of IGFBP-3 leads to higher bioavailability of IGF-I in the tubular fluid, which may contribute to the development of diabetic nephropathy.[145]

THERAPEUTIC IMPLICATIONS

GH therapy is an established therapy for short stature and growth retardation associated with CRF in children.[146–148] GH therapy in pharmacologic doses (ie, 0.05 mg/kg

Table 2
Schematic depiction of short- and long-term changes in the renal GH/IGF axis in experimental diabetes

Renal Expression	Short-term Diabetes	Long-term Diabetes
GHR mRNA	Unchanged	Unchanged
GHBP mRNA	Unchanged	Increased
IGF-I mRNA	Unchanged or decreased	Decreased
IGF-I	Increased	Unchanged
IGF-I receptor	Unchanged	?
IGF-I receptor mRNA	Unchanged	Increased
IGF-II/Man-6-P receptor	Increased	?
IGF-II/Man-6-P receptor mRNA	Increased	Unchanged
IGFBP-1 mRNA	Increased	Increased
IGFBP-2 mRNA	Unchanged	Unchanged
IGFBP-3 mRNA	Unchanged	Unchanged
IGFBP-4 mRNA	Decreased	Decreased
IGFBP-5 mRNA	Increased	Increased

Abbreviations: ?, not done; GHBP, growth hormone binding protein; GHR, growth hormone receptor; IGFBP, insulin-like growth factor binding protein.
Data from Flyvbjerg A, Landau D, Domene H, et al. The role of growth hormone, insulin-like growth factors (IGFs), and IGF-binding proteins in experimental diabetic kidney disease. Metabolism 1995;44:67–71.

body weight per day), increases serum IGF-I levels in children with CRF[149–152] and this increase is positively correlated with longitudinal growth[149]; however, in this article we focus on IGF-I therapy. Treatment with rhIGF-I stimulates linear growth in children with severe IGF-I deficiency owing to GH insensitivity.[153] As described previously, children with chronic renal failure exhibit a severe growth disturbance, mainly because of a functional IGF-I deficiency and GH resistance.[154] From the pathophysiological point, IGF-I therapy should correct the relative IGF deficiency in uremia. Indeed, treatment with exogenous IGF-I was effective in stimulating growth in experimental uremia in subtotally nephrectomized rats[155]; however, combined treatment with rhIGF-I and rhGH has additive effects on the stimulation of longitudinal growth and prevents hypoglycemia that is associated with rhIGF-I therapy alone (**Fig. 7**). In the growth plate of subtotally nephrectomized rats, combined treatment with rhIGF-I and rhGH enlarged hypertrophic chondrocytes and increased growth plate width.[156] Despite these promising results in animals, no data are available on treatment with rhIGF-I alone or in combination with rhGH in growth-retarded children with chronic renal failure. Clearly, rhIGF merits further investigation as a potential drug to improve the growth disorder associated with CKD.

RhIGF-I has also been investigated for treatment of malnutrition and catabolism in patients with ESRD on maintenance hemodialysis, because GH and IGF-I may each affect protein balance by different mechanisms: GH administration to healthy volunteers causes an increase in protein synthesis but does not significantly inhibit proteolysis[157] and the predominant mechanism that mediates the response to IGF-I infusion appears to be inhibition of proteolysis.[158] In one study, for example, in 8 well-nourished adults with end-stage renal failure, rhIGF-I administration at a moderate dose had no effect on protein metabolism, but the combination of a moderate dose of rhIGF-I and rhGH was followed by a significant anabolic response.[159] This strategy

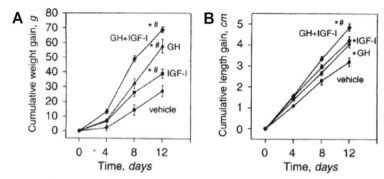

Fig. 7. Effect of combined treatment for 12 days with maximally effective doses of rhGH and of rhIGF-I on weight gain and length gain in uremic animals. Both 10 IU rhGH/kg/d and 4 mg rhIGF-I/kg/d increased mean cumulative weight gain (*A*) and length gain (*B*) compared with solvent controls. Coadministration of both hormones increased weight gain and length gain more than each single hormone. The growth-stimulating effect was nearly additive if one analyzes the growth-stimulating effects above baseline. Symbols are ◆, GH + IGF-I; ▲, GH; ■, IGF-I; ●, control. Data are given as means ± SEM. *Significant versus vehicle; #significant versus the other treatment modalities. (*Reprinted from* Kovacs GT, Oh J, Kovacs J, et al. Growth promoting effects of growth hormone and IGF-I are additive in experimental uremia. Kidney Int 1996;49:1413–21; with permission.)

may have the advantage of limiting the potential side effects of a higher dose of rhIGF-I and might be more suitable for an extended period of use in frail malnourished patients on dialysis.

In healthy volunteers, IGF-I therapy promptly increases GFR and affects renal plasma flow.[97] High-dose IGF-I therapy enhances GFR also in patients with end-stage chronic renal failure, but after stopping treatment the clearance values return to baseline.[160] The renal size does not change under IGF-I therapy. Serum IGFBP-3 drops in response to rhIGF-I therapy, whereas IGFBP-1 and IGFBP-2 levels increase during therapy, changes that affect the bioavailability of IGF-I; therefore, tachyphylaxis occurs. Side effects, such as Bell palsy, pericarditis, and gingival hypertrophy, prompted discontinuation of rhIGF-I therapy in this study.[161] In addition, concerns have been raised that IGF-I therapy in humans is not without risk regarding the development of malignancy.[162] To prevent tachyphylaxis, another study was conducted over a 24-week observation period in patients with advanced CKD who were not diabetic, who received rhIGF-I in a dosage of 50 μg/kg 4 days per week.[163] Although this intermittent rhIGF-I therapy elevated total serum IGF-I and prevented any fall in serum IGFBP-3, it failed to increase GFR in these patients with advanced CKD. This lack of efficacy was attributed to the presence of renal IGF-I resistance in CKD.[163]

SUMMARY

Components of the IGF system are expressed in the kidney in a heterogeneous manner. IGF-I is involved in the regulation of kidney development and growth, renal hemodynamics, and the regulation of certain tubular functions. The regulation of renal IGF-I levels is complex and includes changes of locally produced IGF-I, changes of IGF-I trapped from the circulation owing to altered type 1 IGF-receptor and IGFBP expression, and increased proteolysis of IGFBPs. Furthermore, IGF-I contributes to the pathomechanism of several renal diseases, such as diabetic nephropathy. It is a major determinant of recovery in acute renal failure. Complex disturbances of the IGF system, which result in a functional IGF deficiency, play an important pathophysiological role in growth failure associated with CRF in children and in protein catabolism associated with ESRD. Although in experimental uremia, combined therapy of rhIGF-I and rhGH was superior compared with rhGH therapy alone regarding the stimulation of longitudinal growth, clinical studies in children with uremic growth failure have not yet been performed. Clinical studies with rhIGF-I for enhancement of recovery after acute renal failure have been unsuccessful. Also in the setting of CRF, clinical studies with rhIGF-I for stimulation of GFR have been unsuccessful. Hence, the therapeutic use of rhIGF-I in patients with renal diseases appears rather unlikely.

REFERENCES

1. Baxter RC. Insulin-like growth factor (IGF)-binding proteins: interactions with IGFs and intrinsic bioactivities. Am J Physiol Endocrinol Metab 2000;278: E967–76.
2. Jones JI, Clemmons DR. Insulin-like growth factors and their binding proteins: biological actions. Endocr Rev 1995;16:3–34.
3. Schneider MR, Wolf E, Hoeflich A, et al. IGF-binding protein-5: flexible player in the IGF system and effector on its own. J Endocrinol 2003;172:423–40.
4. Parrizas M, Saltiel AR, LeRoith D. Insulin-like growth factor 1 inhibits apoptosis using the phosphatidylinositol 3'-kinase and mitogen-activated protein kinase pathways. J Biol Chem 1997;272:154–61.
5. Tsakiridis T, Tsiani E, Lekas P, et al. Insulin, insulin-like growth factor-I and platelet-derived growth factor activate extracellular signal-regulated kinase by distinct pathways in muscle cells. Biochem Biophys Res Commun 2001;288: 205–11.
6. Grey A, Chen Q, Xu X, et al. Parallel phosphatidylinositol-3 kinase and p42/44 mitogen-activated protein kinase signaling pathways subserve the mitogenic and antiapoptotic actions of insulin-like growth factor I in osteoblastic cells. Endocrinology 2003;144:4886–93.
7. Petley T, Graff K, Jiang W, et al. Variation among cell types in the signaling pathways by which IGF-I stimulates specific cellular responses. Horm Metab Res 1998;31:70–6.
8. Rabkin R, Brody M, Lu LH, et al. Expression of the genes encoding the rat renal insulin-like growth factor-I system. J Am Soc Nephrol 1995;6:1511–8.
9. Chin E, Bondy C. Insulin-like growth factor system gene expression in the human kidney. J Clin Endocrinol Metab 1992;75:962–8.
10. Rabkin R. Insulin-like growth factor-I treatment of acute renal failure. J Lab Clin Med 1995;125:684–5.
11. Flyvbjerg A. Putative pathophysiological role of growth factors and cytokines in experimental diabetic kidney disease. Diabetologia 2000;43:1205–23.
12. Flyvbjerg A. Potential use of growth hormone receptor antagonist in the treatment of diabetic kidney disease. Growth Horm IGF Res 2001;11(Suppl A): S115–9.
13. Rabkin R, Fervenza FC. Renal hypertrophy and kidney disease in diabetes. Diabetes Metab Rev 1996;12:217–41.
14. Tisher C, Madsen K. Anatomy of the kidney. In: Brenner B, Recotr F, editors. The kidney. Philadelphia: W.B. Saunders Co; 1985. p. 3–60.
15. Osthanondh V, Potter E. Development of the human kidney as shown by microdissection. III. Formation and interrelationship of collecting tubules and nephrons. Arch Pathol 1963;76:290.

16. Osthanondh V, Potter E. Development of the human kidney as shown by microdissection. II. Renal pelvis, calyces, and papillae. Arch Pathol 1963;76:227.

17. Hammerman MR, Ryan G, Miller SB. Expression of insulin-like growth factor in adult and embryonic kidney. Miner Electrolyte Metab 1992;18:253–5.

18. Rogers SA, Ryan G, Hammerman MR. Insulin-like growth factors I and II are produced in the metanephros and are required for growth and development in vitro. J Cell Biol 1991;113:1447–53.

19. Liu ZZ, Kumar A, Wallner EL, et al. Trophic effect of insulin-like growth factor-I on metanephric development: relationship to proteoglycans. Eur J Cell Biol 1994; 65:378–91.

20. Rogers SA, Ryan G, Hammerman MR. Metanephric transforming growth factor-α is required for renal organogenesis in vitro. Am J Physiol 1992;262:F533–9.

21. Hammerman MR, Rogers SA, Ryan G. Growth factors and kidney development. Pediatr Nephrol 1993;7:616–20.

22. Kanwar YS, Liu ZZ, Wada J. Insulin-like growth factor-I receptor in metanephric development. Contrib Nephrol 1994;107:168–73.

23. Cascieri MA, Chicchi GG, Bayne ML. Characterization of the biological activity of IGF-I analogs with reduced affinity for IGF receptors and binding proteins. Adv Exp Med Biol 1991;293:23–30.

24. Mathews LS, Hammer RE, Behringer RR, et al. Growth enhancement of transgenic mice expressing human insulin-like growth factor I. Endocrinology 1988; 123:2827–33.

25. Quaife CJ, Mathews LS, Pinkert CA, et al. Histopathology associated with elevated levels of growth hormone and insulin-like growth factor I in transgenic mice. Endocrinology 1989;124:40–8.

26. Doi T, Striker LJ, Gibson CC, et al. Glomerular lesions in mice transgenic for growth hormone and insulin-like growth factor-I. I. Relationship between increased glomerular size and mesangial sclerosis. Am J Pathol 1990;137: 541–52.

27. Guler HP, Zapf J, Scheiwiller E, et al. Recombinant human insulin-like growth factor I stimulates growth and has distinct effects on organ size in hypophysectomised rats. Proc Natl Acad Sci U S A 1988;85:4889–93.

28. Rogers SA, Powell-Braxton L, Hammerman MR. Insulin-like growth factor I regulates renal development in rodents. Dev Genet 1999;24:293–8.

29. Sjogren K, Liu JL, Blad K, et al. Liver-derived insulin-like growth factor I (IGF-I) is the principal source of IGF-I in blood but is not required for postnatal body growth in mice. Proc Natl Acad Sci U S A 1999;96:7088–92.

30. Svensson J, Tivesten A, Sjogren K, et al. Liver-derived IGF-I regulates kidney size, sodium reabsorption, and renal IGF-II expression. J Endocrinol 2007; 193:359–66.

31. Wallenius K, Sjogren K, Peng XD, et al. Liver-derived IGF-I regulates GH secretion at the pituitary level in mice. Endocrinology 2001;142:4762–70.

32. Wolf E, Kramer R, Blum WF, et al. Consequences of postnatally elevated insulin-like growth factor-II in transgenic mice: endocrine changes and effects on body and organ growth. Endocrinology 1994;135:1877–86.

33. Blackburn A, Schmitt A, Schmidt P, et al. Actions and interactions of growth hormone and insulin-like growth factor-II: body and organ growth of transgenic mice. Transgenic Res 1997;6:213–22.

34. Moerth C, Schneider MR, Renner-Mueller I, et al. Postnatally elevated levels of insulin-like growth factor-II (IGF-II) fail to rescue the dwarfism of IGF-I deficient mice except kidney weight. Endocrinology 2007;148:441–51.

35. Matsell DG, Delhanty PJ, Stepaniuk O, et al. Expression of insulin-like growth factor and binding protein genes during nephrogenesis. Kidney Int 1994;46: 1031–42.

36. O'Mahoney J, Brandon MR, Adams TE. Development and tissue-specific regulation of ovine insulin-like growth factor II (IGF-II) mRNA expression. Mol Cell Endocrinol 1991;78:87–96.

37. Liu ZZ, Wada J, Alvares K, et al. Distribution and relevance of insulin-like growth factor-I receptor in metanephric development. Kidney Int 1993;44:1242–50.

38. Wada J, Liu ZZ, Alvares K, et al. Cloning of cDNA for the alpha subunit of mouse insulin-like growth factor I receptor and the role of the receptor in metanephric development. Proc Natl Acad Sci U S A 1993;90:10360–4.

39. Delhanty PJ, Hill DJ, Shimasaki S, et al. Insulin-like growth factor binding protein-4, -5 and -6 mRNAs in the human fetus: localization to sites of growth and differentiation? Growth Regul 1993;3:8–11.

40. Delhanty PJ, Han VK. The expression of insulin-like growth factor (IGF)-binding protein-2 and IGF-II genes in the tissues of the developing ovine fetus. Endocrinology 1993;132:41–52.

41. Rajkumar K, Barron D, Lewitt MS, et al. Growth retardation and hyperglycemia in insulin-like growth factor binding protein-1 transgenic mice. Endocrinology 1995;136:4029–34.

42. Doublier S, Amri K, Seurin D, et al. Overexpression of human insulin-like growth factor binding protein-1 in the mouse leads to nephron deficit. Pediatr Res 2001; 49:660–6.

43. Doublier S, Seurin D, Fouqueray B, et al. Glomerulosclerosis in mice transgenic for human insulin-like growth factor-binding protein-1. Kidney Int 2000;57: 2299–307.

44. Hoeflich A, Nedbal S, Blum WF, et al. Growth inhibition in giant growth hormone transgenic mice by overexpression of insulin-like growth factor-binding protein-2. Endocrinology 2001;142:1889–98.

45. Modric T, Silha JV, Shi Z, et al. Phenotypic manifestations of insulin-like growth factor-binding protein-3 overexpression in transgenic mice. Endocrinology 2001;142:1958–67.

46. Murphy LJ, Molnar P, Lu X, et al. Expression of human insulin-like growth factor-binding protein-3 in transgenic mice. J Mol Endocrinol 1995;15:293–303.

47. Bienvenu G, Seurin D, Grellier P, et al. Insulin-like growth factor binding protein-6 transgenic mice: postnatal growth, brain development, and reproduction abnormalities. Endocrinology 2004;145:2412–20.

48. Salih DA, Tripathi G, Holding C, et al. Insulin-like growth factor-binding protein 5 (Igfbp5) compromises survival, growth, muscle development, and fertility in mice. Proc Natl Acad Sci U S A 2004;101:4314–9.

49. Schimpff RM, Donnadieu M, Duval M. Serum somatomedin activity measured as sulphation factor in peripheral, hepatic and renal veins of mongrel dogs: basal levels. Acta Endocrinol (Copenh) 1980;93:67–72.

50. Mathews LS, Norstedt G, Palmiter RD. Regulation of insulin-like growth factor I gene expression by growth hormone. Proc Natl Acad Sci U S A 1986;83: 9343–7.

51. Fujinaka H, Katsuyama K, Yamamoto K, et al. Expression and localization of insulin-like growth factor binding proteins in normal and proteinuric kidney glomeruli. Nephrology (Carlton) 2010;15:700–9.

52. Bondy CA, Chin E, Zhou J. Significant species differences in local IGF-I and -II gene expression. Adv Exp Med Biol 1993;343:73–7.

53. Chin E, Michels K, Bondy CA. Partition of insulin-like growth factor (IGF)-binding sites between the IGF-I and IGF-II receptors and IGF-binding proteins in the human kidney. J Clin Endocrinol Metab 1994;78:156–64.

54. Andersson G, Jennische E. IGF-I immunoreactivity is expressed by regenerating renal tubular cells after ischaemic injury in the rat. Acta Physiol Scand 1988;132:453–7.

55. Matejka GL, Jennische E. IGF-I binding and IGF-I mRNA expression in the postischemic regenerating rat kidney. Kidney Int 1992;42:1113–23.

56. Kobayashi S, Clemmons DR, Venkatachalam MA. Colocalization of insulin-like growth factor-binding protein with insulin-like growth factor I. Am J Physiol 1991;261:F22–8.

57. Hise MK, Mantzouris NM, Lahn JS, et al. Low-protein diet regulates a proximal nephron insulin-like growth factor binding protein. Am J Kidney Dis 1994;23:849–55.

58. Chin E, Zhou J, Bondy CA. Renal growth hormone receptor gene expression: relationship to renal insulin-like growth factor system. Endocrinology 1992; 131:3061–6.

59. Chin E, Zhou J, Bondy CA. Anatomical relationships in the patterns of insulin-like growth factor (IGF)-I, IGF binding protein-1, and IGF-I receptor gene expression in the rat kidney. Endocrinology 1992;130:3237–45.

60. Evan AP, Henry DP, Connors BA, et al. Analysis of insulin-like growth factors (IGF)-I, and -II, type II IGF receptor and IGF-binding protein-2 mRNA and peptide levels in normal and nephrectomised rat kidney. Kidney Int 1995;48:1517–29.

61. Rabkin R, Haussman M. Renal metabolism of hormones. In: Becker KL, editor. Principles and practice of endocrinology and metabolism. Philadelphia: Lippincott; 2000. p. 1895–901.

62. Zumkeller W, Hall K. Immunoreactive insulin-like growth factor II in urine. Acta Endocrinol (Copenh) 1990;123:499–503.

63. Gargosky SE, Hasegawa T, Tapanainen P, et al. Urinary insulin-like growth factors (IGF) and IGF-binding proteins in normal subjects, growth hormone deficiency, and renal disease. J Clin Endocrinol Metab 1993;76:1631–7.

64. Flyvbjerg A, Nielsen S, Sheikh MI, et al. Luminal and basolateral uptake and receptor binding of IGF-I in rabbit renal proximal tubules. Am J Physiol 1993; 265:F624–33.

65. Li W, Fawcett J, Widmer HR, et al. Nuclear transport of insulin-like growth factor-I and insulin-like growth factor binding protein-3 in opossum kidney cells. Endocrinology 1997;138:1763–6.

66. Hasegawa Y, Cohen P, Yorgin P, et al. Characterization of urinary insulin-like growth factor binding proteins. J Clin Endocrinol Metab 1992;74:830–5.

67. Garin E, Grant M, Silverstein J. Insulin-like growth factors in patients with active nephrotic syndrome. Am J Dis Child 1989;143:865–7.

68. Hirschberg R, Kopple JD. Evidence that insulin-like growth factor I increases renal plasma flow and glomerular filtration rate in fasted rats. J Clin Invest 1989;83:326–30.

69. Baumann U, Eisenhauer T, Hartmann H. Increase of glomerular filtration rate and renal plasma flow by insulin-like growth factor-I during euglycaemic clamping in anaesthetized rats. Eur J Clin Invest 1992;22:204–9.

70. Hirschberg R, Brunori G, Kopple JD, et al. Effects of insulin-like growth factor I on renal function in normal men. Kidney Int 1993;43:387–97.

71. Guler HP, Eckardt KU, Zapf J, et al. Insulin-like growth factor I increases glomerular filtration rate and renal plasma flow in man. Acta Endocrinol (Copenh) 1989;121:101–6.

72. Hirschberg R, Kopple JD, Blantz RC, et al. Effects of recombinant human insulin-like growth factor I on glomerular dynamics in the rat. J Clin Invest 1991;87:1200–6.

73. Haylor J, Singh I, el Nahas AM. Nitric oxide synthesis inhibitor prevents vasodilatation by insulin-like growth factor I. Kidney Int 1991;39:333–5.

74. Tsukahara H, Gordienko DV, Tönshoff B, et al. Direct demonstration of insulin-like growth factor-I-induced nitric oxide production by endothelial cells. Kidney Int 1994;45:598–604.

75. Tönshoff B, Kaskel FJ, Moore LC. Effects of insulin-like growth factor I on the renal juxtamedullary microvasculature. Am J Physiol 1998;274:F120–8.

76. Hirschberg R. Die aminosäure- und hormoninduzierte Modulation der Nierenfunktion und ihre mögliche Bedeutung für die Progression der chronischen Niereninsuffizienz. Berlin: Free University of Berlin; 1988.

77. Feld S, Hirschberg R. Growth hormone, the insulin-like growth factor system, and the kidney. Endocr Rev 1996;17:423–80.

78. Hirschberg R. Effects of growth hormone and IGF-I on glomerular ultrafiltration in growth hormone-deficient rats. Regul Pept 1993;48:241–50.

79. Laron Z, Klinger B. IGF-I treatment of adult patients with Laron syndrome: preliminary results. Clin Endocrinol (Oxf) 1994;41:631–8.

80. Giordano M, DeFronzo RA. Acute effect of human recombinant insulin-like growth factor I on renal function in humans. Nephron 1995;71:10–5.

81. Corvilain J, Abramow M, Bergans A. Some effects of human growth hormone on renal hemodynamics and on tubular phosphate transport in man. J Clin Invest 1962;41:1230–5.

82. Mulroney SE, Lumpkin MD, Haramati A. Antagonist to GH-releasing factor inhibits growth and renal Pi reabsorption in immature rats. Am J Physiol 1989; 257:F29–34.

83. Hirschberg R. IGF-I is ultrafiltered into the urinary space and may exert biological effects in proximal tubules in the nephrotic syndrome [abstract]. J Am Soc Nephrol 1993;4:771.

84. van Renen MJ, Hogg RJ, Sweeney AL, et al. Accelerated growth in short children with chronic renal failure treated with both strict dietary therapy and recombinant growth hormone. Pediatr Nephrol 1992;6:451–8.

85. Quigley R, Baum M. Effects of growth hormone and insulin-like growth factor I on rabbit proximal convoluted tubule transport. J Clin Invest 1991;88:368–74.

86. Caverzasio J, Bonjour JP. IGF-1 and phosphate homeostasis during growth. Nephrologie 1992;13:109–13.

87. Caverzasio J, Bonjour JP. Growth factors and renal regulation of phosphate transport. Pediatr Nephrol 1993;7:802–6.

88. Ernest S, Coureau C, Escoubet B. Deprivation of phosphate increases IGF-II mRNA in MDCK cells but IGFs are not involved in phosphate transport adaptation to phosphate deprivation. J Endocrinol 1995;145:325–31.

89. Bengtsson BA, Edén S, Lönn L, et al. Treatment of adults with growth hormone (GH) deficiency with recombinant human GH. J Clin Endocrinol Metab 1993;76: 309–17.

90. Jabri N, Schalch DS, Schwartz SL, et al. Adverse effects of recombinant human insulin-like growth factor I in obese insulin-resistant type II diabetic patients. Diabetes 1994;43:369–74.

91. Clemmons DR. Use of growth hormone and insulin-like growth factor I in catabolism that is induced by negative energy balance. Horm Res 1993;40: 62–7.

92. Beck JC, McGarry EE, Dyrenfurth I, et al. The metabolic effects of human and monkey growth hormone in man. Ann Intern Med 1958;49:1090–105.

93. Brenner B, Meyer T, Hostetter T. Dietary protein intake and the progressive nature of kidney disease: the role of hemodynamically mediated glomerular injury in the pathogenesis of progressive glomerular sclerosis in aging, renal ablation, and intrinsic renal disease. N Engl J Med 1982;307:652–9.

94. Gallego M, Chai Q, Marrero M, et al. Stimulation of Na channels by IGF-I in A6 cells. Possible role of tyrosine phosphorylation [abstract]. J Am Soc Nephrol 1995;6:337.

95. Moller S, Juul A, Becker U, et al. Concentrations, release, and disposal of insulin-like growth factor (IGF)-binding proteins (IGFBP), IGF-I, and growth hormone in different vascular beds in patients with cirrhosis. J Clin Endocrinol Metab 1995;80:1148–57.

96. Doi T, Striker LJ, Quaife C, et al. Progressive glomerulosclerosis develops in transgenic mice chronically expressing growth hormone and growth hormone releasing factor but not in those expressing insulinlike growth factor-1. Am J Pathol 1988;131:398–403.

97. Ritz E, Tönshoff B, Worgall S, et al. Influence of growth hormone and insulin-like growth factor-I on kidney function and kidney growth. Pediatr Nephrol 1991;5: 509–12.

98. Mehls O, Irzynjec T, Ritz E, et al. Effects of rhGH and rhIGF-1 on renal growth and morphology. Kidney Int 1993;44:1251–8.

99. Pesce CM, Striker LJ, Peten E, et al. Glomerulosclerosis at both early and late stages is associated with increased cell turnover in mice transgenic for growth hormone. Lab Invest 1991;65:601–5.

100. Stiles AD, Sosenko IR, D'Ercole AJ, et al. Relation of kidney tissue somatomedin-C/insulin-like growth factor I to postnephrectomy renal growth in the rat. Endocrinology 1985;117:2397–401.

101. Flyvbjerg A, Orskov H, Nyborg K, et al. Kidney IGF-I accumulation occurs in four different conditions with rapid initial kidney growth in rats. In: Spencer EM, editor. Modern concepts of insulin-like growth factors. New York: Elsevier: Science Publishing Co; 1991. p. 207–17.

102. Lajara R, Rotwein P, Bortz JD, et al. Dual regulation of insulin-like growth factor I expression during renal hypertrophy. Am J Physiol 1989;257:F252–61.

103. Fagin JA, Melmed S. Relative increase in insulin-like growth factor I messenger ribonucleic acid levels in compensatory renal hypertrophy. Endocrinology 1987; 120:718–24.

104. Hise MK, Lahn JS, Shao ZM, et al. Insulin-like growth factor-I receptor and binding proteins in rat kidney after nephron loss. J Am Soc Nephrol 1993;4: 62–8.

105. Hise MK, Li L, Mantzouris N, et al. Differential mRNA expression of insulin-like growth factor system during renal injury and hypertrophy. Am J Physiol 1995; 269:F817–24.

106. Fervenza FC, Tsao T, Hsu F, et al. Intrarenal insulin-like growth factor-1 axis after unilateral nephrectomy in rat. J Am Soc Nephrol 1999;10(1):43–50.

107. Haylor J, Hickling H, El Eter E, et al. JB3, an IGF-I receptor antagonist, inhibits early renal growth in diabetic and uninephrectomized rats. J Am Soc Nephrol 2000;11:2027–35.

108. Haylor JL, McKillop IH, Oldroyd SD, et al. IGF-I inhibitors reduce compensatory hyperfiltration in the isolated rat kidney following unilateral nephrectomy. Nephrol Dial Transplant 2000;15:87–92.

109. Haramati A, Lumpkin MD, Mulroney SE. Early increase in pulsatile growth hormone release after unilateral nephrectomy in adult rats. Am J Physiol 1994; 266:F628–32.

110. Phan V, Brophy PD, Fleming GM. Acute renal failure. In: Geary DF, Schaefer F, editors. Comprehensive pediatric nephrology. Philadelphia: Elsevier; 2008. p. 607–9.

111. Ding H, Qing PY, Gao XL, et al. Time dependent changes in the expression of insulin-like growth factor I (IGF-I) and IGF-I receptor (IGF-I R) in tissue of rats with acute renal failure (ARF) [abstract]. J Am Soc Nephrol 1995;6:461.

112. Tsao T, Wang J, Fervenza FC, et al. Renal growth hormone-insulin-like growth factor-I system in acute renal failure. Kidney Int 1995;47:1658–68.

113. Hirschberg R, Kopple J, Lipsett P, et al. Multicenter clinical trial of recombinant human insulin-like growth factor I in patients with acute renal failure. Kidney Int 1999;55:2423–32.

114. Clark R, Mortensen D, Rabkin R. Recovery from acute ischaemic renal failure is accelerated by des-(1-3)-insulin-like growth factor-I. Clin Sci 1994;86:709–14.

115. Ding H, Kopple JD, Cohen A, et al. Recombinant human insulin-like growth factor-I accelerates recovery and reduces catabolism in rats with ischemic acute renal failure. J Clin Invest 1993;91:2281–7.

116. Miller SB, Martin DR, Kissane J, et al. Insulin-like growth factor I accelerates recovery from ischemic acute tubular necrosis in the rat. Proc Natl Acad Sci U S A 1992;89:11876–80.

117. Noguchi S, Kashihara Y, Ikegami Y, et al. Insulin-like growth factor-I ameliorates transient ischemia-induced acute renal failure in rats. J Pharmacol Exp Ther 1993;267:919–26.

118. Franklin SC, Moulton M, Sicard GA, et al. Insulin-like growth factor I preserves renal function postoperatively. Am J Physiol 1997;272:F257–9.

119. Samaan NA, Freeman RM. Growth hormone levels in severe renal failure. Metabolism 1970;19:102–13.

120. Pimstone BL, Le Roith D, Epstein S, et al. Disappearance rates of serum growth hormone after intravenous somatostatin in renal and liver disease. J Clin Endocrinol Metab 1975;41:392–5.

121. Davidson M, Fisher M, Dabir-Vaziri N, et al. Effect of protein intake and dialysis on the abnormal growth hormone, glucose, and insulin homeostasis in uremia. Metabolism 1976;25:455–64.

122. Tönshoff B, Powell DR, Zhao D, et al. Decreased hepatic insulin-like growth factor (IGF)-I and increased IGF binding protein-1 and -2 gene expression in experimental uremia. Endocrinology 1997;138:938–46.

123. Chan W, Valerie KC, Chan JCM. Expression of insulin-like growth factor-1 in uremic rats: growth hormone resistance and nutritional intake. Kidney Int 1993;43:790–5.

124. Tönshoff B, Eden S, Weiser E, et al. Reduced hepatic growth hormone (GH) receptor gene expression and increased plasma GH binding protein in experimental uremia. Kidney Int 1994;45:1085–92.

125. Schaefer F, Chen Y, Tsao T, et al. Impaired JAK-STAT signal transduction contributes to growth hormone resistance in chronic uremia. J Clin Invest 2001;108:467–75.

126. Phillips LS, Fusco AC, Unterman TG, et al. Somatomedin inhibitor in uremia. J Clin Endocrinol Metab 1984;59:764–72.

127. Blum WF, Ranke MB, Kietzmann K, et al. Growth hormone resistance and inhibition of somatomedin activity by excess of insulin-like growth factor binding protein in uraemia. Pediatr Nephrol 1991;5:539–44.

128. Frystyk J, Ivarsen P, Skjaerbaek C, et al. Serum-free insulin-like growth factor I correlates with clearance in patients with chronic renal failure. Kidney Int 1999;56:2076–84.

129. Tönshoff B, Blum WF, Wingen AM, et al. Serum insulin-like growth factors (IGFs) and IGF binding proteins 1, 2, and 3 in children with chronic renal failure: relationship to height and glomerular filtration rate. J Clin Endocrinol Metab 1995;80: 2684–91.

130. Ulinski T, Mohan S, Kiepe D, et al. Serum insulin-like growth factor binding protein (IGFBP)-4 and IGFBP-5 in children with chronic renal failure: relationship to growth and glomerular filtration rate. Pediatr Nephrol 2000;14:589–97.

131. Holly JM, Claffey DC, Cwyfan-Hughes SC, et al. Proteases acting on IGFBPs: their occurrence and physiological significance. Growth Regul 1993;3:88–91.

132. Lee DY, Park SK, Yorgin PD, et al. Alteration in insulin-like growth factor-binding proteins (IGFBPs) and IGFBP-3 protease activity in serum and urine from acute and chronic renal failure. J Clin Endocrinol Metab 1994;79:1376–82.

133. Kiepe D, Ulinski T, Powell DR, et al. Differential effects of IGFBP-1, -2, -3, and -6 on cultured growth plate chondrocytes. Kidney Int 2002;62:1591–600.

134. Kiepe D, Andress DL, Mohan S, et al. Intact IGF-binding protein-4 and -5 and their respective fragments isolated from chronic renal failure serum differentially modulate IGF-I actions in cultured growth plate chondrocytes. J Am Soc Nephrol 2001;12:2400–10.

135. Gbadegesin R, Smoyer W. Nephrotic syndrome. In: Geary DF, Schaefer F, editors. Comprehensive pediatric nephrology. Philadelphia: Elsevier; 2008. p. 205–12.

136. Haffner D, Tönshoff B, Blum WF, et al. Insulin-like growth factors (IGFs) and IGF binding proteins, serum acid-labile subunit and growth hormone binding protein in nephrotic children. Kidney Int 1997;52:802–10.

137. Hirschberg R, Kaysen GA. Insulin-like growth factor I and its binding proteins in the experimental nephritic syndrome. Endocrinology 1995;136:1565–71.

138. Flyvbjerg A, Landau D, Domene H, et al. The role of growth hormone, insulin-like growth factors (IGFs), and IGF-binding proteins in experimental diabetic kidney disease. Metabolism 1995;44:67–71.

139. Flyvbjerg A, Bornfeldt KE, Marshall SM, et al. Kidney IGF-I mRNA in initial renal hypertrophy in experimental diabetes in rats. Diabetologia 1990;33: 334–8.

140. Flyvbjerg A, Frystyk J, Osterby R, et al. Kidney IGF-1 and renal hypertrophy in GH deficient dwarf rats. Am J Physiol 1992;262:E956–62.

141. Werner H, Shen-Orr Z, Stannard B, et al. Experimental diabetes increases insulin-like growth factor I and II receptor concentration and gene expression in kidney. Diabetes 1990;39:1490–7.

142. Landau D, Chin E, Bondy C, et al. Expression of insulin-like growth factor binding proteins in the rat kidney: effects of long-term diabetes. Endocrinology 1995;136:1835–42.

143. Baelde HJ, Eikmans M, Doran PP, et al. Gene expression profiling in glomeruli from human kidneys with diabetic nephropathy. Am J Kidney Dis 2004;43: 636–50.

144. Spagnoli A, Chiarelli F, Vorwerk P, et al. Evaluation of the components of insulin-like growth factor (IGF)-IGF binding protein (IGFBP) system in adolescents with type 1 diabetes and persistent microalbuminuria: relationship with increased urinary excretion of IGFBP-3 18 kD N-terminal fragment. Clin Endocrinol (Oxf) 1999;51:587–96.

145. Shinada M, Akdeniz A, Panagiotopoulos S, et al. Proteolysis of insulin-like growth factor-binding protein-3 is increased in urine from patients with diabetic nephropathy. J Clin Endocrinol Metab 2000;85:1163–9.
146. Fine RN, Kohaut E, Brown D, et al. Long-term treatment of growth retarded children with chronic renal insufficiency, with recombinant human growth hormone. Kidney Int 1996;49:781–5.
147. Haffner D, Wühl E, Schaefer F, et al. Factors predictive of the short- and long-term efficacy of growth hormone treatment in prepubertal children with chronic renal failure. The German Study Group for Growth Hormone Treatment in Chronic Renal Failure. J Am Soc Nephrol 1998;9:1899–907.
148. Hokken-Koelega A, Mulder P, De Jong R, et al. Long-term effects of growth hormone treatment on growth and puberty in patients with chronic renal insufficiency. Pediatr Nephrol 2000;14:701–6.
149. Powell DR, Liu F, Baker BK, et al. Modulation of growth factors by growth hormone in children with chronic renal failure. The Southwest Pediatric Nephrology Study Group. Kidney Int 1997;51:1970–9.
150. Tönshoff B, Mehls O, Heinrich U, et al. Growth-stimulating effects of recombinant human growth hormone in children with end-stage renal disease. J Pediatr 1990;4:561–6.
151. Hokken-Koelega AC, Stijnen T, de Muinck Keizer-Schrama SM, et al. Placebo-controlled, double-blind, cross-over trial of growth hormone treatment in prepubertal children with chronic renal failure. Lancet 1991;338:585–90.
152. Powell DR, Durham SK, Liu F, et al. The insulin-like growth factor axis and growth in children with chronic renal failure: a report of the Southwest Pediatric Nephrology Study Group. J Clin Endocrinol Metab 1998;83:1654–61.
153. Chernausek SD, Backeljauw PF, Frane J, et al. GH Insensitivity Syndrome Collaborative Group. Long-term treatment with recombinant insulin-like growth factor (IGF)-I in children with severe IGF-I deficiency due to growth hormone insensitivity. J Clin Endocrinol Metab 2007;92:902–10.
154. Tönshoff B, Kiepe D, Ciarmatori S. Growth hormone/insulin-like growth factor system in children with chronic renal failure. Pediatr Nephrol 2005;20:279–89.
155. Kovács GT, Oh J, Kovács J, et al. Growth promoting effects of growth hormone and IGF-I are additive in experimental uremia. Kidney Int 1996;49:1413–21.
156. Edmondson SR, Baker NL, Oh J, et al. Growth hormone receptor abundance in tibial growth plates of uremic rats: GH/IGF-I treatment. Kidney Int 2000;58:62–70.
157. Horber FF, Haymond MW. Human growth hormone prevents the protein catabolic side effects of prednisone in humans. J Clin Invest 1990;86:265–72.
158. Jacob R, Barrett E, Plewe G, et al. Acute effects of insulin-like growth factor I on glucose and amino acid metabolism in the awake fasted rat. Comparison with insulin. J Clin Invest 1989;83:1717–23.
159. Guebre-Egziabher F, Juillard L, Boirie Y, et al. Short-term administration of a combination of recombinant growth hormone and insulin-like growth factor-I induces anabolism in maintenance hemodialysis. J Clin Endocrinol Metab 2009;94:2299–305.
160. Ike JO, Fervenza FC, Hoffman AR, et al. Early experience with extended use of insulin-like growth factor-1 in advanced chronic renal failure. Kidney Int 1997;51:840–9.
161. Miller SB, Moulton M, O'Shea M, et al. Effects of IGF-I on renal function in end-stage chronic renal failure. Kidney Int 1994;46:201–7.

162. Chan JM, Stampfer MJ, Giovannucci E, et al. Plasma insulin-like growth factor-I and prostate cancer risk: a prospective study. Science 1998;279:563–6.
163. Kuan Y, Surman J, Frystyk J, et al. Lack of effect of IGF-I on the glomerular filtration rate in non-diabetic patients with advanced chronic kidney disease. Growth Horm IGF Res 2009;19:219–25.
164. Kiepe D, Van Der Pas A, Ciarmatori S, et al. Defined carboxy-terminal fragments of insulin-like growth factor (IGF) binding protein-2 exert similar mitogenic activity on cultured rat growth plate chondrocytes as IGF-I. Endocrinology 2008;149:4901–11.
165. Powell DR, Liu F, Baker B, et al. Characterization of insulin-like growth factor binding protein-3 in chronic renal failure serum. Pediatr Res 1993;33:136–43.
166. Durham SK, Mohan S, Liu F, et al. Bioactivity of a 29-kilodalton insulin-like growth factor binding protein-3 fragment present in excess in chronic renal failure serum. Pediatr Res 1997;42:335–41.
167. Powell DR, Durham SK, Brewer ED, et al. Effects of chronic renal failure and growth hormone on serum levels of insulin-like growth factor-binding protein-4 (IGFBP-4) and IGFBP-5 in children: a report of the Southwest Pediatric Nephrology Study Group. J Clin Endocrinol Metab 1999;84:596–601.
168. Ständker L, Braulke T, Mark S, et al. Partial IGF affinity of circulating N- and C-terminal fragments of human insulin-like growth factor binding protein-4 (IGFBP-4) and the disulfide bonding pattern of the C-terminal IGFBP-4 domain. Biochemistry 2000;39:5082–8.
169. Ständker L, Wobst P, Mark S, et al. Isolation and characterization of circulating 13-kDa C-terminal fragments of human insulin-like growth factor binding protein-5. FEBS Lett 1998;441:281–6.
170. Powell DR, Liu F, Baker BK, et al. Insulin-like growth factor-binding protein-6 levels are elevated in serum of children with chronic renal failure: a report of the Southwest Pediatric Nephrology Study Group. J Clin Endocrinol Metab 1997;82:2978–84.

Insulin-Like Growth Factors in the Peripheral Nervous System

Stacey A. Sakowski, PhD[a], Eva L. Feldman, MD, PhD[b],*

KEYWORDS

- Insulin-like growth factor • Peripheral nervous system • Motor neuron
- Sensory neuron • Neurodegeneration • Neurodevelopment

KEY POINTS

- The insulin-like growth factor (IGF) system includes 2 ligands, their respective receptors, and a family of binding proteins that together regulate a variety of cellular responses.
- The IGF system is an appealing target for the treatment of peripheral nervous system (PNS) injury and disease based on its potent effects on neuronal development, physiology, and survival.
- Alterations in the IGF axis following injury or in neurodegenerative diseases affecting the PNS support the development and translation of therapies targeting the IGF system.
- IGFs have potent effects on neurite outgrowth and axonal targeting in development, and they are instrumental in regenerative responses following nerve injury in the PNS.

INTRODUCTION

The insulin-like growth factor (IGF) system comprises 2 ligands with their respective receptors and a variety of binding proteins that regulate the bioavailability and functionality of IGFs.[1] Both IGF ligands, IGF-I and IGF-II, are highly expressed during development and aid in differentiation, migration, and proliferation of developing cells.[2] After birth, the expression and circulating levels of IGF-II fall drastically, whereas IGF-I levels, although lower than observed during development, persist throughout life and have many effects in normal growth, metabolism, regeneration, and survival.[3] The main source of circulating IGF-I is the liver, although IGF-I is produced by most tissues and exhibits an array of endocrine, autocrine, and paracrine effects.[4,5] Most IGF actions are mediated through activation of the type I IGF receptor

This work was supported by the Program for Neurology Research & Discovery and the A. Alfred Taubman Medical Research Institute.

The authors have nothing to disclose.

[a] A. Alfred Taubman Medical Research Institute, University of Michigan, 109 Zina Pitcher Place, 4019 AAT-BSRB, Ann Arbor, MI 48109, USA; [b] Department of Neurology, University of Michigan, 109 Zina Pitcher Place, 5017 AAT-BSRB, Ann Arbor, MI 48109, USA

* Corresponding author.

E-mail address: efeldman@umich.edu

Endocrinol Metab Clin N Am 41 (2012) 375–393

doi:10.1016/j.ecl.2012.04.020

0889-8529/12/$ – see front matter © 2012 Elsevier Inc. All rights reserved.

endo.theclinics.com

(IGF-IR). IGF-I binding results in intracellular phosphorylation of the IGF-IR, which then induces a cascade of phosphorylation events that includes activation of insulin receptor substrate proteins and subsequent activation of the p44/42 mitogen-activated protein kinase (MAPK), phosphatidylinositol 3-kinase (PI3K)/Akt, and Raf-1 kinase/14-3-3 pathways, among others.[4–6] The bioavailability of IGFs in the circulation is further regulated by 6 high-affinity IGF binding proteins (IGFBPs). IGFBPs stabilize circulating IGFs, but also modulate the availability of IGFs and have some distinct actions in the absence of IGFs.[4,5]

The impact of the IGF system in tissues, such as skeletal muscle, bone, kidney, reproductive organs, and the vascular system, is well characterized and numerous reviews are available.[2,5,6] In addition to these pleiotropic roles in normal non-neuronal physiology, however, IGFs also exhibit neurotrophic, neurogenic, and neuroprotective actions.[3,7–9] These effects are well documented in the central nervous system (CNS), where studies on auditory neurons and brain tissues have elicited profound insight into the integral role IGFs play in development, growth, and survival of these neuronal populations.[3,7–10] However, limited overviews are available on IGF effects in the peripheral nervous system (PNS).[11] Given the recent interest in targeting the IGF system for the treatment of PNS injury and diseases, this review summarizes what is currently know about the effects of the IGF system on the PNS during health and disease, and reflects on IGF therapeutic efficacy in recent and ongoing preclinical and clinical studies in neurologic conditions in the PNS.

THE IGF SYSTEM IN THE PNS
IGFs in PNS Development and Maturation

Insight into the roles of IGFs in CNS development are the result of numerous studies characterizing the effects of IGF overexpression, IGF knockout, or IGF-IR knockout on neuronal growth, neurogenesis, neuroplasticity, synaptogenesis, myelination, neuronal apoptosis, and cognition.[3,9,11] The IGF system, however, also plays an integral role in the development of the sensory and motor neurons (MNs) that constitute the PNS (**Fig. 1**A). During embryonic development in mice, IGF-II mRNA expression is observed in neural crest cells that differentiate into neuronal populations, including sensory, dorsal root ganglia (DRG), and sympathetic neurons.[12,13] IGF-II expression is also observed in brain stem glia and non-neuronal floor plate cells of the developing neural tube,[14,15] and IGF-I mRNA is detected in neural crest cells and the floor plate of the cervicothoracic spinal cord in embryonic rats.[14,16,17] Expression studies in embryonic rats also demonstrate IGF-I and IGF-IR in developing ganglia and nerve target zones,[18] and further studies support the presence of IGF-I and IGF-II in target zones, but not in the developing peripheral axons themselves.[19] Together, these data support a role for the IGF system in nerve sprouting and targeting during PNS development.

The IGF system coordinates neurite outgrowth and axon guidance throughout the development and maturation of neuromuscular and sensory systems in the PNS (see **Fig. 1**A). Neurite outgrowth during both motor and sensory axon development has been linked to IGF-I, IGF-II, and signaling via the IGF-IR.[10,20,21] In vitro studies demonstrate that focal adhesion kinase and paxillin, 2 proteins involved in the extension of neurites, are upregulated in response to IGF-I treatment.[22] These effects are associated with activation of the PI3K and MAPK pathways, and are prevented in the presence of factors that inhibit IGF-I/IGF-IR binding.[22–24] IGF-IR activation of the PI3K and MAPK pathways, and downstream activation of proteins that modulate actin dynamics, such as rac and LIM kinase, also result in enhanced motility in 2

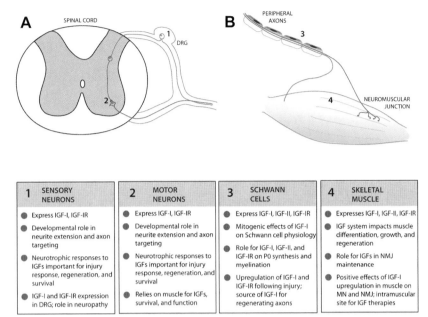

1	SENSORY NEURONS	2	MOTOR NEURONS	3	SCHWANN CELLS	4	SKELETAL MUSCLE
	● Express IGF-I, IGF-IR		● Express IGF-I, IGF-IR		● Express IGF-I, IGF-II, IGF-IR		● Expresses IGF-I, IGF-II, IGF-IR
	● Developmental role in neurite extension and axon targeting		● Developmental role in neurite extension and axon targeting		● Mitogenic effects of IGF-I on Schwann cell physiology		● IGF system impacts muscle differentiation, growth, and regeneration
	● Neurotrophic responses to IGFs important for injury response, regeneration, and survival		● Neurotrophic responses to IGFs important for injury response, regeneration, and survival		● Role for IGF-I, IGF-II, and IGF-IR on P0 synthesis and myelination		● Role for IGFs in NMJ maintenance
	● IGF-I and IGF-IR expression in DRG; role in neuropathy		● Relies on muscle for IGFs, survival, and function		● Upregulation of IGF-I and IGF-IR following injury; source of IGF-I for regenerating axons		● Positive effects of IGF-I upregulation in muscle on MN and NMJ; intramuscular site for IGF therapies

Fig. 1. The IGF system in PNS tissues. (*A*) Neuronal cells in the PNS include *sensory neurons* (*1, pink*) and *MNs* (*2, blue*). MN cell bodies, found in the ventral horn of the spinal cord, send axonal projections through the ventral root to establish NMJs and coordinate muscle movement. Sensory neuron cell bodies are found in DRG, and receive sensory input from peripheral tissues to relay signals to neurons in the dorsal spinal cord. Both sensory and MNs express IGF-I, IGF-II (mostly during development), and IGF-IR and rely on the IGF system for development, response to injury, regeneration, and survival. (*B*) Neuronal cells in the PNS are closely associated with *Schwann cells* (*3*) and *muscle* (*4*). Schwann cells express IGF-I, IGF-II, and IGF-IR to support peripheral axons and support P0 synthesis and myelination. They also provide IGF-I to regenerating axons. IGFs produced in skeletal muscle support muscle differentiation, growth, and regeneration, and play an integral role in NMJ maintenance. Intramuscular delivery, and subsequent retrograde transport, also offers a source for IGF delivery and gene therapy application.

in vitro neuroblastoma cell lines.[25,26] In vivo models recapitulate these observations, as cultured embryonic DRG explants from chick and rat both exhibit amplified neurite extension following IGF-I treatment.[27,28] Effects are similar to those observed with nerve growth factor application, and were attenuated by inhibiting the PI3K or MAPK pathways.[20] Similarly, in vitro and in vivo studies demonstrate that corticospinal MNs extend axons in the presence of IGF-I, and this response can be inhibited by blocking PI3K or MAPK signaling or IGF-IR activation.[21] Together, these studies strongly support the role of the IGF system in neurite extension and peripheral axon projection for both motor and sensory axons.

As indicated by the expression of IGFs in nerve target zones during development, the IGF system also plays a profound role in axon targeting. Studies using olfactory neurons, which express both IGF-I and IGF-IR during development, have provided insight into the chemoattractant potential of IGFs. IGF-I and IGF-IR knockout mice exhibit profound defects in axonal projections to the olfactory bulb, which is compounded when both IGF-I and IGF-IR are knocked out.[10] Furthermore, primary olfactory neuron cultures target axonal projections toward IGF-I gradients in growth cone turning assays.[10] These observations, along with the known expression of IGFs in the ventral floor plate of the developing spinal cord[15–17] where commissural axons are subjected to multiple guidance cues, support the role of the IGF system in axon guidance during development of the PNS.

Sustained Roles for IGFs in the PNS

The responses of both MNs and sensory neurons to IGF-I and IGF-II persist into adulthood, and IGF-I expression is observed in adult spinal cord ventral horn, sympathetic ganglia, and DRG, and in peripheral axons and associated Schwann cells (see **Fig. 1**).[11,29] Similar to the developing PNS, sensory and MNs both respond to IGF stimulation with enhanced neurite outgrowth in the adult PNS.[30] This long-term effect on sustained neurite outgrowth is in addition to the effects on growth cone motility observed during development, and are associated with activation of MAPK signaling.[31] The activation of signaling pathways that promote neuronal survival are also paramount to the role of IGFs in the adult PNS, and IGF-I activation of PI3K, MAPK, and 14-3-3 have been associated with enhanced survival in neuronal cells.[6,9] For example, activation of these pathways phosphorylates and inactivates the proapoptotic protein Bad, and activation of PI3K promotes increased transcription of antiapoptotic proteins, such as Bcl-2.[32,33] IGF-I–induced phosphorylation of the forkhead transcription factor and IGF-IR–directed activation of RACK1 also modulate neuronal survival.[32,34] Notably, the IGF system is the only growth factor system that has neurotrophic properties for both sensory and MNs.[31,35–37]

The neuroprotective properties of the IGF system are important for the PNS response to injury, and beneficial effects of IGF signaling have linked to regeneration and survival of MNs, sensory neurons, Schwann cells, and sympathetic nerves.[3,31] Following crush injury of the sciatic nerve in rats, IGF-I accumulates in axons and Schwann cells shortly after injury, likely owing to anterograde transport from MN cell bodies in the spinal cord and sensory neurons in DRG.[38] This is accompanied by a modest increase in IGF-I distal to the injury that is probably attributed to Schwann cells,[38] and increases in both IGF-I and IGF-II mRNA have been observed in the distal axon.[39] Elevated IGF mRNAs are observed at 6 days after crush, or persist for more than 20 days following nerve transection.[40] Similarly, IGF-I protein expression peaks at 2 weeks after transection and is still detectable elevated after 4 weeks.[41–44] This is paralleled with a significant upregulation of IGF-IR in Schwann cells.[41] Furthermore, IGF-I application to nerve crush sites in rats is associated with enhanced rates of sensory functional recovery following nerve crush,[45] and IGF-I has also been linked to MN survival and the maintenance of neuromuscular junctions (NMJs) following sciatic nerve transection.[46–48] Increased levels of IGF-II, which are observed in axons within a week of injury, are also elevated 20 days following crush injury in muscle.[40,49] Although both IGF-I and IGF-II are upregulated following nerve injury, these data reflect more predominant upregulation for IGF-I in nerve and IGF-II in muscle. IGF-II treatment, however, has demonstrated neuroprotective properties in a frog nerve crush model.[50]

The observed increases in IGF levels following nerve injury play a significant role in the ability of both sensory and MNs to regenerate, and multiple in vitro and in vivo studies have demonstrated a profound effect of IGFs on axonal regeneration following injury. Cultured transected sciatic nerves exhibit significant increases in the length of regenerating axons in the presence of IGF-I; however, IGF-I does not appear to solicit the same chemoattractant properties for regenerating axons as it does in developing axons.[10,43] In a rat sciatic nerve injury model, axonal regeneration was drastically enhanced in the presence of IGF-I,[51] and IGF-II treatment is effective in promoting regeneration after nerve grafting in a rat sciatic nerve transection model.[51,52] Vector-mediated upregulation of IGF-I also enhances motor endplate and regenerating axon numbers, and prevents muscle atrophy associated with denervation.[53–55] Furthermore, nerve grafting in combination with IGF-I treatment also improves NMJ innervation following transection.[56] Finally, neuroprotective effects of IGFs are demonstrated in rodents and patients following spinal cord injury, supporting similar potential approaches in the PNS. Rats treated with Limaprost, a prostaglandin E2 analog that induces calcitonin gene–related peptide and subsequent production of IGF-I from sensory neurons, improves neuronal survival and motor function following spinal cord injury.[57] Similarly, intravenous IGF-I administration resulting in increased serum IGF-I levels improved outcomes in a small study of patients with traumatic brain injury.[58] Overall, multiple lines of evidence indicate that the IGF system participates in tissue maintenance, injury response, regeneration and remodeling of both sensory and motor systems, and represents a promising therapeutic prospect for PNS injury.

The IGF System in Associated Peripheral Tissues

Sensory and MNs in the PNS are closely associated with and dependent on interactions with non-neuronal cells, including Schwann cells and muscle (see **Fig. 1**B). As previously mentioned, Schwann cells provide a source for IGF-I upregulation following injury that supplements neuronal alterations in local IGF levels resulting from axonal transport.[38,39,41–44] Following nerve transection in rats, Schwann cells upregulate IGF-I and IGF-IR to facilitate axonal regeneration, after which sustained upregulation of IGF-I by invading macrophages, which along with Schwann cell production of IGFBP5, functions to enhance the neuroprotective response to injury in this model.[41] The IGF system, however, also supports general Schwann cell physiology. In culture, Schwann cells rely on the mitogenic effects of IGF-I and forskolin, and IGF-I protects cultured Schwann cells from serum withdrawal via activation of PI3K-mediated survival pathways.[59–61] IGF-II, however, has no observed mitogenic properties in vitro, but evidence does support a role for IGF-I, IGF-II, and insulin in the upregulation of the P0 myelin protein.[59,61] In fact, IGF-I activation of PI3K signaling pathways facilitates myelination in cultured Schwann cells by stimulating the synthesis of fatty acids, enhancing motility, and increasing process extension.[62,63] Furthermore, IGF-I induces myelination of DRG neurons in culture that structurally resembles in vivo myelinated fibers, complete with nodes of Ranvier.[64] Taken together, these data demonstrate that Schwann cells express IGFs and IGF-IR, and participate in the maintenance and regeneration of the PNS during development, normal physiology, and response to injury.

The intricate interplay between MNs and muscle at the NMJ specifies the importance of skeletal muscle in the development and maintenance of the motor system. Although IGFs play a direct role in skeletal muscle differentiation, growth, and regeneration,[2] both MNs and muscle produce IGF-I, IGF-II, and IGF-IR, and the 2 tissues rely heavily on each other for survival and function.[2,65] As previously mentioned, upregulation of IGFs are linked to axonal targeting in development.[10] Following NMJ formation, IGF-I expression in muscle decreases, while growth-associated protein (GAP) expression in axons, which is associated with axon sprouting, correlatively decreases.[66,67] Subsequent long-term maintenance of distal axons and NMJs depends on IGF neurotrophic support, and with aging, the loss of motor endplate innervation and numbers coincide with gradual decreases in IGF-I levels.[68] IGF-I expression in muscle, however, through the direct injection of IGF-I or vectors that produce a muscle-specific form of IGF-I, attenuates the loss of GAP expression in neurons and can promote sprouting and regeneration.[66,69] Along these lines, recent studies in mouse models of the MN disease spinal muscular atrophy (SMA) demonstrate the efficacy of muscle-specific IGF-I upregulation on survival and muscle fiber size.[70] Muscle-specific IGF-I expression in SMA mice has also been linked to activation of Akt signaling in muscle, as well as in MN cell bodies in the spinal cord; these mice exhibited improved motor performance, diminished pathologic features, and increased survival, demonstrating that alterations of the IGF system in muscle can have a profound impact on the PNS.[71] Studies also indicate that disuse muscle atrophy and the associated decrease in muscular IGF-I levels induce compensatory upregulation of IGF-IR in MN cell bodies in the spinal cord.[72,73] Furthermore, upregulation of IGF-I in MNs via retrograde transport of vectors through motor axons following intramuscular injection also prevents neuromuscular loss with aging and enhances NMJ innervation.[74] Together, these data demonstrate that alterations of the IGF system in muscle, or through muscle-targeted therapeutic approaches, represent an appealing avenue for the treatment of NMJ and MN degeneration.

IGFs IN PNS DISEASES

The neurotrophic, neurogenic, and neuroprotective actions of IGFs have fostered interest in the use of IGF therapies for the treatment of neurodegenerative diseases. CNS disorders, such as Parkinson disease, Alzheimer disease, Huntington disease, and traumatic brain injury, exhibit alterations in the IGF axis during pathogenesis, and therapies targeting the IGF system offer neuroprotection.[3,7] In the PNS, IGFs have similar potential to offer neuroprotection in conditions that affect both sensory and motor neuronal systems. Here, we discuss and examine the IGF system in the pathogenesis and treatment of diabetic neuropathy and amyotrophic lateral sclerosis (ALS).

Targeting the IGF System in Neuropathy

Deficient IGF-I expression in mice induces abnormal nerve conduction velocities in both sensory and MNs.[75] These defects can be rescued with IGF-I treatment,[75] and highlight the potential therapeutic efficacy of the IGF system in neuropathy. Diabetic neuropathy is one of the most prevalent and debilitating complications associated with diabetes, and involves distal-to-proximal dysfunction in sensory, autonomic, and motor neuronal systems characterized by hyperalgesia and eventual loss of sensation.[76] Hyperglycemia resulting from alterations in insulin production or insulin sensitivity in diabetes is associated with damage to vasculature and increases neuronal apoptosis, and is also correlated with multiple defects in the IGF system.[76–79] In patients with diabetic neuropathy, circulating IGF-I and IGF-IR levels are decreased, and increased levels of IGFBP1 are also observed, suggesting further limitations on the amount of available free IGF-I.[80,81] Decreased circulating IGF-I levels are also observed in type 1 diabetic rats; IGF-I and IGF-II expression is decreased in peripheral nerves and reduced IGF-I and IGF-IR levels are found in DRG.[78,82,83] Similar findings are observed in the liver, adrenal glands, and spinal cords of these rats, although insulin treatment is capable of partially restoring IGF levels.[84,85] In rats with type 2 diabetes, decreased levels of IGF-II are observed in brain, spinal cord, and peripheral nerves; however, IGF-I levels are normal in these rats.[83,85] Alternatively, increased IGF-I and IGF-IR mRNA levels are observed in sural nerves from patients with diabetic neuropathy, perhaps indicating the induction of the injury response in affected nerves in these patients.[86] Together, these studies demonstrate that defects in the IGF axis are present in diabetes, thus supporting the potential therapeutic efficacy of IGFs.

Multiple lines of evidence demonstrate that increased expression of IGF-I prevents neuropathy in diabetic rodents. In a mouse model of type 1 diabetes, IGF-I treatment improves both motor and sensory defects.[87] In these mice, muscle atrophy and demyelination is attenuated in MNs, and Schwann cell vacuolization and sensory neuron demyelination is mitigated following plasmid or viral-mediated IGF-I overexpression in the liver. Type 1 diabetic rats, which exhibit nerve dysfunction and decreased levels of IGF-I in the sciatic nerve, also show improvements in diabetic neuropathy onset following intramuscular delivery of a compound that upregulates IGF-I levels in sciatic nerve.[88] Diabetic rats subjected to nerve crush injury also exhibit improvements in nerve regeneration following subcutaneous or mini-pump administration of IGF-I.[89,90] Furthermore, subcutaneous IGF-I or IGF-II is associated with improvements in hyperalgesia and nerve regeneration in rats, and IGF-I treatment prevents the onset of diabetic autonomic neuropathy.[90,91] These observations are associated with improvements in neurite outgrowth, which is hindered by high glucose, and attenuation of hyperglycemia-induced neuronal apoptosis.[90–92] Alterations in the distribution of IGF-IR are also observed in the PNS in diabetic rats, but normal distribution is restored with IGF-I administration.[93]

Observations in cellular and rodent diabetes models have provided insight into some of the mechanisms behind IGF-I therapeutic efficacy. Alterations in insulin production and subsequent alterations in the IGF axis indicate that diabetes can impair the natural response to neuronal injury. As previously mentioned, nerve injury stimulates an influx of IGF-I and upregulation of IGF-IR at the site of injury[38,44]; however, no increase in IGF-IR levels are observed and the IGF-I response at the site of injury is delayed in diabetic rats.[94] Direct application of IGF-I at the crush site improves regeneration in these rats.[78] In vitro data indicate an interesting effect on survival and IGF-I levels in neuronal cells subjected to fluctuating high glucose levels, a condition mimicking a neuronal environment that may be observed in patients with poorly controlled diabetes. In these cells, intermittent high glucose impairs IGF-I and IGFBP2 release, decreases expression of a prosurvival gene, and induces apoptosis.[95] Further mechanistic insight into IGF neuroprotective potential is obtained from studies using embryonic DRG cultures to model neuropathy. In vivo, reductions in IGF-I and IGF-IR are observed in small DRG neurons.[82] In culture, IGF-I treatment prevents hyperglycemia-induced neuronal death through activation of PI3K pathways to block caspase-3 activation.[96] IGF-I also prevents mitochondrial defects associated with hyperglycemia.[97]

Targeting the IGF System in ALS

ALS is a fatal neurodegenerative disease characterized by the progressive degeneration of upper and lower MNs. Although the exact mechanisms of ALS remain unknown, defects in axonal transport, glutamate toxicity, and loss of neurotrophic support are likely players in disease pathogenesis.[98] The multiple tissues affected by ALS, including MNs, astrocytes, Schwann cells, and muscle, all normally express IGF-I.[99] In the spinal cords of patients with ALS, however, decreased levels of free IGF-I; increased levels of IGFBPs 2, 5, and 6; and increased IGF-IR density in gray matter are observed.[77] Increased IGF-I and IGF-II binding to IGF-IR is also present in the spinal cord, although total IGF levels remain stable, indicating a deficiency in free bioavailable IGF-I.[99–102] In fact, free IGF-I in patients with ALS is reduced by 53% compared with healthy matched controls in one study.[102] IGF-I expression is also abnormal in the skeletal muscle of patients with ALS.[103] Together, these data demonstrate disturbances in the IGF axis in patients with ALS that represent a shift in the bioavailability of free IGFs, and support the examination of targeted IGF therapies in ALS.

A vast amount of cellular data are available supporting the efficacy and mechanisms of therapies targeting the IGF axis for the treatment of ALS.[104] The treatment of primary embryonic MNs with IGF-I prevents glutamate-induced activation of caspase-3 via MAPK and PI3K activation,[105] and activation of PI3K signaling following growth factor treatment also prevents caspase-3 activation in primary MNs expressing the familial ALS mutant protein, G93A-SOD1.[106] IGF-I–induced MAPK and PI3K signaling enhances neurite outgrowth in postnatal corticospinal MN cultures as well.[21] Furthermore, IGF-I upregulation using an adenoviral-associated viral (AAV) vector not only protects transfected MNs against glutamate toxicity, but also protects neighboring cells, thus demonstrating neuroprotection in both an autocrine and paracrine manner.[107] IGF-I is also neuroprotective against glutamate toxicity in organotypic slice cultures from ALS rodent models.[108,109]

Rodent models of MN degeneration offer additional insight into the therapeutic potential of IGF therapies.[104] As previously mentioned, IGF-I treatment has positive effects on MN loss in SMA mice[70,71,110] and prevents MN loss following sciatic nerve transection.[51,53–55] In the *wobbler* mouse, a model of lower MN degeneration, subcutaneous IGF-I treatment improves motor function.[111] Examination of an ALS mouse model indicates that mutant SOD1 expression in Schwann cells induces diminished IGF-I levels in nerves that enhance disease progression,[112] and that increased IGF-I expression is observed in astrocytes in the spinal cord.[113] Subcutaneous administration of IGF-I in ALS mice, however, demonstrates no significant impact on survival.[104] Thus, the application of IGF-I in ALS mice has been approached using multiple alternative tactics to more efficiently deliver IGF-I to degenerating MNs. Intrathecal IGF-I delays symptom onset and improves survival through activation of PI3K and MAPK pathways.[114] Gene therapy and muscle-targeted treatments have also been tested and use retrograde transport through MN axons to deliver AAV–IGF-I vectors or IGF-I produced in muscle to MN cell bodies in the spinal cord. Expression of a muscle-specific isoform of IGF-I in ALS mice delayed symptom onset and improved MN and overall survival.[115] Similarly, retrograde delivery of AAV–IGF-I following intramuscular injection delays symptom onset and increases the lifespan of ALS mice.[116–119] Alternatively, administration of AAV–IGF-I therapies via the ventricular system delayed motor symptoms and improved survival in ALS mice,[120] and intraspinal injection of AAV–IGF-I protected MNs and improved motor behavior in male ALS rats.[121] Intramuscular administration of an IGF-I splice variant in ALS mice was also effective in improving motor symptoms and survival.[122] Finally, intraspinal transplantation of neural stem cells engineered to overexpress IGF-I results in MN protection in ALS mice.[123] Overall, MOST cellular and animal studies examining IGF-I efficacy in ALS models support translational studies to patients with ALS.

Clinical Translation of IGF-I Therapies in the PNS

The pleiotropic neuroprotective properties of IGFs in the PNS make them promising agents to treat disorders involving neuronal death and axonal degeneration. The clinical application of IGFs for neuropathy for the most part still remains in preclinical stages (**Table 1**). Mechanistic rationale and preclinical support for trials investigating IGF-I therapies in diabetic neuropathy are available from in vitro and in vivo studies, but only one small trial has been completed to date. This trial examined the efficacy of IGF-I for the treatment of a small fiber neuropathy and showed no effect of the treatment.[124] In the trial, subcutaneous IGF-I was administered twice daily for 6 months in 40 patients with painful idiopathic small fiber painful neuropathy. The treatment was well tolerated, but no effects on pain or sensory and autonomic function were observed.[124] Additional studies, however, have been proposed or are under way that examine the efficacy of IGF-I in patients with neuropathy (for example, http://mayoresearch.mayo.edu/mayo/research/cellular_neurobiology/research.cfm), and should provide valuable insight into the prospects of translating preclinical IGF-I treatments to patients.

Based on the resounding preclinical data supporting the IGF-I efficacy in ALS models,[104] larger advances in the clinical translation of IGF therapies for ALS have been examined or are currently under way (see **Table 1**). Two Phase III clinical trials investigating the efficacy of subcutaneous IGF-I treatment in patients with ALS, however, showed conflicting results.[125–127] A US trial involving 266 patients with ALS who received 0.05 or 0.1 mg/kg subcutaneous IGF-I daily for 9 months exhibited a modest but significant 26% decrease in the rate of disease progression,[126] although a parallel European trial involving 183 patients receiving daily 0.1 mg/kg subcutaneous IGF-I injections did not demonstrate any significant differences between the treatment groups.[125] These conflicting results provoked a third trial, where the efficacy of daily subcutaneous injections of 0.05 mg/kg IGF-I for 2 years was examined in 330 patients with ALS.[127] Similar to the European study group, the third trial did not demonstrate a significant effect on disease symptom progression.[127]

The results of the trials examining subcutaneous IGF-I administration in patients with ALS emphasize the need to consider what is known about the IGF axis in the PNS and spinal cord. IGFs are not readily transported through the blood brain barrier[3]; therefore, developing an approach to more efficiently deliver IGFs to MNs is warranted. Systemic delivery has proven efficacy to promote regeneration of MNs; however, little to no functional recovery is observed. This is likely attributable to sequestration of IGF-I by endogenous IGFBPs, the instability of free circulating IGF-I, or an inability of systemic IGF-I to reach MNs.[2,3,9,104] Therefore, approaches that elicit autocrine/paracrine IGF-I production in MNs may be key for successful outcomes in patients. As previously mentioned, numerous approaches have been tested in rodent ALS models and show robust neuroprotection, including gene therapy, intramuscular upregulation of IGFs, and intrathecal or intraspinal delivery of IGF therapies.[114–121] Gene therapy approaches using AAV–IGF-I have the benefit of an accessible administration site via intramuscular delivery and retrograde transport of the vector allowing for autocrine/paracrine actions of IGF-I produced by MNs.[116,118–120] The previous trials demonstrate that IGF-I is safe and well tolerated in an ALS patient population, and the clinical safety of AAV vectors is also established; therefore, translation to ALS patient populations is warranted.[116] The Robert Packard ALS Center at Johns Hopkins proposed a trial examining an AAV–IGF-I therapy in patients with ALS, although results and the status of the trial have not been reported to our knowledge at this time.[3] Direct intrathecal administration of IGF-I has also been examined in a small study involving 9 patients with ALS.[128] IGF-I (3 µg/kg) was administered every 2 weeks for 40 weeks and promoted modest improvements in motor symptom progression rates. A trial in which growth hormone treatment was used to achieve systemic upregulation of serum IGF-I was also completed, although no significant treatment effect was observed.[129] Alternatively, intraspinal transplantation of neural progenitor cells provides a cellular source of trophic factors, including IGF-I, that could support MN populations in the ALS spinal cord. Extensive preclinical support for this approach includes the identification of cellular mechanisms of neuroprotection, examination of efficacy in rodent ALS models, and development and validation of a device to safely deliver neural stem cells into the human spinal cord.[130–132] This strategy is currently being investigated in a Phase 1 trial, and results to this point indicate that the approach is safe.[133]

Table 1
Clinical trials examining IGF-I in the PNS

	Treatment	Details	±	Conclusion	Reference
Amyotrophic lateral sclerosis	0.05 or 0.1 mg/kg subcutaneous daily IGF-I for 9 months	North American ALS/IGF-I Study Group; Phase III, randomized, double-blind, placebo-controlled study; included 266 patients; Primary outcome measure was disease symptom progression measure by Appel ALS rating; Secondary outcome measure included a Sickness Impact Profile	+	IGF-I slowed progression of functional impairment and decline in quality of life with no adverse effects	Lai et al,[126] 1997
	0.1 mg/kg subcutaneous daily IGF-I for 9 months	European ALS/IGF-I Study Group; Phase III, randomized, double-blind, placebo-controlled study; Included 183 patients; Primary outcome measure was disease symptom progression measure by Appel ALS rating; Secondary outcome measure included a Sickness Impact Profile	–	No significant difference between treatment groups; IGF-I appears safe and well-tolerated	Borasio et al,[125] 1998
	0.5 or 3 μg/kg body weight intrathecal IGF-I every 2 weeks for 40 weeks	Double-blind study; Included 48 patients; Outcome measures included Norris scale rate of decline for bulbar and limb functions and FVC	+	Intrathecal administration had modest but significant effects on bulbar Norris scale function and FVC	Nagano et al,[128] 2005
	0.05 mg/kg body weight subcutaneous IGF-I	Great Lakes ALS Consortium; Phase III, randomized, double-blind, placebo-	–	No difference was observed between treatment and	Sorenson et al,[127] 2008

	twice daily for 2 years	controlled study; Included 330 patients; Primary outcome measure included manual muscle testing score; Secondary outcome measures included tracheostomy-free survival and rate of ALSFRS change		control groups after the 2-year study	
	2–8 IU subcutaneous GH every other day to achieve target 435–580 ng/mL serum IGF-I levels for 12 months	Phase II, randomized, double-blind, placebo-controlled study; Included 40 patients; Primary outcome measure was neuronal loss in motor cortex; Secondary outcome measures were mortality and ALSFRS	–	No affect on rate of motor neuron loss in motor cortex or on ALSFRS between groups	Sacca et al,[129] 2012
Neuropathy	0.05 mg/kg subcutaneous IGF-I twice daily for 6 months	Included 40 patients with painful idiopathic small fiber neuropathy; Primary outcome measure of pain; Secondary outcome measures included sensory and autonomic function	–	No pain improvement	Windebank et al,[124] 2004

Abbreviations: ALS, amyotrophic lateral sclerosis; ALSFRS, ALS Functional Rating Score; FVC, forced vital capacity; GH, growth hormone; IGF-I, insulin-like growth factor-I.

SUMMARY

The IGF system is an appealing target for the treatment of PNS injury and disease based on its potent effects on neuronal development, physiology, and survival.[11] Alterations in the IGF axis following injury or in neurodegenerative diseases affecting the PNS support the development and translation of therapies targeting the IGF system. IGFs have potent effects on neurite outgrowth and axonal targeting in development, and they are instrumental in regenerative responses following nerve injury in the PNS. Furthermore, preclinical data in cellular and rodent PNS disease models have supported the translation of IGF therapies for conditions affecting the sensory and motor systems.[11] To build on the recent advances in IGF therapies for PNS disorders, however, it is important to understand the status of the IGF axis in various pathologic states to ensure delivery of IGFs to the desired cellular targets. Further knowledge of what alterations exist in various PNS disorders and the neuroprotective mechanisms associated with treatments targeting the IGF system will be needed to successfully develop IGF therapies for the treatment of PNS injury and disease.

ACKNOWLEDGMENTS

The authors thank Mrs Judith Bentley for excellent secretarial support during the preparation of this manuscript and Dr J. Simon Lunn for graphical support. This work was supported by the Program for Neurology Research & Discovery and the A. Alfred Taubman Medical Research Institute.

REFERENCES

1. Duan C. Specifying the cellular responses to IGF signals: roles of IGF-binding proteins. J Endocrinol 2002;175(1):41–54.
2. Duan C, Ren H, Gao S. Insulin-like growth factors (IGFs), IGF receptors, and IGF-binding proteins: roles in skeletal muscle growth and differentiation. Gen Comp Endocrinol 2010;167(3):344–51.
3. Russo VC, Gluckman PD, Feldman EL, et al. The insulin-like growth factor system and its pleiotropic functions in brain. Endocr Rev 2005;26(7):916–43.
4. Duan C, Xu Q. Roles of insulin-like growth factor (IGF) binding proteins in regulating IGF actions. Gen Comp Endocrinol 2005;142(1–2):44–52.
5. Le Roith D. The insulin-like growth factor system. Exp Diabesity Res 2003;4(4):205–12.
6. Martin JL, Baxter RC. Signalling pathways of insulin-like growth factors (IGFs) and IGF binding protein-3. Growth Factors 2011;29(6):235–44.
7. Bibollet-Bahena O, Cui QL, Almazan G. The insulin-like growth factor-1 axis and its potential as a therapeutic target in central nervous system (CNS) disorders. Cent Nerv Syst Agents Med Chem 2009;9(2):95–109.
8. D'Ercole AJ, Ye P, Calikoglu AS, et al. The role of the insulin-like growth factors in the central nervous system. Mol Neurobiol 1996;13(3):227–55.
9. Torres-Aleman I. Toward a comprehensive neurobiology of IGF-I. Dev Neurobiol 2010;70(5):384–96.
10. Scolnick JA, Cui K, Duggan CD, et al. Role of IGF signaling in olfactory sensory map formation and axon guidance. Neuron 2008;57(6):847–57.
11. Sullivan KA, Kim B, Feldman EL. Insulin-like growth factors in the peripheral nervous system. Endocrinology 2008;149(12):5963–71.
12. Lee JE, Pintar J, Efstratiadis A. Pattern of the insulin-like growth factor II gene expression during early mouse embryogenesis. Development 1990;110(1):151–9.

13. Stylianopoulou F, Efstratiadis A, Herbert J, et al. Pattern of the insulin-like growth factor II gene expression during rat embryogenesis. Development 1988;103(3): 497–506.
14. Rotwein P, Burgess SK, Milbrandt JD, et al. Differential expression of insulin-like growth factor genes in rat central nervous system. Proc Natl Acad Sci U S A 1988;85(1):265–9.
15. Wood TL, Brown AL, Rechler MM, et al. The expression pattern of an insulin-like growth factor (IGF)-binding protein gene is distinct from IGF-II in the midgestational rat embryo. Mol Endocrinol 1990;4(8):1257–63.
16. Santos A, Yusta B, Fernandez-Moreno MD, et al. Expression of insulin-like growth factor-I (IGF-I) receptor gene in rat brain and liver during development and in regenerating adult rat liver. Mol Cell Endocrinol 1994;101(1–2):85–93.
17. Schuller AG, van Neck JW, Lindenbergh-Kortleve DJ, et al. Gene expression of the IGF binding proteins during post-implantation embryogenesis of the mouse; comparison with the expression of IGF-I and -II and their receptors in rodent and human. Adv Exp Med Biol 1993;343:267–77.
18. Ayer-le Lievre C, Stahlbom PA, Sara VR. Expression of IGF-I and -II mRNA in the brain and craniofacial region of the rat fetus. Development 1991;111(1):105–15.
19. Bondy CA, Werner H, Roberts CT Jr, et al. Cellular pattern of insulin-like growth factor-I (IGF-I) and type I IGF receptor gene expression in early organogenesis: comparison with IGF-II gene expression. Mol Endocrinol 1990;4(9):1386–98.
20. Kimpinski K, Mearow K. Neurite growth promotion by nerve growth factor and insulin-like growth factor-1 in cultured adult sensory neurons: role of phosphoinositide 3-kinase and mitogen activated protein kinase. J Neurosci Res 2001; 63(6):486–99.
21. Ozdinler PH, Macklis JD. IGF-I specifically enhances axon outgrowth of corticospinal motor neurons. Nat Neurosci 2006;9(11):1371–81.
22. Leventhal PS, Shelden EA, Kim B, et al. Tyrosine phosphorylation of paxillin and focal adhesion kinase during insulin-like growth factor-I-stimulated lamellipodial advance. J Biol Chem 1997;272(8):5214–8.
23. Kim B, Leventhal PS, Saltiel AR, et al. Insulin-like growth factor-I-mediated neurite outgrowth in vitro requires mitogen-activated protein kinase activation. J Biol Chem 1997;272(34):21268–73.
24. Leventhal PS, Feldman EL. Insulin-like growth factors as regulators of cell motility signaling mechanisms. Trends Endocrinol Metab 1997;8(1):1–6.
25. Meyer G, Kim B, van Golen C, et al. Cofilin activity during insulin-like growth factor I-stimulated neuroblastoma cell motility. Cell Mol Life Sci 2005;62(4): 461–70.
26. Meyer GE, Shelden E, Kim B, et al. Insulin-like growth factor I stimulates motility in human neuroblastoma cells. Oncogene 2001;20(51):7542–50.
27. Bothwell M. Insulin and somatemedin MSA promote nerve growth factor-independent neurite formation by cultured chick dorsal root ganglionic sensory neurons. J Neurosci Res 1982;8(2–3):225–31.
28. Xiang Y, Ding N, Xing Z, et al. Insulin-like growth factor-1 regulates neurite outgrowth and neuronal migration from organotypic cultured dorsal root ganglion. Int J Neurosci 2011;121(2):101–6.
29. Hansson HA, Nilsson A, Isgaard J, et al. Immunohistochemical localization of insulin-like growth factor I in the adult rat. Histochemistry 1988;89(4):403–10.
30. Caroni P, Schneider C, Kiefer MC, et al. Role of muscle insulin-like growth factors in nerve sprouting: suppression of terminal sprouting in paralyzed muscle by IGF-binding protein 4. J Cell Biol 1994;125(4):893–902.

31. Feldman EL, Sullivan KA, Kim B, et al. Insulin-like growth factors regulate neuronal differentiation and survival. Neurobiol Dis 1997;4(3–4):201–14.
32. Pugazhenthi S, Boras T, O'Connor D, et al. Insulin-like growth factor I-mediated activation of the transcription factor cAMP response element-binding protein in PC12 cells. Involvement of p38 mitogen-activated protein kinase-mediated pathway. J Biol Chem 1999;274(5):2829–37.
33. Bai H, Pollman MJ, Inishi Y, et al. Regulation of vascular smooth muscle cell apoptosis. Modulation of bad by a phosphatidylinositol 3-kinase-dependent pathway. Circ Res 1999;85(3):229–37.
34. Kiely PA, Sant A, O'Connor R. RACK1 is an insulin-like growth factor 1 (IGF-1) receptor-interacting protein that can regulate IGF-1-mediated Akt activation and protection from cell death. J Biol Chem 2002;277(25):22581–9.
35. Carro E, Trejo JL, Nunez A, et al. Brain repair and neuroprotection by serum insulin-like growth factor I. Mol Neurobiol 2003;27(2):153–62.
36. Oorschot DE, McLennan IS. The trophic requirements of mature motoneurons. Brain Res 1998;789(2):315–21.
37. Torres-Aleman I. Serum growth factors and neuroprotective surveillance: focus on IGF-1. Mol Neurobiol 2000;21(3):153–60.
38. Hansson HA, Rozell B, Skottner A. Rapid axoplasmic transport of insulin-like growth factor I in the sciatic nerve of adult rats. Cell Tissue Res 1987;247(2):241–7.
39. Hansson HA, Dahlin LB, Lowenadler B, et al. Transient increase in insulin-like growth factor I immunoreactivity in rat peripheral nerves exposed to vibrations. Acta Physiol Scand 1988;132(1):35–41.
40. Glazner GW, Morrison AE, Ishii DN. Elevated insulin-like growth factor (IGF) gene expression in sciatic nerves during IGF-supported nerve regeneration. Brain Res 1994;25(3–4):265–72.
41. Cheng HL, Randolph A, Yee D, et al. Characterization of insulin-like growth factor-I and its receptor and binding proteins in transected nerves and cultured Schwann cells. J Neurochem 1996;66(2):525–36.
42. Hansson HA, Dahlin LB, Danielsen N, et al. Evidence indicating trophic importance of IGF-I in regenerating peripheral nerves. Acta Physiol Scand 1986;126(4):609–14.
43. Nachemson AK, Lundborg G, Hansson HA. Insulin-like growth factor I promotes nerve regeneration: an experimental study on rat sciatic nerve. Growth Factors 1990;3(4):309–14.
44. Zochodne DW, Cheng C. Neurotrophins and other growth factors in the regenerative milieu of proximal nerve stump tips. J Anat 2000;196(Pt 2):279–83.
45. Emel E, Ergun SS, Kotan D, et al. Effects of insulin-like growth factor-I and platelet-rich plasma on sciatic nerve crush injury in a rat model. J Neurosurg 2011;114(2):522–8.
46. Iwasaki Y, Ikeda K. Prevention by insulin-like growth factor-I and riluzole in motor neuron death after neonatal axotomy. J Neurol Sci 1999;169(1–2):148–55.
47. Li L, Oppenheim RW, Lei M, et al. Neurotrophic agents prevent motoneuron death following sciatic nerve section in the neonatal mouse. J Neurobiol 1994;25(7):759–66.
48. Vergani L, Di Giulio AM, Losa M, et al. Systemic administration of insulin-like growth factor decreases motor neuron cell death and promotes muscle reinnervation. J Neurosci Res 1998;54(6):840–7.
49. Eustache I, Seyfritz N, Gueritaud JP. Effects of insulin-like growth factors on organotypic cocultures of embryonic rat brainstem slices and skeletal muscle fibers. Brain Res Dev Brain Res 1994;81(2):284–92.

50. Edbladh M, Fex-Svenningsen A, Ekstrom PA, et al. Insulin and IGF-II, but not IGF-I, stimulate the in vitro regeneration of adult frog sciatic sensory axons. Brain Res 1994;641(1):76–82.
51. Kanje M, Skottner A, Sjoberg J, et al. Insulin-like growth factor I (IGF-I) stimulates regeneration of the rat sciatic nerve. Brain Res 1989;486(2):396–8.
52. Tiangco DA, Papakonstantinou KC, Mullinax KA, et al. IGF-I and end-to-side nerve repair: a dose-response study. J Reconstr Microsurg 2001;17(4):247–56.
53. Kerns JM, Shott S, Brubaker L, et al. Effects of IGF-I gene therapy on the injured rat pudendal nerve. Int Urogynecol J Pelvic Floor Dysfunct 2003;14(1):2–7 [discussion: 8].
54. Shiotani A, O'Malley BW Jr, Coleman ME, et al. Reinnervation of motor endplates and increased muscle fiber size after human insulin-like growth factor I gene transfer into the paralyzed larynx. Hum Gene Ther 1998;9(14):2039–47.
55. Shiotani A, O'Malley BW Jr, Coleman ME, et al. Human insulinlike growth factor 1 gene transfer into paralyzed rat larynx: single vs multiple injection. Arch Otolaryngol Head Neck Surg 1999;125(5):555–60.
56. Thanos PK, Tiangco DA, Terzis JK. Enhanced reinnervation of the paralyzed orbicularis oculi muscle after insulin-like growth factor-I (IGF-I) delivery to a nerve graft. J Reconstr Microsurg 2001;17(5):357–62.
57. Umemura T, Harada N, Kitamura T, et al. Limaprost reduces motor disturbances by increasing the production of insulin-like growth factor I in rats subjected to spinal cord injury. Transl Res 2010;156(5):292–301.
58. Hatton J, Rapp RP, Kudsk KA, et al. Intravenous insulin-like growth factor-I (IGF-I) in moderate-to-severe head injury: a Phase II safety and efficacy trial. Neurosurg Focus 1997;2(5):ECP1 [discussion: 1 p following ECP1].
59. Cheng HL, Feldman EL. Insulin-like growth factor-I (IGF-I) and IGF binding protein-5 in Schwann cell differentiation. J Cell Physiol 1997;171(2):161–7.
60. Schumacher M, Jung-Testas I, Robel P, et al. Insulin-like growth factor I: a mitogen for rat Schwann cells in the presence of elevated levels of cyclic AMP. Glia 1993;8(4):232–40.
61. Stewart HJ, Bradke F, Tabernero A, et al. Regulation of rat Schwann cell Po expression and DNA synthesis by insulin-like growth factors in vitro. Eur J Neurosci 1996;8(3):553–64.
62. Cheng HL, Steinway ML, Russell JW, et al. GTPases and phosphatidylinositol 3-kinase are critical for insulin-like growth factor-I-mediated Schwann cell motility. J Biol Chem 2000;275(35):27197–204.
63. Liang G, Cline GW, Macica CM. IGF-1 stimulates de novo fatty acid biosynthesis by Schwann cells during myelination. Glia 2007;55(6):632–41.
64. Russell JW, Cheng HL, Golovoy D. Insulin-like growth factor-I promotes myelination of peripheral sensory axons. J Neuropathol Exp Neurol 2000;59(7):575–84.
65. Delbono O. Neural control of aging skeletal muscle. Aging Cell 2003;2(1):21–9.
66. Caroni P, Becker M. The downregulation of growth-associated proteins in motoneurons at the onset of synapse elimination is controlled by muscle activity and IGF1. J Neurosci 1992;12(10):3849–61.
67. Caroni P, Grandes P. Nerve sprouting in innervated adult skeletal muscle induced by exposure to elevated levels of insulin-like growth factors. J Cell Biol 1990;110(4):1307–17.
68. Messi ML, Clark HM, Prevette DM, et al. The lack of effect of specific overexpression of IGF-1 in the central nervous system or skeletal muscle on pathophysiology in the G93A SOD-1 mouse model of ALS. Exp Neurol 2007;207(1):52–63.

69. Alila H, Coleman M, Nitta H, et al. Expression of biologically active human insulin-like growth factor-I following intramuscular injection of a formulated plasmid in rats. Hum Gene Ther 1997;8(15):1785–95.

70. Bosch-Marce M, Wee CD, Martinez TL, et al. Increased IGF-1 in muscle modulates the phenotype of severe SMA mice. Hum Mol Genet 2011;20(9):1844–53.

71. Palazzolo I, Stack C, Kong L, et al. Overexpression of IGF-1 in muscle attenuates disease in a mouse model of spinal and bulbar muscular atrophy. Neuron 2009;63(3):316–28.

72. Suliman IA, Lindgren JU, Elhassan AM, et al. Effects of short- and long-term rat hind limb immobilization on spinal cord insulin-like growth factor-I and its receptor. Brain Res 2001;912(1):17–23.

73. Suliman IA, Lindgren JU, Gillberg PG, et al. Alteration of spinal cord IGF-I receptors and skeletal muscle IGF-I after hind-limb immobilization in the rat. Neuroreport 1999;10(6):1195–9.

74. Payne AM, Zheng Z, Messi ML, et al. Motor neuron targeting of IGF-1 prevents specific force decline in ageing mouse muscle. J Physiol 2006;570(Pt 2): 283–94.

75. Gao WQ, Shinsky N, Ingle G, et al. IGF-I deficient mice show reduced peripheral nerve conduction velocities and decreased axonal diameters and respond to exogenous IGF-I treatment. J Neurobiol 1999;39(1):142–52.

76. Vincent AM, Callaghan BC, Smith AL, et al. Diabetic neuropathy: cellular mechanisms as therapeutic targets. Nat Rev Neurol 2011;7(10):573–83.

77. Houston MS, Holly JM, Feldman EL, editors. IGF and nutrition in health and disease. Totowa (NJ): Humana Press Inc; 2005. Nutrition and Health.

78. Ishii DN. Implication of insulin-like growth factors in the pathogenesis of diabetic neuropathy. Brain Res Brain Res Rev 1995;20(1):47–67.

79. Sima AA, Li ZG, Zhang W. The insulin-like growth factor system and neurological complications in diabetes. Exp Diabesity Res 2003;4(4):235–56.

80. Capoluongo E, Pitocco D, Santonocito C, et al. Association between serum free IGF-I and IGFBP-3 levels in type-I diabetes patients affected with associated autoimmune diseases or diabetic complications. Eur Cytokine Netw 2006; 17(3):167–74.

81. Migdalis IN, Kalogeropoulou K, Kalantzis L, et al. Insulin-like growth factor-I and IGF-I receptors in diabetic patients with neuropathy. Diabet Med 1995;12(9): 823–7.

82. Craner MJ, Klein JP, Black JA, et al. Preferential expression of IGF-I in small DRG neurons and down-regulation following injury. Neuroreport 2002;13(13): 1649–52.

83. Wuarin L, Namdev R, Burns JG, et al. Brain insulin-like growth factor-II mRNA content is reduced in insulin-dependent and non-insulin-dependent diabetes mellitus. J Neurochem 1996;67(2):742–51.

84. Ishii DN, Guertin DM, Whalen LR. Reduced insulin-like growth factor-I mRNA content in liver, adrenal glands and spinal cord of diabetic rats. Diabetologia 1994;37(11):1073–81.

85. Zhuang HX, Wuarin L, Fei ZJ, et al. Insulin-like growth factor (IGF) gene expression is reduced in neural tissues and liver from rats with non-insulin-dependent diabetes mellitus, and IGF treatment ameliorates diabetic neuropathy. J Pharmacol Exp Ther 1997;283(1):366–74.

86. Grandis M, Nobbio L, Abbruzzese M, et al. Insulin treatment enhances expression of IGF-I in sural nerves of diabetic patients. Muscle Nerve 2001;24(5): 622–9.

87. Chu Q, Moreland R, Yew NS, et al. Systemic insulin-like growth factor-1 reverses hypoalgesia and improves mobility in a mouse model of diabetic peripheral neuropathy. Mol Ther 2008;16(8):1400–8.
88. Jian-bo L, Cheng-ya W, Jia-wei C, et al. The preventive efficacy of methylcobalamin on rat peripheral neuropathy influenced by diabetes via neural IGF-1 levels. Nutr Neurosci 2010;13(2):79–86.
89. Ishii DN, Lupien SB. Insulin-like growth factors protect against diabetic neuropathy: effects on sensory nerve regeneration in rats. J Neurosci Res 1995;40(1): 138–44.
90. Zhuang HX, Snyder CK, Pu SF, et al. Insulin-like growth factors reverse or arrest diabetic neuropathy: effects on hyperalgesia and impaired nerve regeneration in rats. Exp Neurol 1996;140(2):198–205.
91. Schmidt RE, Dorsey DA, Beaudet LN, et al. Insulin-like growth factor I reverses experimental diabetic autonomic neuropathy. Am J Pathol 1999;155(5): 1651–60.
92. Ekstrom AR, Kanje M, Skottner A. Nerve regeneration and serum levels of insulin-like growth factor-I in rats with streptozotocin-induced insulin deficiency. Brain Res 1989;496(1–2):141–7.
93. Russell JW, Feldman EL. Insulin-like growth factor-I prevents apoptosis in sympathetic neurons exposed to high glucose. Horm Metab Res 1999; 31(2–3):90–6.
94. Xu G, Sima AA. Altered immediate early gene expression in injured diabetic nerve: implications in regeneration. J Neuropathol Exp Neurol 2001;60(10): 972–83.
95. Giannini S, Benvenuti S, Luciani P, et al. Intermittent high glucose concentrations reduce neuronal precursor survival by altering the IGF system: the involvement of the neuroprotective factor DHCR24 (Seladin-1). J Endocrinol 2008; 198(3):523–32.
96. Leinninger GM, Backus C, Uhler MD, et al. Phosphatidylinositol 3-kinase and Akt effectors mediate insulin-like growth factor-I neuroprotection in dorsal root ganglia neurons. FASEB J 2004;18:1544–6.
97. Leinninger GM, Backus C, Sastry AM, et al. Mitochondria in DRG neurons undergo hyperglycemic mediated injury through Bim, Bax and the fission protein Drp1. Neurobiol Dis 2006;23(1):11–22.
98. Ilieva H, Polymenidou M, Cleveland DW. Non-cell autonomous toxicity in neurodegenerative disorders: ALS and beyond. J Cell Biol 2009;187(6):761–72.
99. Kerkhoff H, Hassan SM, Troost D, et al. Insulin-like and fibroblast growth factors in spinal cords, nerve roots and skeletal muscle of human controls and patients with amyotrophic lateral sclerosis. Acta Neuropathol 1994;87:411–21.
100. Dore S, Krieger C, Kar S, et al. Distribution and levels of insulin-like growth factor (IGF-I and IGF-II) and insulin receptor binding sites in the spinal cords of amyotrophic lateral sclerosis (ALS) patients. Brain Res 1996;41(1–2):128–33.
101. Torres-Aleman I, Barrios V, Berciano J. The peripheral insulin-like growth factor system in amyotrophic lateral sclerosis and in multiple sclerosis. Neurology 1998;50:772–6.
102. Wilczak N, de Vos RA, De Keyser J. Free insulin-like growth factor (IGF)-I and IGF binding proteins 2, 5, and 6 in spinal motor neurons in amyotrophic lateral sclerosis. Lancet 2003;361:1007–11.
103. Lunetta C, Serafini M, Prelle A, et al. Impaired expression of insulin-like growth factor-1 system in skeletal muscle of amyotrophic lateral sclerosis patients. Muscle Nerve 2012;45(2):200–8.

104. Sakowski SA, Schuyler AD, Feldman EL. Insulin-like growth factor-I for the treatment of amyotrophic lateral sclerosis. Amyotroph Lateral Scler 2009;10(2): 63–73.
105. Vincent AM, Mobley BC, Hiller A, et al. IGF-I prevents glutamate-induced motor neuron programmed cell death. Neurobiol Dis 2004;16:407–16.
106. Lunn JS, Sakowski SA, Kim B, et al. Vascular endothelial growth factor prevents G93A-SOD1-induced motor neuron degeneration. Dev Neurobiol 2009;69(13): 871–84.
107. Vincent AM, Feldman EL, Song DK, et al. Adeno-associated viral-mediated insulin-like growth factor delivery protects motor neurons in vitro. Neuromolecular Med 2004;6:79–86.
108. Bilak MM, Corse AM, Kuncl RW. Additivity and potentiation of IGF-I and GDNF in the complete rescue of postnatal motor neurons. Amyotroph Lateral Scler Other Motor Neuron Disord 2001;2:83–91.
109. Corse AM, Bilak MM, Bilak SR, et al. Preclinical testing of neuroprotective neurotrophic factors in a model of chronic motor neuron degeneration. Neurobiol Dis 1999;6:335–46.
110. Shababi M, Glascock J, Lorson CL. Combination of SMN trans-splicing and a neurotrophic factor increases the life span and body mass in a severe model of spinal muscular atrophy. Hum Gene Ther 2011;22(2):135–44.
111. Hantai D, Akaaboune M, Lagord C, et al. Beneficial effects of insulin-like growth factor I on wobbler mouse motoneuron disease. J Neurol Sci 1995;129:122–6.
112. Lobsiger CS, Boillee S, McAlonis-Downes M, et al. Schwann cells expressing dismutase active mutant SOD1 unexpectedly slow disease progression in ALS mice. Proc Natl Acad Sci U S A 2009;106(11):4465–70.
113. Chung YH, Joo KM, Shin CM, et al. Immunohistochemical study on the distribution of insulin-like growth factor I (IGF-I) receptor in the central nervous system of SOD1(G93A) mutant transgenic mice. Brain Res 2003;994(2):253–9.
114. Nagano I, Ilieva H, Shiote M, et al. Therapeutic benefit of intrathecal injection of insulin-like growth factor-1 in a mouse model of amyotrophic lateral sclerosis. J Neurol Sci 2005;235(1–2):61–8.
115. Dobrowolny G, Giacinti C, Pelosi L, et al. Muscle expression of a local Igf-1 isoform protects motor neurons in an ALS mouse model. J Cell Biol 2005;168:193–9.
116. Boillee S, Cleveland DW. Gene therapy for ALS delivers. Trends Neurosci 2004; 27(5):235–8.
117. Kabashi E, Bercier V, Lissouba A, et al. FUS and TARDBP but not SOD1 interact in genetic models of amyotrophic lateral sclerosis. PLoS Genet 2011;7(8): e1002214.
118. Kaspar BK, Erickson D, Schaffer D, et al. Targeted retrograde gene delivery for neuronal protection. Mol Ther 2002;5:50–6.
119. Kaspar BK, Llado J, Sherkat N, et al. Retrograde viral delivery of IGF-1 prolongs survival in a mouse ALS model. Science 2003;301:839–42.
120. Dodge JC, Treleaven CM, Fidler JA, et al. AAV4-mediated expression of IGF-1 and VEGF within cellular components of the ventricular system improves survival outcome in familial ALS mice. Mol Ther 2010;18(12):2075–84.
121. Franz CK, Federici T, Yang J, et al. Intraspinal cord delivery of IGF-I mediated by adeno-associated virus 2 is neuroprotective in a rat model of familial ALS. Neurobiol Dis 2009;33(3):473–81.
122. Riddoch-Contreras J, Yang SY, Dick JR, et al. Mechano-growth factor, an IGF-I splice variant, rescues motoneurons and improves muscle function in SOD1(G93A) mice. Exp Neurol 2009;215(2):281–9.

123. Park S, Kim HT, Yun S, et al. Growth factor-expressing human neural progenitor cell grafts protect motor neurons but do not ameliorate motor performance and survival in ALS mice. Exp Mol Med 2009;41(7):487–500.

124. Windebank AJ, Sorenson EJ, Civil R, et al. Role of insulin-like growth factor-I in the treatment of painful small fiber predominant neuropathy. J Peripher Nerv Syst 2004;9(3):183–9.

125. Borasio GD, Robberecht W, Leigh PN, et al. A placebo-controlled trial of insulin-like growth factor-I in amyotrophic lateral sclerosis. European ALS/IGF-I Study Group. Neurology 1998;51(2):583–6.

126. Lai EC, Felice KJ, Festoff BW, et al. Effect of recombinant human insulin-like growth factor-I on progression of ALS. A placebo-controlled study. The North America ALS/IGF-I Study Group. Neurology 1997;49:1621–30.

127. Sorenson EJ, Windbank AJ, Mandrekar JN, et al. Subcutaneous IGF-1 is not beneficial in 2-year ALS trial. Neurology 2008;71(22):1770–5.

128. Nagano I, Shiote M, Murakami T, et al. Beneficial effects of intrathecal IGF-1 administration in patients with amyotrophic lateral sclerosis. Neurol Res 2005; 27(7):768–72.

129. Sacca F, Quarantelli M, Rinaldi C, et al. A randomized controlled clinical trial of growth hormone in amyotrophic lateral sclerosis: clinical, neuroimaging, and hormonal results. J Neurol 2012;259(1):132–8.

130. Boulis NM, Federici T, Glass JD, et al. Translational stem cell therapy for amyotrophic lateral sclerosis. Nat Rev Neurol 2011;8(3):172–6.

131. Lunn JS, Sakowski SA, Federici T, et al. Stem cell technology for the study and treatment of motor neuron diseases. Regen Med 2011;6(2):201–13.

132. Lunn JS, Sakowski SA, Hur J, et al. Stem cell technology for neurodegenerative diseases. Ann Neurol 2011;70(3):353–61.

133. Glass JD, Boulis NM, Johe K, et al. Lumbar intraspinal injection of neural stem cells in patients with ALS: results of a phase I trial in 12 patients. Stem Cells 2012. DOI: 10.1002/stem.1079. [Epub ahead of print].

Insulin-Like Growth Factor-1 and Central Neurodegenerative Diseases

Ignacio Torres Aleman, PhD[a,b],*

KEYWORDS

• Neurodegeneration • Aging • Neurotrophic input

KEY POINTS

• During the past decades, insulin-like growth factor 1 (IGF-1) has enjoyed a reputation as a prototype neuroprotective factor.
• The ample neuroprotective profile displayed by IGF-1 led to the suggestion that a common determinant of neurodegeneration could be loss of IGF-1 input.
• Recent experiments suggest that IGF-1 may be detrimental in Alzheimer disease and possibly other age-related diseases.
• The use of IGF-1 receptor blockers to treat neurodegenerative conditions associated with old age is now advocated.
• However, the use of IGF-1 or its mimetics still seems appropriate in neurodegenerative diseases in which IGF-1 resistance and/or deficiency occurs.

During the past decades, insulin-like growth factor 1 (IGF-1) has enjoyed a reputation as a prototype neuroprotective factor. Its therapeutic use has been proposed for a multitude of neurologic conditions, and in several instances clinical trials have been conducted. Although none have yet led to its clinical use, its beneficial effects in several of them support further analysis of its therapeutic potential. The ample neuroprotective profile displayed by IGF-1 led to the suggestion that a common determinant of neurodegeneration could be loss of IGF-1 input. Pathologic mechanisms involved in neurodegeneration, such as oxidative stress, inflammation, or excitotoxicity, elicit IGF-1 resistance. A similar mechanism may underlie endoplasmic reticulum stress or autophagy. However, recent experiments suggest that IGF-1 may be detrimental in Alzheimer disease and possibly other age-related diseases. These observations have rapidly modified the view of IGF-1 as a neuroprotective factor. Now, the use

Work in the laboratory has been supported by the Spanish Ministry of Science, Ciberned, and Madrid Local government.
The author has nothing to disclose.
[a] Department of Functional and Systems Neuroscience, Cajal Institute, Avda Doctor Arce 37, Madrid 28002, Spain; [b] Ciberned, Madrid, Spain
* Cajal Institute, Avda Doctor Arce 37, Madrid 28002, Spain.
E-mail address: torres@cajal.csic.es

of IGF-1 receptor (IGF-1R) blockers to treat neurodegenerative conditions associated with old age is advocated. As new insights into the significance of IGF-1 in neurodegenerative diseases unfold, for a highly pleiotropic factor such as IGF-1, the context under which its actions are examined is crucial. Hence, the use of IGF-1 or its mimetics still seems appropriate in neurodegenerative diseases in which IGF-1 resistance and/or deficiency occurs.

INTRODUCTION

Many growth factors that play important regulatory roles during development turn into key determinants of brain homeostasis in adulthood. Consequently, pathologic disturbance of homeostasis may be assumed to include altered growth factor function in the brain. A bias to consider growth factors as beneficial modulators of brain diseases has been based on the cumulative evidence of the neuroprotective actions of most of them. However, ambivalent roles of growth factors such as tumor necrosis factor α (TNF-α)[1,2] indicate a considerable degree of complexity in their biologic role in brain physiology and pathology. Therefore, their role should not be viewed in an oversimplistic way as beneficial or detrimental. A good example of this complexity is provided by the current controversy surrounding the role of IGF-1 in neurodegenerative diseases.[3] This article addresses both sides of the controversy, discussing the positive and negative actions documented for this pleiotropic growth factor in relation to this devastating group of diseases. Because IGF-1 acts both systemically and centrally to regulate brain function,[4] bidirectional interactions of the brain with the periphery must be considered the appropriate frame when determining IGF-1 actions in neurodegenerative diseases. In other words, when accounting for the role of IGF-1 in brain diseases, one must bear in mind that systemic and brain IGF-1 are functionally interconnected,[5] reflecting the existing cross-talk between the brain and the periphery, as exemplified by insulin actions in the brain.

IGF-1, AGING, AND NEURODEGENERATION

Because many neurodegenerative diseases are associated with old age, factors associated with aging may either trigger or unveil pathologic processes that until then were restrained by a balance between damage and repair (ie, homeostasis). What the cause of this imbalance is unclear, although many theories have been proposed. Aging research is therefore becoming a flourishing field not only for its association to so-called modern diseases but also because an increasing aging population in the world is making this condition of prominent interest to health agencies.[6] Unfortunately, research into aging is in its infancy and the field is still at a stage of formulating hypotheses and data gathering.

A major thrust in understanding the biologic underpinnings of aging was undoubtedly provided by the genetic analyses of aging that showed that longevity is genetically modulated. This latter aspect is where IGF and insulin signaling (IIS) become important through their proposed involvement in regulating protein homeostasis.[7] In mammals, the biologic role of this family of hormones is well delineated, with insulin and IGFs, particularly IGF-1, playing a vital role in energy homeostasis and in somatic growth and tissue remodeling, respectively; however, in more primitive organisms, which have a single insulin-like receptor and multiple insulin-like peptides, the role of each of the numerous insulin peptides is blurred.[8] In invertebrates, such as worms and insects, IIS is clearly associated with aging in a negative fashion.[9] In mammals, such as mice and humans, this negative association has also been shown,[9] but the evidence is not as convincing as in the case of simpler organisms.[10] As elimination of the IGF-1R is lethal in mammals,[11] the studies have been performed in mutants partially lacking the receptor or lacking signaling molecules, such as insulin receptor substrates (IRS), that do not exclusively affect IIS because they are shared by multiple signaling pathways. Currently, it is widely accepted that reduced IIS delays aging from worms to humans.

An important variation introduced in mammals is to consider growth hormone (GH) an additional determinant of aging because of its physiologic connection to IGF-1.[10] The emphasis placed on the GH/IGF-1 axis as a key regulator of mammalian aging is somewhat coupled with downplaying the role of insulin, although a variant of the insulin receptor is linked to longevity in humans.[12] Therefore, current aging research favors the notion that IGF-1 plays a negative role, which inevitably leads to the assumption that this growth factor will also contribute to age-associated diseases. This link has already been proposed in animal models of familiar Alzheimer disease.[13] This association is discussed in greater detail.

ROLE OF IGF-1 IN PATHOLOGIC CASCADES ASSOCIATED WITH NEURODEGENERATION

Although the origins of most neurodegenerative diseases remain widely unknown, except for a few linked to monogenic mutations,[14] they share many important characteristics, and in all probability, the underlying pathologic cascades may also be common to many of them. In other words, the triggering mechanisms of neuronal death may vary among different diseases, but the ultimate death-effector processes will be the same (**Fig. 1**). Theoretically, one may take advantage of this situation by directing drug-seeking efforts toward these universal death mechanisms while overlooking the myriad causes. For instance, tackling oxidative stress will be far easier than each of the mechanisms that may lead to it. Naturally, each disease will recruit a specific set of death mechanisms, and these common death mechanisms may in turn retroactivate proximal causes of diseases, as illustrated by inflammation, that trigger more Aβ production.[15] A direct connection with IGF-1 in this regard is the proposal that these common pathologic processes in turn share a common mechanism: they all trigger neuronal IGF-1 resistance.[16] Intriguingly, resistance is almost always produced through interfering with IRS coupling to the IGF-1 receptor, and therefore this mechanism may also be amenable to selective drug targeting.

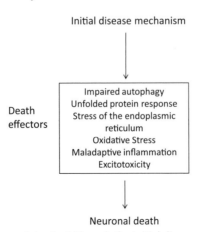

Fig. 1. Many roads to neuronal death. Although the initial disease mechanism is likely to be different for each type of neurodegenerative process, triggers of disease may converge on a few pathologic processes that mediate cell death. These cell-death effectors may all alter IGF-1 function to negate trophic support to affected neurons.

INFLAMMATION

Inflammation arises to resolve tissue disturbances after infection or injury, but if it becomes chronic, it is usually detrimental; maladaptive inflammation is linked to disease. Currently, it is widely accepted that chronic inflammation plays a prominent role in the most important neurodegenerative diseases. Microglia, the resident macrophages of the brain, and astrocytes are the major cell effectors in the brain contributing to inflammation, although the process also includes vascular cells and neurons as proximal bystanders of ongoing insult. Therefore, glial cells are the main target of inquiry in neuroinflammatory mechanisms, and a great deal is already known about inflammatory signaling in these two types of glial cells.[17] Although each disease will trigger inflammation through different pathways,[18] and inflammation should be considered a disease progression factor, recent evidence indicates that attenuation of inflammation is sufficient not only to slow progress but also to revert pathology in Alzheimer disease, such as seen in mice.[19] If confirmed, this type of observation opens the possibility of treating neurodegenerative diseases with drugs targeting inflammatory processes. But for this to occur, the processes involved must be better understood, because administration of anti-inflammatory drugs to patients with Alzheimer disease has been fruitless.[20]

Proinflammatory cytokines have been linked to diabetic insulin resistance through inhibiting signaling downstream of the insulin receptor.[21] Because the IGF-1 receptor shares signaling mechanisms with the insulin receptor, investigators then determined that TNF-α also inhibited IGF-1 signaling in neurons through inhibiting phosphorylation of IRS-2 by the IGF-1R.[22] Whether TNF-α in neurons stimulates SOCS proteins to interfere with IRS phosphorylation through the IGF-1R, as previously seen with the insulin receptor,[21] is not known. At any rate, this initial observation in neurons allowed the hypothesis that development of resistance to IGF-1 may underlie all of the major pathogenic routes in the central nervous system.[16] The existence of this mechanism suggests that neuroinflammation is deleterious at least partly because it negates IGF-1 neuroprotection.

Excitotoxicity

Unchecked glutamatergic neurotransmission leads to neuronal damage through a pathologic cascade that is initiated by intracellular Ca^{++} excess.[23] This type of neuronal death is believed to occur after brain trauma or ischemic injury, among other prominent conditions. Overstimulation of glutamatergic receptors seems to trigger IGF-1 resistance by uncoupling downstream signaling through IRS. Specifically, phosphorylation of IRS-1 in serine residues by protein kinase C (PKC; probably the ξ isoform) underlies the action of high levels of glutamate on IGF-1 signaling in neurons.[24] Even relatively low levels of glutamate, acting through ionotropic N-methyl-D-aspartate (NMDA) receptors, have been reported to inhibit IGF-1 signaling in neurons.[25] Again, these observations suggest IGF-1 resistance as an underlying mechanism of cell death in conditions such as brain ischemia. Administration of an orally active PKC inhibitor significantly decreased ischemic lesions in the rat brain.[24] Therefore, addressing the existence of IGF-1 resistance after brain ischemia may open new therapeutic opportunities. IGF-1 is a potent neuroprotective agent against brain ischemia.[26]

Oxidative Stress

Although generation of free radicals is linked to normal cell metabolic oxidation, the numerous mechanisms that have evolved to check excess reactive oxygen species

(ROS) usually protect the cells from unspecific damage by these highly reactive chemical species. Moreover, a moderate level of oxidative radicals is now known to be required for normal cell function, because ROS display signaling properties of physiologic relevance.[27] However, it is considered that when the balance between generation and disposal of ROS is disrupted and excess ROS accumulate, cellular damage through DNA, lipid, and protein oxidation occur. In fact, excess oxidative stress is the most favored mechanism to explain the wear and tear process normally associated with aging that underlies macromolecular damage[28] (although see report by Yang and Hekimi[29]) and is likely linked to neuronal demise during brain ischemia, Alzheimer dementia, amyotrophic lateral sclerosis, and other neurodegenerative processes. Again, the precedent of insulin resistance triggered by oxidative excess[30] supported the notion that a similar process is elicited for IGF-1 signaling to neurons. The authors found that ROS uncouples IRS phosphorylation by the IGF-1R through activation of MAPK p38, and at the same time stimulates JNK to phosphorylate FOXO3.[31] Therefore, the deleterious effects of excess oxidative stress on neurons probably also involves induced resistance to IGF-1. Albeit somewhat indirectly, recent evidence supports this possibility, because neuronal insulin resistance has been reported to develop in diabetic rats prone to brain ischemic insult.[32]

Autophagy

Among the various intracellular pathways of protein turnover, autophagy eliminates cytosolic proteins and recycles cellular organelles. Autophagy is of great relevance in neurodegeneration, because it seems to be affected in various diseases, particularly in Alzheimer, Parkinson, and Huntington diseases. Suppression of basal autophagy in neurons perturbs protein homeostasis sufficient to generate neurodegeneration.[33,34] Impaired autophagy may occur at multiple steps, and each is linked to different types of neurodegenerative processes.[35] Accumulation of intraneuronal autophagosomes is usually a hallmark of impaired autophagy in Alzheimer disease and other conditions. Conversely, aberrant autophagy may lead to neuronal death, because autophagy constitutes an alternative pathway to cell death.[35] Thus, as with every other homeostatic system, the role of autophagy in neurodegeneration is context-dependent. Although overactivation may be beneficial to eliminate unwanted organelles/proteins, it may also lead to a "self-eating" process. For neurons, mostly postmitotic cells, accumulation of damaged proteins and organelles over their lifespan probably demands an exquisite fine-tuning of autophagy. However, regulatory mechanisms of autophagy in neurons are not yet well understood.

The main regulator of autophagy is the mammalian target of rapamycin (mTOR) pathway, which is downstream of IGF-1, although mTOR-independent routes also exist. IGF-1 reportedly inhibits autophagy through stimulation of mTOR (but see later discussion). In patients in whom autophagy is deleterious, IGF-1 may be beneficial.[36] In turn, inhibition of mTOR with rapamycin ameliorates neurodegenerative processes associated with protein accumulation, such as those produced by triplet repeat diseases, indicating a protective role of autophagy.[37] However, stimulation of the IGF-1 pathway stimulates autophagy-mediated clearance of mutant huntingtin aggregates even though mTOR is active, indicating an mTOR-independent action of IGF-1.[38] Therefore, depending on the role played by autophagy in a given disease, and whether IGF-1 acts through mTOR-dependent or mTOR-independent pathways, it may be detrimental or beneficial. Whether disturbed autophagy leads to IGF-1 resistance as part of its deleterious actions in neurodegeneration is currently entirely speculative. Because normal autophagy inhibits mTOR,[39] and this kinase in turn modulates IGF-1 signaling through Akt,[40] a putative feedback loop between autophagic activity and IGF-1 signaling is theoretically possible.

Endoplasmic Reticulum Stress and the Unfolded Protein Response

The endoplasmic reticulum (ER) forms part of the protein synthesis machinery and secretory pathway of the cell. Under normal conditions, proteins are trafficked through this organelle as part of their normal maturation. Under higher protein synthesis demand, the ER may experience stress that is in turn finely modulated, because this situation forms part of normal cell physiology.[41] A common response to ER stress is the unfolded protein response (UPR), a signaling pathway from the ER to the nucleus that is recruited also under normal ER function.[41] The purpose of the UPR is to normalize ER activity, and to this end, it diminishes protein translation, upregulates ER chaperones, and increases degradation of unfolded proteins.[42] If abnormally high levels of misprocessed proteins accumulate at the ER, they may lead, if unresolved, to altered cell function and ultimately cell death.[43] The UPR is considered to be involved in many neurodegenerative diseases (eg, Parkinson, amyotrophic lateral sclerosis, prionopathies), and is usually interpreted as a sign of altered protein homeostasis associated with these pathologies.

In addition to accumulation of abnormal proteins, different alterations in cell function impact the ER, including mitochondrial stress[44] or autophagy,[45] providing a link between these disturbances and the UPR. This function probably results from the central role of the ER in cellular homeostasis, which links this organelle to any other types of cell dysfunction. Therefore, as seen with oxidative stress and inflammation, the UPR may also constitute a common pathway of cell death in many neurodegenerative diseases.

Insulin resistance has been shown to arise as a consequence of ER stress. Activation of JNK by ER stress leads to inhibition of IRS phosphorylation by the insulin receptor.[46] Because until now all cellular alterations that lead to insulin resistance have been shown to also generate IGF-1 resistance, it is plausible that ER stress will provoke it. However, this possibility remains to be explored. Regardless, ER stress and IGF-1 signaling are functionally connected. Thus, an association between the UPR and IGF-1 may be established through its reported upregulation of ER chaperones, such as GRP78 or CHOP, that lead to increased cell survival,[47–49] or the enhanced nuclear translocation of the UPR transcriptional activator XBP1 by PI3K, which helps resolve the UPR.[50] In turn, XBP1 induces expression of IGF-1 and promotes Akt phosphorylation as part of its downstream effects toward normalizing protein folding and degradation.[51] In addition, AATF, an antiapoptotic protein of the UPR, stimulates Akt1 and in this way promotes cell survival.[52] Furthermore, a cell context–dependent action of IGF-1 signaling has been shown in cells under hypoxic conditions, whereby IGF-1 turns into a potentiator of ER stress to promote cell death.[53] In summary, ER stress and IGF-1 function are interconnected, but whether ER stress is associated with IGF-1 resistance remains a theoretical possibility that merits further attention.

IS IGF-1 BENEFICIAL OR DETRIMENTAL IN NEURODEGENERATIVE DISEASES?

The earlier observations suggest that pathologic mechanisms commonly associated with neurodegeneration may ultimately arise from IGF-1 resistance as part of their deleterious actions on neurons. However, if IGF-1 is considered as detrimental in age-associated diseases,[54] then resistance may be interpreted as an adaptive defensive mechanism, at least in neurodegenerative diseases associated with old age. Until now, all available evidence indicates the opposite: IGF-1 administration has been proven beneficial in many neurodegenerative conditions, and no reports indicate that IGF-1 administration is harmful. It is worth highlighting that, in this regard, the observed down-regulation of the GH/IGF-1 system associated with normal aging and premature senescence was proposed as a defensive mechanism against age-associated disturbances.[55] However, in a recent study with a mouse model of premature aging, administration of IGF-1 resulted in a dramatic alleviation of the aging phenotype.[56] In addition, the authors recently reported that, in mice, serum levels of IGF-1 before brain ischemia have a negative relationship with brain damage: the lower the levels, the smaller the lesion.[57] However, low serum IGF-1 levels after ischemia are associated with poorer prognosis,[58] and, more importantly, administration of IGF-1 after brain ischemia is neuroprotective.[26] Finally, either resistance to IGF-1[59–62] and/or IGF-1 deficiency[63,64] have been reported in patients with Alzheimer disease, whereas administration of IGF-1 to Alzheimer mice models alleviated pathology,[65,66] although these beneficial effects have not been replicated by others.[67] In view of these discrepancies, whether changes in brain IGF-1 function in Alzheimer disease are adaptive or detrimental to progress of the pathology is currently difficult to determine.

The possibility exists that a hormonal system that started as an integrator of growth responses to food availability in invertebrates became a modulator of longevity, expanded during vertebrate evolution into a much wider and complex network, becoming in this way a modulator of cell homeostasis.[4] Although very useful from an operational point of view, reductionist approaches purporting the IIS as a conserved regulatory system in aging from worms to humans[68] are probably an oversimplification. As with every other homeostatic mechanism, the context in which IGF-1 function is examined is key to understanding its function. Even within mammalian species, such as mice and humans, important differences have been found regarding IGF-1 in prolongevity manipulations, such as diet restriction.[69] A key issue is then to determine whether high or low IGF-1 activity will be positive or negative in a given context.

The current controversy on the role of IGF-I in Alzheimer disease, albeit parsimoniously, suggests a role for this growth factor in this important disease. The controversy stems from observations made in aging research. Researchers reasoned that age-related diseases, such as neurodegenerative diseases, will also benefit from reduced IIS,[70] at least partly through increased resistance to oxidative stress,[71] although recent data question a deleterious role of oxidative stress in aging.[29] Thus, mice null for the IGF-1R in forebrain neurons or full-body heterozygous IGF-1R mice showed improved pathology when cross-bred with transgenic mice with Alzheimer disease.[13,72] These observations agree with a similar protection found in IRS2 mutants.[73] However, blockade of IGF-1R specifically in the choroid plexus epithelium led to brain amyloidosis and Alzheimer disease pathology in wild-type rodents.[74] This finding conforms with reduced brain Aβ clearance when IGF-1 function is reduced.[66] In turn, reduced Aβ clearance is considered the cause of brain amyloidosis in Alzheimer disease.[75]

Furthermore, IGF-1 not only controls Aβ clearance but is also involved in amyloid precursor protein (APP) metabolism, controlling the amyloidogenic and nonamyloidogenic pathways.[76,77] Genetic down-regulation of the IGF-1R during development may produce an adjustment in APP metabolism, ultimately resulting in reduced Aβ production. In this regard, mice with Alzheimer disease that are heterozygous for the IGF-1 receptor have been noted to have lower levels of soluble Aβ,[13] an observation compatible with reduced production of Aβ. However, because APP metabolism was not measured in these mice, this possibility is entirely theoretical. In addition, the IGF-1R may functionally interact with APP metabolism, because it is also a substrate of the APP secretase complex.[78]

This putative functional connection would be reminiscent of the relationship between Aβ and insulin through the insulin-degrading enzyme (IDE), a protease shared by both molecules that, in the presence of high levels of Aβ, is diverted from its insulin target, generating hyperinsulinemia. This competitive mechanism has been proposed to form part of the pathologic cascade in Alzheimer disease.[79,80] Similarly, absence of the IGF-1R may divert the secretase complex toward its APP target, resulting in altered APP metabolism. In turn, absence of presenilin 1, which forms part of the Aβ secretase complex,[81] results in lower IGF-1[82] and IDE levels.[83] In this regard, it is important to point out that mutant Alzheimer disease–like mice usually display IGF-1 deficiency[66] and/or resistance[84] (as human patients, see earlier discussion). Therefore, when analyzing the effects of the IGF-1R in mouse models of Alzheimer disease that already show altered IGF-1 function, overall IGF-1 function must be determined before assuming that the observed phenotype (ie, amelioration of Alzheimer disease pathology) is caused by reduced IGF-1 action.

Alternative explanations[85] include that reduction/deletion of brain IGF-1 receptors may elicit compensatory responses in related systems (ie, brain insulin receptors). Compensatory and/or redundant mechanisms in null mutants is a common pitfall of these animals models and should therefore be investigated in IGF-1R hemizygous mice. Elimination of the IGF-1 receptor may also address other functions of this receptor that are currently poorly characterized, such as its role in the cell nucleus[86] or apoptotic pathways.[87] The latter opens an entirely new way of looking at insulin/IGF-1 receptor

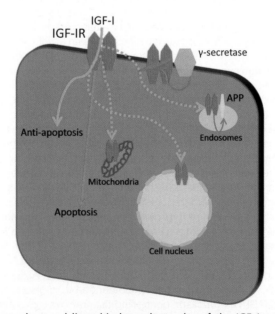

Fig. 2. Ligand-dependent and ligand-independent roles of the IGF-1 receptor. Canonical signaling by IGF-1 through the IGF-1R (*solid brown line*) leads to antiapoptotic responses (and/or anabolic routes) in target cells. Noncanonical signaling by IGF-1 (*dashed lines*) includes the mitochondria and the cell nucleus as signaling organelles of as yet uncertain significance. Another pathway leads to modulation of APP metabolism (probably at the endosomal compartment) in a complex manner. In turn, the IGF-1 receptor participates in proapoptotic signaling independently of IGF-1, and is cleaved by γ-secretase, a proamyloidogenic APP protease, at the cell membrane. The latter two processes are currently of unknown significance.

function, because absence of these receptors produces resistance to apoptosis. Whether this antiapoptotic effect of IGF-1R/IR deletion plays a role in the neuroprotective effects of reduced IGF-1R in mice with Alzheimer disease should also be considered. However, the important point raised by these observations is that elimination of the IGF-1R does not equate to elimination of IGF-1 actions only.

For the opposite observation, that administration of IGF-1 to mice with Alzheimer disease ameliorates pathology, the explanation seems more straightforward. Brain amyloidosis has been shown to elicit insulin resistance by down-regulation of insulin receptors through a CamKII-dependent pathway[88] or through phosphorylation of IRS via JNK.[89] In all probability, amyloidosis will also produce IGF-1 resistance,[59,90,91] because Aβ also interferes with IGF-1 signaling.[91] Thus, administration of IGF-1 will reduce IGF-1 resistance in Alzheimer disease. Because IGF-1 is widely neuroprotective and actively participates in APP/Aβ metabolism, allowing IGF-1 actions in the Alzheimer disease brain will increase its resilience to ongoing insult. When IGF-1 resistance or IGF-1 deficiency is observed, such as in cerebellar ataxia[92–96] and diabetes,[97] respectively, the use of IGF-1 has proven beneficial.[98,99]

SUMMARY

The previously undisputed neuroprotective role of IGF-1 has been challenged by recent observations in IGF-1R–defective mutants. As new ligand-dependent and ligand-independent roles for the IGF-1R are emerging (**Fig. 2**), new insights into the biologic role of brain IGF-1R and its connection with serum and brain IGF-1 function are urgently required. In the meantime, treatment of specific neurodegenerative diseases with IGF-1 may still be explored using adequate preclinical procedures.[100]

REFERENCES

1. Allan SM, Rothwell NJ. Cytokines and acute neurodegeneration. Nat Rev Neurosci 2001;2(10):734–44.
2. Beattie EC, Stellwagen D, Morishita W, et al. Control of synaptic strength by glial TNFalpha. Science 2002;295(5563):2282–5.
3. Freude S, Schilbach K, Schubert M. The role of IGF-1 receptor and insulin receptor signaling for the pathogenesis of Alzheimer's disease: from model organisms to human disease. Curr Alzheimer Res 2009;6(3):213–23.
4. Torres-Aleman I. Toward a comprehensive neurobiology of IGF-I. Dev Neurobiol 2010;70(5):384–96.
5. Nishijima T, Piriz J, Duflot S, et al. Neuronal activity drives localized blood-brain-barrier transport of serum insulin-like growth factor-I into the CNS. Neuron 2010; 67(5):834–46.
6. Christensen K, Doblhammer G, Rau R, et al. Ageing populations: the challenges ahead. Lancet 2009;374(9696):1196–208.
7. Douglas PM, Dillin A. Protein homeostasis and aging in neurodegeneration. J Cell Biol 2010;190(5):719–29.
8. Kleemann GA, Murphy CT. The endocrine regulation of aging in Caenorhabditis elegans. Mol Cell Endocrinol 2009;299(1):51–7.
9. Kenyon CJ. The genetics of ageing. Nature 2010;464(7288):504–12.
10. Bartke A. The somatotropic axis and aging: mechanisms and persistent questions about practical implications. Exp Gerontol 2009;44(6–7):372–4.
11. Liu JP, Baker J, Perkins AS, et al. Mice carrying null mutations of the genes encoding insulin-like growth factor I (Igf-1) and type 1 IGF receptor (Igf1r). Cell 1993;75(1):59–72.

12. Kojima T, Kamei H, Aizu T, et al. Association analysis between longevity in the Japanese population and polymorphic variants of genes involved in insulin and insulin-like growth factor 1 signaling pathways. Exp Gerontol 2011;39(11–12):1595–8.

13. Cohen E, Paulsson JF, Blinder P, et al. Reduced IGF-1 signaling delays age-associated proteotoxicity in mice. Cell 2009;139(6):1157–69.

14. Gusella JF, MacDonald ME. Molecular genetics: unmasking polyglutamine triggers in neurodegenerative disease. Nat Rev Neurosci 2000;1(2):109–15.

15. Sastre M, Walter J, Gentleman SM. Interactions between APP secretases and inflammatory mediators. J Neuroinflammation 2008;5:25.

16. Trejo JL, Carro E, Garcia-Galloway E, et al. Role of insulin-like growth factor I signaling in neurodegenerative diseases. J Mol Med 2004;82(3):156–62.

17. Mrak RE, Griffin WS. Glia and their cytokines in progression of neurodegeneration. Neurobiol Aging 2005;26(3):349–54.

18. Glass CK, Saijo K, Winner B, et al. Mechanisms underlying inflammation in neurodegeneration. Cell 2010;140(6):918–34.

19. Fernandez AM, Jimenez S, Mecha M, et al. Regulation of the phosphatase calcineurin by insulin-like growth factor I unveils a key role of astrocytes in Alzheimer's pathology. Mol Psychiatry 2011. DOI: 10.1038/mp.2011.128.

20. Imbimbo BP. An update on the efficacy of non-steroidal anti-inflammatory drugs in Alzheimer's disease. Expert Opin Investig Drugs 2009;18(8):1147–68.

21. Grimble RF. Inflammatory status and insulin resistance. Curr Opin Clin Nutr Metab Care 2002;5(5):551–9.

22. Venters HD, Tang Q, Liu Q, et al. A new mechanism of neurodegeneration: a proinflammatory cytokine inhibits receptor signaling by a survival peptide. Proc Natl Acad Sci U S A 1999;96(17):9879–84.

23. Arundine M, Tymianski M. Molecular mechanisms of calcium-dependent neurodegeneration in excitotoxicity. Cell Calcium 2003;34(4–5):325–37.

24. Garcia-Galloway E, Arango C, Pons S, et al. Glutamate excitotoxicity attenuates insulin-like growth factor-i prosurvival signaling. Mol Cell Neurosci 2003;24(4):1027–37.

25. Zheng WH, Quirion R. Glutamate acting on NMDA receptors attenuates IGF-1 receptor tyrosine phosphorylation and its survival signaling properties in rat hippocampal neurons. J Biol Chem 2009;284(2):855–61.

26. Guan J, Bennet L, Gluckman PD, et al. Insulin-like growth factor-1 and post-ischemic brain injury. Prog Neurobiol 2003;70(6):443–62.

27. Goldstein BJ, Mahadev K, Wu X. Redox paradox: insulin action is facilitated by insulin-stimulated reactive oxygen species with multiple potential signaling targets. Diabetes 2005;54(2):311–21.

28. Droge W. Oxidative stress and aging. Adv Exp Med Biol 2003;543:191–200.

29. Yang W, Hekimi S. A mitochondrial superoxide signal triggers increased longevity in caenorhabditis elegans. PLoS Biol 2010;8(12):e1000556.

30. Houstis N, Rosen ED, Lander ES. Reactive oxygen species have a causal role in multiple forms of insulin resistance. Nature 2006;440(7086):944–8.

31. Davila D, Torres-Aleman I. Neuronal death by oxidative stress involves activation of FOXO3 through a two-arm pathway that activates stress kinases and attenuates insulin-like growth factor I signaling. Mol Biol Cell 2008;19(5):2014–25.

32. Kim B, Sullivan KA, Backus C, et al. Cortical neurons develop insulin resistance and blunted Akt signaling: a potential mechanism contributing to enhanced ischemic injury in diabetes. Antioxid Redox Signal 2011;14(10):1829–39.

33. Hara T, Nakamura K, Matsui M, et al. Suppression of basal autophagy in neural cells causes neurodegenerative disease in mice. Nature 2006;441(7095):885–9.

34. Komatsu M, Waguri S, Chiba T, et al. Loss of autophagy in the central nervous system causes neurodegeneration in mice. Nature 2006;441(7095):880–4.

35. Lee JA. Autophagy in neurodegeneration: two sides of the same coin. BMB Rep 2009;42(6):324–30.

36. Bains M, Zaegel V, Mize-Berge J, et al. IGF-I stimulates Rab7-RILP interaction during neuronal autophagy. Neurosci Lett 2011;488(2):112–7.

37. Ravikumar B, Vacher C, Berger Z, et al. Inhibition of mTOR induces autophagy and reduces toxicity of polyglutamine expansions in fly and mouse models of Huntington disease. Nat Genet 2004;36(6):585–95.

38. Yamamoto A, Cremona ML, Rothman JE. Autophagy-mediated clearance of huntingtin aggregates triggered by the insulin-signaling pathway. J Cell Biol 2006;172(5):719–31.

39. Feng Z, Levine AJ. The regulation of energy metabolism and the IGF-1/mTOR pathways by the p53 protein. Trends Cell Biol 2010;20(7):427–34.

40. Haruta T, Uno T, Kawahara J, et al. A rapamycin-sensitive pathway down-regulates insulin signaling via phosphorylation and proteasomal degradation of insulin receptor substrate-1. Mol Endocrinol 2000;14(6):783–94.

41. Rutkowski DT, Arnold SM, Miller CN, et al. Adaptation to ER stress is mediated by differential stabilities of pro-survival and pro-apoptotic mRNAs and proteins. PLoS Biol 2006;4(11):e374.

42. Engin F, Hotamisligil GS. Restoring endoplasmic reticulum function by chemical chaperones: an emerging therapeutic approach for metabolic diseases. Diabetes Obes Metab 2010;12(Suppl 2):108–15.

43. Shore GC, Papa FR, Oakes SA. Signaling cell death from the endoplasmic reticulum stress response. Curr Opin Cell Biol 2011;23(2):143–9.

44. Bouman L, Schlierf A, Lutz AK, et al. Parkin is transcriptionally regulated by ATF4: evidence for an interconnection between mitochondrial stress and ER stress. Cell Death Differ 2011;18(5):769–82.

45. Matus S, Nassif M, Glimcher LH, et al. XBP-1 deficiency in the nervous system reveals a homeostatic switch to activate autophagy. Autophagy 2009;5(8):1226–8.

46. Ozcan U, Cao Q, Yilmaz E, et al. Endoplasmic reticulum stress links obesity, insulin action, and type 2 diabetes. Science 2004;306(5695):457–61.

47. Novosyadlyy R, Kurshan N, Lann D, et al. Insulin-like growth factor-I protects cells from ER stress-induced apoptosis via enhancement of the adaptive capacity of endoplasmic reticulum. Cell Death Differ 2008;15(8):1304–17.

48. Pfaffenbach KT, Lee AS. The critical role of GRP78 in physiologic and pathologic stress. Curr Opin Cell Biol 2011;23(2):150–6.

49. Rubovitch V, Shahar A, Werner H, et al. Does IGF-1 administration after a mild traumatic brain injury in mice activate the adaptive arm of ER stress? Neurochem Int 2011;8(4):443–6.

50. Park SW, Zhou Y, Lee J, et al. The regulatory subunits of PI3K, p85[alpha] and p85[beta], interact with XBP-1 and increase its nuclear translocation. Nat Med 2010;16(4):429–37.

51. Hu MC, Gong HY, Lin GH, et al. XBP-1, a key regulator of unfolded protein response, activates transcription of IGF1 and Akt phosphorylation in zebrafish embryonic cell line. Biochem Biophys Res Commun 2007;359(3):778–83.

52. Ishigaki S, Fonseca SG, Oslowski CM, et al. AATF mediates an antiapoptotic effect of the unfolded protein response through transcriptional regulation of AKT1. Cell Death Differ 2010;17(5):774–86.

53. Endo H, Murata K, Mukai M, et al. Activation of insulin-like growth factor signaling induces apoptotic cell death under prolonged hypoxia by enhancing endoplasmic reticulum stress response. Cancer Res 2007;67(17):8095–103.

54. Puglielli L. Aging of the brain, neurotrophin signaling, and Alzheimer's disease: is IGF1-R the common culprit? Neurobiol Aging 2008;29(6):795–811.

55. Monnat RJ Jr. From broken to old: DNA damage, IGF1 endocrine suppression and aging. DNA Repair 2007;6(9):1386–90.

56. Marino G, Ugalde AP, Fernandez AF, et al. Insulin-like growth factor 1 treatment extends longevity in a mouse model of human premature aging by restoring somatotroph axis function. Proc Natl Acad Sci U S A 2010;107(37):16268–73.

57. Endres M, Piriz J, Gertz K, et al. Serum insulin-like growth factor I and ischemic brain injury. Brain Res 2007;1185:328–35.

58. Schwab S, Spranger M, Krempien S, et al. Plasma insulin-like growth factor I and IGF binding protein 3 levels in patients with acute cerebral ischemic injury. Stroke 1997;28(9):1744–8.

59. Moloney AM, Griffin RJ, Timmons S, et al. Defects in IGF-1 receptor, insulin receptor and IRS-1/2 in Alzheimer's disease indicate possible resistance to IGF-1 and insulin signalling. Neurobiol Aging 2010;31(2):224–43.

60. Salehi Z, Mashayekhi F, Naji M. Insulin like growth factor-1 and insulin like growth factor binding proteins in the cerebrospinal fluid and serum from patients with Alzheimer's disease. Biofactors 2008;33(2):99–106.

61. Tham A, Nordberg A, Grissom FE, et al. Insulin-like growth factors and insulin-like growth factor binding proteins in cerebrospinal fluid and serum of patients with dementia of the Alzheimer type. J Neural Transm Park Dis Dement Sect 1993;5(3):165–76.

62. Vardy ER, Rice PJ, Bowie PC, et al. Increased circulating insulin-like growth factor-1 in late-onset Alzheimer's disease. J Alzheimers Dis 2007;12(4):285–90.

63. Rivera EJ, Goldin A, Fulmer N, et al. Insulin and insulin-like growth factor expression and function deteriorate with progression of Alzheimer's disease: link to brain reductions in acetylcholine. J Alzheimers Dis 2005;8(3):247–68.

64. Watanabe T, Miyazaki A, Katagiri T, et al. Relationship between serum insulin-like growth factor-1 levels and Alzheimer's disease and vascular dementia. J Am Geriatr Soc 2005;53(10):1748–53.

65. Carro E, Trejo JL, Gerber A, et al. Therapeutic actions of insulin-like growth factor I on APP/PS2 mice with severe brain amyloidosis. Neurobiol Aging 2006;27(9):1250–7.

66. Carro E, Trejo JL, Gomez-Isla T, et al. Serum insulin-like growth factor I regulates brain amyloid-beta levels. Nat Med 2002;8(12):1390–7.

67. Lanz TA, Salatto CT, Semproni AR, et al. Peripheral elevation of IGF-1 fails to alter Abeta clearance in multiple in vivo models. Biochem Pharmacol 2008;75(5):1093–103.

68. Kenyon C. A conserved regulatory system for aging. Cell 2001;105(2):165–8.

69. Redman LM, Martin CK, Williamson DA, et al. Effect of caloric restriction in non-obese humans on physiological, psychological and behavioral outcomes. Physiol Behav 2008;94(5):643–8.

70. Pehar M, O'Riordan KJ, Burns-Cusato M, et al. Altered longevity-assurance activity of p53:p44 in the mouse causes memory loss, neurodegeneration and premature death. Aging Cell 2010;9(2):174–90.

71. Holzenberger M, Dupont J, Ducos B, et al. IGF-1 receptor regulates lifespan and resistance to oxidative stress in mice. Nature 2003;421(6919):182–7.

72. Freude S, Hettich MM, Schumann C, et al. Neuronal IGF-1 resistance reduces Abeta accumulation and protects against premature death in a model of Alzheimer's disease. FASEB J 2009;23:3315.

73. Killick R, Scales G, Leroy K, et al. Deletion of Irs2 reduces amyloid deposition and rescues behavioural deficits in APP transgenic mice. Biochem Biophys Res Commun 2009;386(1):257–62.

74. Carro E, Trejo JL, Spuch C, et al. Blockade of the insulin-like growth factor I receptor in the choroid plexus originates Alzheimer's-like neuropathology in rodents: new cues into the human disease? Neurobiol Aging 2006;27(11):1618–31.

75. Mawuenyega KG, Sigurdson W, Ovod V, et al. Decreased clearance of CNS β-amyloid in Alzheimer's disease. Science 2010;330(6012):1774.

76. Adlerz L, Holback S, Multhaup G, et al. IGF-1-induced processing of the amyloid precursor protein family is mediated by different signaling pathways. J Biol Chem 2007;282(14):10203–9.

77. Shineman DW, Dain AS, Kim ML, et al. Constitutively active Akt inhibits trafficking of amyloid precursor protein and amyloid precursor protein metabolites through feedback inhibition of phosphoinositide 3-kinase. Biochemistry 2009; 48(17):3787–94.

78. McElroy B, Powell JC, McCarthy JV. The insulin-like growth factor 1 (IGF-1) receptor is a substrate for gamma-secretase-mediated intramembrane proteolysis. Biochem Biophys Res Commun 2007;358(4):1136–41.

79. Farris W, Mansourian S, Chang Y, et al. Insulin-degrading enzyme regulates the levels of insulin, amyloid beta-protein, and the beta-amyloid precursor protein intracellular domain in vivo. Proc Natl Acad Sci U S A 2003;100(7):4162–7.

80. Fishel MA, Watson GS, Montine TJ, et al. Hyperinsulinemia provokes synchronous increases in central inflammation and beta-amyloid in normal adults. Arch Neurol 2005;62(10):1539–44.

81. Selkoe DJ, Wolfe MS. Presenilin: running with scissors in the membrane. Cell 2007;131(2):215–21.

82. Nakajima M, Watanabe S, Okuyama S, et al. Restricted growth and insulin-like growth factor-1 deficiency in mice lacking presenilin-1 in the neural crest cell lineage. Int J Dev Neurosci 2009;27(8):837–43.

83. Qin W, Jia J. Down-regulation of insulin-degrading enzyme by presenilin 1 V97L mutant potentially underlies increased levels of amyloid beta 42. Eur J Neurosci 2008;27(9):2425–32.

84. Lopez-Lopez C, Dietrich MO, Metzger F, et al. Disturbed cross talk between insulin-like growth factor I and AMP-activated protein kinase as a possible cause of vascular dysfunction in the amyloid precursor protein/presenilin 2 mouse model of Alzheimer's disease. J Neurosci 2007;27(4):824–31.

85. Piriz J, Muller A, Trejo JL, et al. IGF-I and the aging mammalian brain. Exp Gerontol 2011;46(2–3):96–9.

86. Sehat B, Tofigh A, Lin Y, et al. SUMOylation mediates the nuclear translocation and signaling of the IGF-1 receptor. Sci Signal 2010;3(108):ra10.

87. Boucher J, Macotela Y, Bezy O, et al. A kinase-independent role for unoccupied insulin and IGF-1 receptors in the control of apoptosis. Sci Signal 2010;3(151): ra87.

88. De Felice FG, Vieira MN, Bomfim TR, et al. Protection of synapses against Alzheimer's-linked toxins: insulin signaling prevents the pathogenic binding of Aβ oligomers. Proc Natl Acad Sci U S A 2009;106(6):1971–6.

89. Ma QL, Yang F, Rosario ER, et al. Beta-amyloid oligomers induce phosphorylation of tau and inactivation of insulin receptor substrate via c-Jun N-terminal

kinase signaling: suppression by omega-3 fatty acids and curcumin. J Neurosci 2009;29(28):9078–89.

90. Carro E, Torres-Aleman I. The role of insulin and insulin-like growth factor I in the molecular and cellular mechanisms underlying the pathology of Alzheimer's disease. Eur J Pharmacol 2004;490(1–3):127–33.

91. Gasparini L, Xu H. Potential roles of insulin and IGF-1 in Alzheimer's disease. Trends Neurosci 2003;26(8):404–6.

92. Busiguina S, Fernandez AM, Barrios V, et al. Neurodegeneration is associated to changes in serum insulin-like growth factors. Neurobiol Dis 2000;7(6 Pt B): 657–65.

93. Gatchel JR, Watase K, Thaller C, et al. The insulin-like growth factor pathway is altered in spinocerebellar ataxia type 1 and type 7. Proc Natl Acad Sci U S A 2008;105(4):1291–6.

94. Peretz S, Jensen R, Baserga R, et al. ATM-dependent expression of the insulin-like growth factor-I receptor in a pathway regulating radiation response. Proc Natl Acad Sci U S A 2001;98(4):1676–81.

95. Saute JA, da Silva AC, Muller AP, et al. Serum insulin-like system alterations in patients with spinocerebellar ataxia type 3. Mov Disord 2011;26(4):731–5.

96. Torres-Aleman I, Barrios V, Lledo A, et al. The insulin-like growth factor I system in cerebellar degeneration. Ann Neurol 1996;39(3):335–42.

97. Acerini CL, Dunger DB. Insulin-like growth factor-I for the treatment of type 1 diabetes. Diabetes Obes Metab 2000;2(6):335–43.

98. Arpa J, Sanz-Gallego I, Medina-Baez J, et al. Subcutaneous insulin-like growth factor-1 treatment in spinocerebellar ataxias: an open label clinical trial. Mov Disord 2011;26(2):358–9.

99. Clemmons DR, Moses AC, Sommer A, et al. Rh/IGF-I/rhIGFBP-3 administration to patients with type 2 diabetes mellitus reduces insulin requirements while also lowering fasting glucose. Growth Horm IGF Res 2005;15(4):265–74.

100. Jucker M. The benefits and limitations of animal models for translational research in neurodegenerative diseases. Nat Med 2010;16(11):1210–4.

Insulin-Like Growth Factors in the Gastrointestinal Tract and Liver

John F. Kuemmerle, MD[a,b],*

KEYWORDS

- IGF • IGF binding proteins • Growth hormone • Gastrointestinal tract • Liver

KEY POINTS

- The majority of IGF-1 in circulation is synthesized in the liver and circulates bound to IGFBPs. In this context, IGF-1 is an endocrine growth factor.
- IGF-1 and IGFBPs are also produced in abundance by peripheral tissues of the GI tract. In this context, IGF-1 is a paracrine/autocrine regulator of GI and liver physiology.
- IGF-1, IGFBP-3 and IGFBP-5 are important pathophysiologic mediators of intestinal fibrosis in inflammatory bowel disease.
- Epigenetic regulation of IGFs including IGF-2 is an important risk factor for development of gastrointestinal and liver neoplasia.

OVERVIEW AND DISCOVERY OF INSULIN-LIKE GROWTH FACTORS

The insulin-like growth factor (IGF) family includes 3 structurally related ligands, insulin, IGF-1, and IGF-2, and 2 high-affinity cell surface receptors, the IGF-1 receptor (IGF-1R) and the IGF-2 receptor (IGF-2R). Although the insulin receptor (IR) shares significant, approximately 70%, sequence homology with the IGF-1 receptor, it possesses a distinct ligand affinity profile. The IGF binding proteins (IGFBPs) are important physiologic regulators of the interaction of IGFs with their receptors within the gastrointestinal tract and liver. The growth hormone (GH) is structurally unrelated to IGFs, but its actions are mediated primarily through the regulation of synthesis and secretion of IGF-1 by the liver; hence, GH and its biology are intimately intertwined with IGF-1 and its biology and are referenced in this article.

The IGF system functions as a leading endocrine, paracrine, and autocrine regulatory axis for cellular proliferation, survival, and apoptosis in the gastrointestinal tract. In

Supported by DK-49691 from the National Institutes of Diabetes, Digestive and Kidney Diseases.
[a] Department of Medicine, Medical College of Virginia Campus, Virginia Commonwealth University, Richmond, VA 23298-0341, USA; [b] Department of Physiology and Biophysics, Medical College of Virginia Campus, Virginia Commonwealth University, Richmond, VA 23298-0341, USA
* Division of Gastroenterology, Medical College of Virginia Campus, Virginia Commonwealth University, PO Box 980341, 1220 East Broad Street, Molecular Medicine Research Building 5-036, Richmond, VA 23298-0341.
E-mail address: john.kuemmerle@vcu.edu

Endocrinol Metab Clin N Am 41 (2012) 409–423
doi:10.1016/j.ecl.2012.04.018
0889-8529/12/$ – see front matter © 2012 Elsevier Inc. All rights reserved.

addition, it has general activities relating to energy metabolism, body size, carcinogenesis, and various organ-specific functions. There have been several comprehensive reviews regarding these activities.[1–9]

INSULIN-LIKE GROWTH FACTOR GENES AND PROTEINS IN THE GASTROINTESTINAL TRACT AND LIVER

IGF-1 and IGF-2 are 2 closely related members of the insulin superfamily of peptide hormones. IGF-1 and IGF-2 are 67% identical single-polypeptide chains that share an amino acid identity of approximately 40% with insulin. Unlike insulin, IGFs are not produced and stored solely in the beta cells of the pancreatic islets. They are synthesized and secreted by many cells in the body, including cells of the gastrointestinal tract and liver, in a highly regulated manner.

The IGF-1 gene is located on human chromosome 12q22–q23. The genomic sequence is large, spanning more than 80-kB DNA, including 6 exons.[10] At least 4 transcriptional start sites have been identified, and IGF-1 messenger RNA species range from about 1 to 8 kB. Complex, tissue-specific alternate splicing patterns have been observed, but the biological significance of these variants has not been clearly delineated for gastrointestinal tissues.[11] For human pro-IGF-1, 2 primary translation products exist: IGF-1Ea and IGF-1Eb. The most commonly recognized mature IGF-1, IGF-1Ea, is a 70–amino acid secreted protein. The existence of a putative peptide derived from alternative splicing that yields the IGF-1Ec variant, mechanogrowth factor (MGF), remains speculative.[12] However, evidence suggests that MGF plays a role in the pathophysiologic response of the gastrointestinal smooth muscle to inflammation and injury.[13]

The majority of IGF-1 in the peripheral circulation is synthesized in the liver under the control of GH and circulates bound to IGFBPs, primarily IGFBP-3 and the acid-labile subunit (ALS) as a ternary complex. In this context, IGF-1 is an endocrine hormone growth factor that stimulates somatic growth and exerts feedback to the pituitary to downregulate GH synthesis. Most growth-stimulating activities of GH can be mimicked by IGF-1. Peripheral tissues in the gastrointestinal tract are also abundant sources of IGF-1, particularly intestinal smooth muscle, that acts in an autocrine and paracrine manner to regulate cell growth and survival. Although GH regulates IGF production in the liver and other tissues under normal circumstances (see later) and in disease states, for example, malnutrition and Crohn disease, a relative GH-insensitive state exists, whereby the stimulatory effects of GH on IGF-1 expression and secretion are markedly reduced and IGF-1 expression is regulated by other factors. IGF-1 binds to IGF-1R with high affinity and to IGF-2R with a lower affinity.

The human IGF-2 gene is located on chromosome 11p15.5. Like the IGF-1 precursor, the IGF-2 precursor is large and multiple splice variants have been described, many of which are developmentally regulated and contain gut-specific promoters.[14] A pro-IGF-2–containing a COOH-terminal precursor sequence is secreted from cells before being processed to the mature 67–amino acid protein.[5] The IGF-2 gene is relatively unique in that it is "imprinted" in 90% of humans, which means that normally one allele is silenced on the basis of parental origin. When maternal IGF-2 silencing is lost (loss of imprinting [LOI]), biallelic IGF-2 expression correlates strongly with the hypomethylation of a differentially methylated region near its promoter and results in increased IGF-2 levels. IGF-2 levels resulting from LOI are increased and are associated with an increased risk for a variety of cancers, including colorectal cancer.[15] More recently, other mechanisms responsible for elevated levels of IGF-2 in colorectal cancer have been identified, including microsatellite instability.[16] IGF-2 binds to both IGF-1R and IGF-1R with high affinity.

INSULIN-LIKE GROWTH FACTOR RECEPTOR GENES AND PROTEINS

The IGF-1 receptor (IGF-1R) gene is located on human chromosome 15q26.3 and is 70% identical to the IR gene.[17] The protein is synthesized as a single polypeptide chain that is cleaved by proteolysis at a tetrabasic amino acid site resulting in α and β subunits. These subunits associate by disulfide bridging into α and β heterodimers that further associate by disulfide bridging forming the mature heterotetrameric $\alpha_2\beta_2$ receptors. Structurally, this overall configuration is identical to the IR; in fact, hybrid IGF-1R and IRs are well recognized.[18] Most biological activities of IGF-1 and IGF-2 in the gastrointestinal tract and liver are mediated by the IGF-1R.

IGF-1 binding results in autophosphorylation of specific cytosolic tyrosine residues within the IGF-1R receptor, activation of its intrinsic tyrosine kinase activity, and phosphorylation of intracellular substrates (**Fig. 1**). IR substrate 1 (IRS-1), a 185-kDa intracellular signaling protein with multiple phosphorylation sites and SH domains permitting docking of multiple intracellular signaling molecules, is a key early mediator of IGF-1R function.[19] The result of IRS-1 phosphorylation is activation of a variety of signaling cascades, including the Ras-Erk1/2 and phosphoinosotide-3 kinase pathways. The IGF-1R also activates the heterotrimeric G protein, G_{i2}, that is coupled to activation of the Erk1/2 pathway.[20] In intestinal smooth muscle, the intensity and duration of IGF-1–stimulated IGF-1R activity is positively regulated by ligand occupancy of $\alpha V\beta 3$ integrin by the resultant temporally regulated translocation of SH2 domain–containing tyrosine phosphatase 2 from $\alpha V\beta 3$ integrin to the IGF-1 receptor.[21] Activation of IGF-1R regulates cellular proliferation and survival, key regulatory activities of IGFs in the gastrointestinal tract.

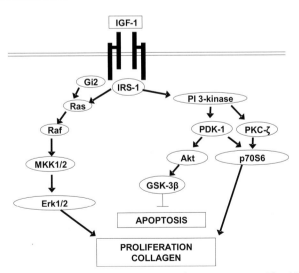

Fig. 1. Signaling cascades activated by the activated IGF-1 receptor. The IGF-1 receptor is located on the basolateral membrane of intestinal epithelial cells and on smooth muscle cells. Ligand binding and activation of the IGF-1 receptor elicit phosphorylation of cytoplasmic tyrosine residues in this receptor tyrosine kinase. Subsequently, binding of scaffolding and docking proteins results in activation of distinct intracellular signaling cascades that regulate proliferation and survival and collagen IαI expression.

The IGF-2R, also referred to as the cation-independent mannose 6-phosphate receptor, bears no structural homology to the IR or IGF-1R.[9] It is located on human chromosome 6q26. The IGF-2R is a single transmembrane polypeptide that binds IGF-2 with a greatly reduced affinity for IGF-1 and insulin. It has 15 cysteine-laden, contiguous, extracellular repeats and a short intracellular sequence with no recognizable signaling motifs.[4] Although the function of IGF-2 signaling is controversial, most experts believe that the signaling downmodulates IGF-2 activity by regulating its endocytosis and intracellular degradation by targeting the proteins to the lysosome. This is relevant to the gastrointestinal tract and is consistent with data showing that IGF-2R is a tumor-suppressor gene, acting as a sink or reservoir for IGF-2, and with the effects of LOI of IGF-2 in colorectal cancer.[6,15,16,22]

IGFBP GENE AND PROTEIN FAMILY IN THE GASTROINTESTINAL TRACT

IGFBPs are a well-characterized family of 6 secreted proteins, designated as IGFBP-1 through IGFBP-6, that bind IGFs with high affinity and display a broad spectrum of biological activity. Extensive information about the gene organization, protein structure, and molecular biology and physiology of IGFBPs can be found in the reviews referenced at the beginning of this article. IGFBPs are potent modulators of IGF activity in the gastrointestinal tract, exerting both positive and negative effects, because they generally have 10- to 100-fold greater affinity for IGFs than for the IGF receptors. Both IGF-1 and IGF-2 bind to all 6 IGFBPs, albeit with different affinity.

The structure of all 6 IGFBPs is similar because of their conserved evolution and can be divided into 3 domains: highly conserved C- and N-terminal domains and a central domain that is unique among IGFBP family members. The C- and N-terminal domains bind IGFs. It is the central domain that is modified by posttranslational modifications and confers functional diversity among IGFBPs.[7] Depending on the experimental setting and IGF function being assessed, IGFBPs may potentiate or inhibit IGF activity in the gastrointestinal tract primarily by altering the interaction of IGF-1 or IGF-2 with the IGF-1R. IGFBPs exert inhibitory effects by binding IGFs into a biologically inaccessible pool, whereas stimulation or potentiation of IGF action occurs by the facilitation of IGFs binding with the IGF-1R. Regulated proteolysis of IGFBPs is a key mechanism for release of IGF and regulating its bioavailability to cells of the gastrointestinal tract.[7] For example, addition of IGFBP-3 to colon cancer cell culture medium decreases bioactivity of IGF-1. Addition of matrix metalloproteinase 7 cleaves IGFBP-3 into 4 fragments, releases IGF-1, and potentiates IGF-1 biological activity.[7] An important function of hepatic-derived IGFBP function is to transport IGFs made in the liver in the circulation and in extracellular fluids. IGFBPs are detectable in plasma and extracellular fluids and are expressed during gastrointestinal tract development and into adult life. The primary hepatic-derived IGFBP is IGFBP-3, which carries approximately 75% of circulating IGF-1 and IGF-2 bound to it and the cocarrier, ALS.[7] IGF-independent activities of IGFBPs (IGFBP-1, IGFBP-3, IGFBP-4 and IGFBP-5) in the gastrointestinal tract are also recognized. These play a role both in gastrointestinal tract physiology and in pathophysiologic events. IGFBP-3 directly activates the transforming growth factor (TGF)-βRI/II receptor complex and initiates Smad signaling in human intestinal smooth muscle cells.[23,24] In intestinal muscle cells, although IGFBP-5 facilitates interaction of IGF-1 with the IGF-1R, it also acts independently of IGF-1 to stimulate proliferation and further increase expression of IGF-1 (**Fig. 2**).[25] Both processes involving IGFBP-3 and IGFBP-5 play a role in muscle hyperplasia in stricturing Crohn disease and also in the concomitant excess collagen production.

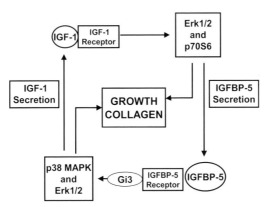

Fig. 2. Positive feedback between IGFBP-5 and IGF-1. The expression and effects of IGF-1 and IGFBP-5 are linked, whereby IGF-1 stimulates IGFBP-5 expression and IGFBP-5, independent of IGF-1, stimulates IGF-1 expression, each reinforcing the expression and effects of the other.

IGFBP-3 and IGFBP-5 also possess COOH-terminal consensus nuclear localization sequences that allow cell entry and the direct nuclear activity of these binding proteins via a β-importin–dependent nuclear translocation mechanism. By this mechanism, IGFBP-3 regulates apoptosis in prostate cancer cells, and IGFBP-5 regulates heterodimerization of retinoid X receptor and vitamin D receptors and modulates vitamin D–dependent differentiation.[26,27] An NH$_2$-terminal sequence is a consensus transactivator domain that has been shown to possess strong IGF-1–independent transactivation activity.[28] The participation of these mechanisms in gastrointestinal tract function has not yet been examined.

BIOLOGY OF THE INSULIN-LIKE GROWTH FACTOR FAMILY IN THE GASTROINTESTINAL TRACT

The gastrointestinal tract is a major target organ of IGF action.[29] One of the most prominent effects is stimulation of intestinal epithelial cell and muscle cell proliferation and maintenance of cell survival by reduction of apoptosis. Other activities relate to the diverse effects of this ligand/receptor family on somatic growth, energy balance, and metabolism of glucose, carbohydrate, and proteins.

INSULIN-LIKE GROWTH FACTOR FAMILY DISTRIBUTION IN THE GASTROINTESTINAL TRACT

The presence and distribution of IGFs and IGF receptors in the gastrointestinal tract has been extensively characterized.[11,14,30–40] IGF-1, IGF-2, and IGFBPs are also present in human breast milk and in gastrointestinal tract secretions.[41–43] A portion of enterally administered ^{125}I-IGF-1 and ^{125}I-IGF-2 can be recovered intact from gastrointestinal tissues of suckling rats, which indicates that the peptide is stable in the milieu of the neonatal stomach and small intestine.[44,45] Although the expression of this ligand receptor system in the gastrointestinal epithelium is clear, a precise understanding of its distribution along the crypt-villus axis and in the epithelial-mesenchymal compartments has not emerged. It is clear that both IGF-1 and IGF-2 bind to intestinal epithelial cells[35,37,39,46,47] and that IGF-1R and IGF-2R are targeted to the basolateral membrane domain of the enterocyte.[48,49] Multiple components of the IGF system, including IGFBPs, are expressed in subepithelial myofibroblasts and lamina propria in the gastrointestinal tract, implying an important role in regulation of epithelial-mesenchymal interactions.[50,51] The intestinotrophic effects of IGF-1 are mediated by glucagon-like peptide 2 (GLP-2)-dependent regulation of myofibroblast IGF-1 expression. In support of this, transgenic mice in which IGF-1 is overexpressed in the intestinal lamina propria under the direction of an alpha smooth muscle actin promoter show increased proliferation of the ileal epithelium.[52]

Several other observations in transgenic mice are worth noting. In mice with a hepatic deletion of IGF-1, the gastrointestinal tract, including the muscularis propria, develops normally. However, while mice overexpressing IGF-1 have a normal gastrointestinal epithelium but expanded submucosa, the muscularis propria is hyperplastic and hypertrophic.[53] C57BL/6J mice heterozygous for IGF-1 [IGF-1($\pm$)] have normal gastrointestinal development but with a thinner submucosal compartment in comparison with wild-type mice in the neonatal period.[54] The hyperplasia and stricturing that occurs during the course of 2,4,6-trinitrobenzene sulfonic acid (TNBS)-induced colitis are markedly attenuated in IGF-1($\pm$) mice (**Fig. 3**).[55] In aggregate, these observations highlight the autocrine role of IGF-1 produced in the gastrointestinal tract, particularly by smooth muscle cells of the gastrointestinal tract, in its growth, development, and response to inflammation.

As noted earlier, most circulating IGF-1 is synthesized in the liver under the regulation of GH. Consequently, hepatocyte levels of IGF-1 are very high. IGFBPs are also synthesized in the liver. However, the normal hepatocyte is not considered a major target for

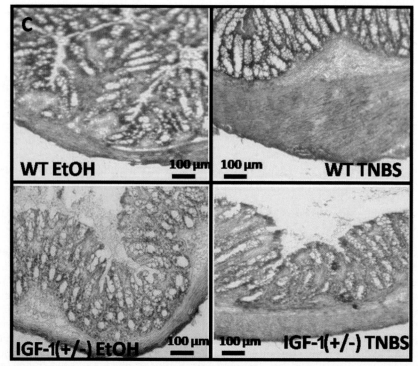

Fig. 3. Inflammation-induced fibrosis is decreased in IGF-1($\pm$) mice. Collagen deposition in smooth muscle layer of vehicle-treated IGF-1($\pm$) mice and its increase in response to TNBS-induced colitis are lower than in wild-type C57BL/6J mice (Masson's trichrome stained sections, original magnification ×10).

IGF action because of the extremely low level of IGF-1R expression.[56] Hepatic stellate cells and myofibroblasts also express IGFBPs and IGF-1.[57] These cells are believed to play a pivotal role in the fibrogenic response to IGFs in the liver.[58]

The expression of IGF-2 and IGF-2R are highly developmentally regulated. IGF-2 RNA transcripts are readily detectable in the intestine during gestation but are much less apparent in the adult rat.[11,32] Similar observations have been made in human stomach and intestine.[40] Similarly, IGF-2R levels are developmentally regulated during rat and human intestinal development.[11,59] IGFBP-2 has high affinity for IGF-2 and tightly regulates IGF-2 availability during fetal and early neonatal growth.[60] Overall these studies indicate that the IGF-2/IGF-2R axis plays an important role in fetal intestinal development.[40,59] A clear pattern of developmental expression of IGF-1/IGFIR has not emerged, but IGF-1 is generally recognized to be the predominant IGF-1 in adults. Fluctuations in expression are observed, and the degree of change is less apparent than that described for IGF-2.[11,39,49,60]

INSULIN-LIKE GROWTH FACTOR STIMULATES CELLULAR PROLIFERATION

IGFs are mitogenic for intestinal epithelial and smooth muscle cells and for hepatic stellate cells in vitro and in vivo. In vitro, IGFs stimulate intestinal epithelial proliferation but, in most instances, less so than other growth factors such as epidermal growth factor (EGF).[60–65] When EGF is provided with IGF-1 or insulin, a synergistic effect on intestinal epithelial proliferation is often observed. Isolated intestinal smooth muscle cells and isolated hepatic stellate cells in vitro also proliferate in response to IGF-1.[66,67]

In vivo evidence of the proliferative effects of IGF on the intestinal epithelium is robust and derives from experimental models using both enteral and parenteral IGF-1. Oral feeding of IGF-1 to neonatal pigs increases indices of small intestinal weight, DNA content, protein content, and villus height in the small intestine.[68] In utero ligation of the esophagus in fetal sheep deprives the intestine from growth regulatory peptides in amniotic fluid. A 10-day infusion of IGF-1 distal to the ligation results in increased small intestinal growth.[69] A small increase in intestinal crypt labeling was seen even after briefly treating mice with intraperitoneal administration of IGF-1.[70] A 14-day parenteral administration of IGF-1 to adult rats increased crypt depth and villus height by 30%.[71] In multiple models, infusion of LR³IGF-1, an N-terminal–extended analogue of IGF-1 that has a reduced affinity for IGFBPs, better stimulates proliferation in the epithelium and muscularis of the small intestine than the parent peptide.[72,73] The effects of IGF-1 in these studies are most prominent in the proximal intestine and are not seen in the pancreas or stomach.

IGF-1 also has important regulatory effects on intestinal growth in pathophysiologic conditions. Adaptive mucosal proliferation in the small intestine of rats that have undergone a partial small intestinal resection is increased by IGF-1.[74–76] Atrophy of the jejunal mucosa in parenterally fed rats is blunted by administration of inclusion of IGF-1 in the parenteral nutrition solution.[77] Small intestinal atrophy occurring in the setting of chronic liver disease or sepsis is also reduced by administration of IGF-1.[78,79] Fibrosis and stricture formation in patients with Crohn disease and in animal models of ileocolitis, including TNBS-induced colitis, are associated with increased IGF-1 expression and increased smooth muscle proliferation.[21] Smooth muscle proliferation and fibrosis from TNBS-induced colitis are significantly diminished in IGF-1(±)-heterozygous mice.[55]

Studies in transgenic mice also demonstrate the proliferative effect of GH or IGFs on the intestinal mucosa. Mice overexpressing GH have increased plasma and intestinal mucosal IGF-1 levels, increased bowel length and mass, but normal intestinal crypt cell proliferation rate, indicative of GH-stimulated survival of intestinal epithelial cells.[80]

In mice overexpressing IGF-1 under an MT-I promoter, circulating GH was undetectable because of negative feedback from IGF-1, allowing determination of the specific effects of GH and IGF-1 on the intestine. MT-IGF-1 mice exhibit a significantly greater small intestinal length and mass, an increased villus height, greater crypt depth, and a higher crypt cell mitotic index in comparison with wild-type mice, but there was no alteration in differentiation.[81] In contrast, transgenic overexpression of IGF-2 has variable effects on mass of the gastrointestinal tract.[82,83] Transgenic overexpression of IGFBP-3 was associated with increased liver mass.[84] Transgenic overexpression of IGFBP-4 coupled with a smooth muscle α-actin promoter (SMP4/SMP8-IGFBP-4) induced hypoplasia of intestinal smooth muscle suggesting that IGFBP-4 acts as an endogenous inhibitor of IGF-1 actions in intestinal smooth muscle. This was confirmed in vitro in human intestinal smooth muscle cells.[85] A detailed analysis of the gastrointestinal effects of IGFBP deletion or overexpression has not been reported.

These studies suggest that IGF-1 and GH, both of which are used extensively in the clinical arena for other indications, may be useful therapeutic agents in patients with short bowel syndrome, and some studies suggest that GH improves intestinal function in patients with short bowel syndrome.[86,87] In animal models and in human studies of short bowel syndrome, intestinal atrophy, or inflammatory bowel disease, IGF-1 is more potent in stimulating intestinal growth than GH. This may be because of induction of suppressor of cytokine signaling 2 by GH but not IGF-1.[88] More recently the role of GLP-2 in this respect has been examined. GLP-2 directly and indirectly, via induction of IGF-1 expression, increases intestinal growth. In IGF-1–null mice, the ability of GLP-2 to increase intestinal growth is lost.[89] New clinical trials using IGF-1 alone and in combination with GLP-2 may offer more encouraging results in subjects with decreased gastrointestinal mucosal function.[90,91]

INSULIN-LIKE GROWTH FACTOR IN PROSURVIVAL

The studies discussed earlier indicate that IGFs increase intestinal growth, in part, by inhibition of apoptosis. MT-IGF-1 transgenic mice have a lower basal level of apoptosis in small intestine crypts and a lower level of apoptosis in response to irradiation.[92] This is consistent with studies showing that IGF-1 inhibits apoptosis in cultured cells.[93]

In vitro and in vivo studies have shown that autocrine IGF-1 in addition to stimulating proliferation inhibits apoptosis (promotes survival) in smooth muscle cells of the muscularis propria of humans and mice.[21,55]

INSULIN-LIKE GROWTH FACTOR IS PROFIBROGENIC

Several lines of investigation have shown the profibrogenic actions of IGFs in the intestinal tract. IGF-1 not only stimulates proliferation and inhibits apoptosis of fibroblasts, myofibroblasts, and smooth muscle cells but also increases collagen expression and production in each of these cells.[94,95] In SMP8-IGF-1 mice, transgenic expression of IGF-1 increases the mass of the muscularis propria and length of the intestine.[53,55] The adaptive response to surgical resection of the small intestine in this same SMP8-IGF-1 mouse is characterized by a marked lengthening of the residual bowel, suggesting that IGF-1 autocrine activity increases the mesenchymal elements in the intestine.[96] In Crohn disease, a human disorder characterized by fibrosis and stricture formation, mucosal IGF-1 and IGF-1R levels are increased relative to normal intestine as are muscularis propria IGF-1, IGFBP-3, and IGFBP-5 levels. In human intestinal muscle, the predominant collagen isotype is collagen Iαl. In these cells and in animal models of Crohn disease (eg, TNBS-induced colitis), the increased IGF-1, IGFBP-3, and

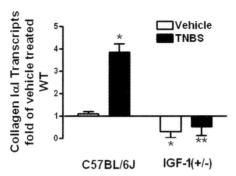

Fig. 4. Inflammation-induced collagen Iαl expression is decreased in IGF-1(±) mice. Collagen Iαl transcripts in smooth muscle cells of vehicle-treated IGF-1(±) mice and its increase in response to TNBS-induced colitis are lower than in wild-type C57BL/6J mice. Transcript levels were measured by real-time polymerase chain reaction using the $2^{-\Delta\Delta Ct}$ method. * Denotes P<.05 vs C57BL/6J vehicle treated animals, ** denotes P<.05 vs C57BL/6J TNBS treated animals.

IGFBP-5 levels (and increased TGF-β1 levels) in the inflamed intestine, individually and in concert, stimulate collagen Iαl expression, leading to increased collagen secretion and fibrosis (**Fig. 4**).[24,25,55,97] A profibrogenic response to IGF-1 in all regions of the gastrointestinal tract is not seen. In the liver, carbon tetrachloride injury in the SMP8-IGF-1 mouse results in reduced collagen synthesis and amelioration of the extent of liver injury.[98]

INSULIN-LIKE GROWTH FACTOR IN GASTROINTESTINAL CANCERS

The prominent effects of IGF ligands mediated via IGF receptors on cellular proliferation and survival suggest that the IGF axis may play an important role in the development of dysplasia and neoplasia. Multiple lines of investigation have supported this view.[6,8] Although circulating IGF-1 levels vary considerably among healthy individuals, population-based studies suggest an overall trend toward increasing cancer risk, including cancers of the gastrointestinal tract, in persons at the high end of the normal range of IGF-1 blood levels. Loss of IGF-2 imprinting results in a modest increase in IGF-2 levels and is now widely accepted as a marker for colorectal cancer risk.[15] Increased expression of IGF-1, IGF-2, and IGF-1R are observed in colorectal cancers.[99] Mice overexpressing IGF-2 treated with 1,2-dimethylhydrazine to induce neoplastic alteration promoted the growth of colonic aberrant crypt foci and increased colonic tumor volume without affecting tumor numbers in comparison with wild-type mice.[100] Transgenic overexpression of IGFBP-2, which has high affinity for IGF-2, reduced the appearance of dysplastic aberrant crypt foci and inhibited tumor growth in the same model.[101]

IGFBP-3 has been shown to promote TGF-β1-mediated epithelial to mesenchymal transition and tumor cell invasion in esophageal cancer.[102] These effects seemed to be mediated independent of IGF-1.

SUMMARY

The liver is a major source of IGFs and IGFBPs that are present in the circulation and have important endocrine activities relating to energy metabolism, body size, carcinogenesis, and various organ-specific functions. Although IGFs have only minor effects on the normal liver itself, production of IGFs and IGFBPs in a tissue-specific manner in the gastrointestinal tract exert important regulatory effects, via autocrine and paracrine mechanisms, on cellular proliferation, survival, and apoptosis. IGFs and IGFBPs play important regulatory roles in the response of both the liver and the gastrointestinal tract to inflammation and in the development of neoplasia.

REFERENCES

1. LeRoith D. Insulin-like growth factor receptors and binding proteins. Baillieres Clin Endocrinol Metab 1996;10:49–73.
2. Rubin R, Baserga R. Insulin-like growth factor-I receptor. Its role in cell proliferation, apoptosis, tumorigenicity. Lab Invest 1995;73:311–31.
3. Jones JI, Clemmons DR. Insulin-like growth factors and their binding proteins: biological actions. Endocr Rev 1995;16:3–34.
4. Nielsen FC. The molecular and cellular biology of insulin-like growth factor II. Prog Growth Factor Res 1992;4:257–90.
5. Sussenbach JS. The gene structure of the insulin-like growth factor family. Prog Growth Factor Res 1989;1:33–48.
6. Pollak MN, Schernhammer ES, Hankinson SE. Insulin-like growth factors and neoplasia. Nat Rev Cancer 2004;4:505–18.
7. Firth SM, Baxter RC. Cellular actions of the insulin-like growth factor binding proteins. Endocr Rev 2002;23:824–54.
8. Foulstone E, Prince S, Zaccheo O, et al. Insulin-like growth factor ligands, receptors, and binding proteins in cancer. J Pathol 2005;205:145–53.
9. Dupont J, Holzenberger M. Biology of insulin-like growth factors in development. Birth Defects Res C Embryo Today 2003;69:257–71.
10. Rotwein P, Pollock KM, Didier DK, et al. Organization and sequence of the human insulin-like growth factor I gene. Alternative RNA processing produces two insulin-like growth factor I precursor peptides. J Biol Chem 1986;261:4828–32.
11. Lund PK, Moats-Staats BM, Hynes MA, et al. Somatomedin-C/insulin-like growth factor-I and insulin-like growth factor-II mRNAs in rat fetal and adult tissues. J Biol Chem 1986;261:14539–44.
12. Matheny RW, Nindl BC, Adamo ML. Minireview: mechano-growth factor: a putative product of the IGF-I gene expression involved in tissue repair and regeneration. Endocrinology 2010;151:865–75.
13. Berg KM, Bowers JG, Kuemmerle JF. The IGF-IEa (IGF-I) and IGF-IEc (MGF) splice variants of the IGF-I gene mediate hypertrophy and hyperplasia of human intestinal smooth muscle. Gastroenterology 2007;132:A-234.
14. Han VK, Lund PK, Lee DC, et al. Expression of somatomedin/insulin-like growth factor messenger ribonucleic acids in the human fetus: identification, characterization, and tissue distribution. J Clin Endocrinol Metab 1988;66:422–9.
15. Cui H, Cruz-Correa M, Giardiello FM, et al. Loss of IGF2 imprinting: a potential marker of colorectal cancer risk. Science 2003;299:1753–5.
16. Cheng YW, Idrees K, Shattock R, et al. Loss of imprinting and marked gene elevation are 2 forms of aberrant IGF2 expression in colorectal cancer. Int J Cancer 2009;127:568–77.
17. Abbott AM, Bueno R, Pedrini MT, et al. Insulin-like growth factor I receptor gene structure. J Biol Chem 1992;267:10759–63.
18. Pandini G, Frasca F, Mineo R, et al. Insulin/insulin-like growth factor I hybrid receptors have different biological characteristics depending on the insulin receptor isoform involved. J Biol Chem 2002;277:39684–95.

19. Izumi T, White MF, Kadowaki T, et al. Insulin-like growth factor I rapidly stimulates tyrosine phosphorylation of a Mr 185,000 protein in intact cells. J Biol Chem 1987;262:1282–7.

20. Kuemmerle JF, Murthy KS. Coupling of the insulin-like growth factor-I receptor tyrosine kinase to Gi2 in human intestinal smooth muscle: Gβγ-dependent mitogen-activated protein kinase activation and growth. J Biol Chem 2001; 276:71787–7194.

21. Flynn RS, Murthy KS, Grider JR, et al. Endogenous IGF-I and alphaVbeta3 integrin ligands regulate increased smooth muscle hyperplasia in stricturing Crohn's disease. Gastroenterology 2010;138:285–93.

22. Li J, Sahagian GG. Demonstration of tumor suppression by mannose 6-phosphate/insulin-like growth factor 2 receptor. Oncogene 2004;23:9359–68.

23. Kuemmerle JF, Murthy KS, Bowers JG. IGFBP-3 activates TGF-beta receptors and directly inhibits growth in human intestinal smooth muscle cells. Am J Physiol Gastrointest Liver Physiol 2004;287:G795–802.

24. Flynn RS, Mahavadi S, Murthy KS, et al. Endogenous IGFBP-3 regulates excess collagen expression in intestinal smooth muscle cells of Crohn's disease strictures. Inflamm Bowel Dis 2011;17:193–201.

25. Flynn RS, Madavadi S, Murthy KS, et al. Insulin-like growth factor-binding protein-5 stimulates growth of human intestinal muscle cells by activation of Gαi3. Am J Physiol Gastrointest Liver Physiol 2009;297:G1232–8.

26. Schedlich LJ, Le Page SL, Firth SM, et al. Nuclear import of insulin-like growth factor-binding protein-3 and -5 is mediated by the importin beta subunit. J Biol Chem 2000;275:23462–70.

27. Schedlich LJ, Marthukaruppan A, O'Han MK, et al. Insulin-like growth factor binding protein-5 interacts with the vitamin D receptor and modulates the vitamin D response in osteoblasts. Mol Endocrinol 2007;21:2378–80.

28. Schedlich LJ, Graham LD, O'Han MK, et al. Molecular basis of the interaction between IGFBP-3 and retinoid X receptor: role in modulation of RAR-signaling. Arch Biochem Biophys 2007;465:359–69.

29. Howarth GS. Insulin-like growth factor-I and the gastrointestinal system: therapeutic indications and safety implications. J Nutr 2003;133:2109–12.

30. Laburthe M, Rouyer-Fessard C, Gammeltoft S. Receptors for insulin-like growth factors I and II in rat gastrointestinal epithelium. Am J Physiol 1988;254:G457–62.

31. Ryan J, Costigan DC. Determination of the histological distribution of insulin like growth factor 1 receptors in the rat gut. Gut 1993;34:1693–7.

32. Brown AL, Graham DE, Nissley SP, et al. Developmental regulation of insulin-like growth factor II mRNA in different rat tissues. J Biol Chem 1986;261: 13144–50.

33. Hoyt EC, Van Wyk JJ, Lund PK. Tissue and development specific regulation of a complex family of rat insulin-like growth factor I messenger ribonucleic acids. Mol Endocrinol 1988;2:1077–86.

34. Heinz-Erian P, Kessler U, Funk B, et al. Identification and in situ localization of the insulin-like growth factor-II/mannose-6-phosphate (IGF-II/M6P) receptor in the rat gastrointestinal tract: comparison with the IGF-I receptor. Endocrinology 1991;129:1769–78.

35. Adamo M, Lowe WL Jr, LeRoith D, et al. Insulin-like growth factor I messenger ribonucleic acids with alternative 5'-untranslated regions are differentially expressed during development of the rat. Endocrinology 1989;124:2737–44.

36. Pillion DJ, Grizzle WE, Yang M, et al. Expression of IGF-II/Man-6-P receptors on rat, rabbit, and human colon epithelial cells. Am J Physiol 1993;264:R1101–10.

37. Pillion DJ, Haskell JF, Atchison JA, et al. Receptors for IGF-I, but not for IGF-II, on proximal colon epithelial cell apical membranes. Am J Physiol 1989;257:E27–34.
38. Termanini B, Nardi RV, Finan TM, et al. Insulinlike growth factor I receptors in rabbit gastrointestinal tract. Characterization and autoradiographic localization. Gastroenterology 1990;99:51–60.
39. Schober DA, Simmen FA, Hadsell DL, et al. Perinatal expression of type I IGF receptors in porcine small intestine. Endocrinology 1990;126:1125–32.
40. Freier S, Eran M, Reinus C, et al. Relative expression and localization of the insulin-like growth factor system components in the fetal, child and adult intestine. J Pediatr Gastroenterol Nutr 2005;40:202–9.
41. Eriksson U, Duc G, Froesch ER, et al. Insulin-like growth factors (IGF) I and II and IGF binding proteins (IGFBPs) in human colostrum/transitory milk during the first week postpartum: comparison with neonatal and maternal serum. Biochem Biophys Res Commun 1993;196:267–73.
42. Donovan SM, Hintz RL, Rosenfeld RG. Insulin-like growth factors I and II and their binding proteins in human milk: effect of heat treatment on IGF and IGF binding protein stability. J Pediatr Gastroenterol Nutr 1991;13:242–53.
43. Chaurasia OP, Marcuard SP, Seidel ER. Insulin-like growth factor I in human gastrointestinal exocrine secretions. Regul Pept 1994;50:113–9.
44. Philipps AF, Rao R, Anderson GG, et al. Fate of insulin-like growth factors I and II administered orogastrically to suckling rats. Pediatr Res 1995;37:586–92.
45. Philipps AF, Kling PJ, Grille JG, et al. Intestinal transport of insulin-like growth factor-I (igf-I) in the suckling rat. J Pediatr Gastroenterol Nutr 2002;35:539–44.
46. Rouyer-Fessard C, Gammeltoft S, Laburthe M. Expression of two types of receptor for insulinlike growth factors in human colonic epithelium. Gastroenterology 1990;98:703–7.
47. Park JH, Vanderhoof JA, Blackwood D, et al. Characterization of type I and type II insulin-like growth factor receptors in an intestinal epithelial cell line. Endocrinology 1990;126:2998–3005.
48. Dahms NM, Seetharam B, Wick DA. Expression of insulin-like growth factor (IGF)-I receptors, IGF-II/cation-independent mannose 6-phosphate receptors (CI-MPRs), and cation-dependent MPRs in polarized human intestinal Caco-2 cells. Biochim Biophys Acta 1996;1279:84–92.
49. Wick DA, Seetharam B, Dahms NM. Basolateral sorting signal of the 300-kDa mannose 6-phosphate receptor. Am J Physiol Gastrointest Liver Physiol 2002; 282:G51–60.
50. Shoubridge CA, Steeb CB, Read LC. IGFBP mRNA expression in small intestine of rat during postnatal development. Am J Physiol Gastrointest Liver Physiol 2001;281:G1378–84.
51. Winesett DE, Ulshen MH, Hoyt EC, et al. Regulation and localization of the insulin-like growth factor system in small bowel during altered nutrient status. Am J Physiol 1995;268:G631–40.
52. Williams KL, Fuller CR, Fagin J, et al. Mesenchymal IGF-I overexpression: paracrine effects in the intestine, distinct from endocrine actions. Am J Physiol Gastrointest Liver Physiol 2002;283:G875–85.
53. Wang J, Niu W, Nikoforov Y, et al. Targeted overexpression of IGF-I evokes distinct patterns of organ remodeling in smooth muscle cell tissue beds of transgenic mice. J Clin Invest 1997;100:1425–39.
54. Herman AC, Carlisle EM, Paxton JB, et al. Insulin-like growth factor-I governs submucosal growth and thickness in the newborn mouse ileum. Pediatr Res 2004;55:507–13.

55. Mahavadi S, Flynn RS, Grider JR, et al. Amelioration of excess collagen Iαl, fibrosis, and smooth muscle growth in TNBS-induced colitis in IGF-I(+/-) mice. Inflamm Bowel Dis 2011;17(3):711–9.

56. Zimmermann EM, Li L, Hoyt EC, et al. Cell-specific localization of insulin-like growth factor binding protein mRNAs in rat liver. Am J Physiol Gastrointest Liver Physiol 2000;278:G447–57.

57. Novosyadlyy R, Tron K, Dudas J, et al. Expression and regulation of the insulin-like growth factor axis components in rat liver myofibroblasts. J Cell Physiol 2004;199:388–98.

58. Scharf JG, Dombrowski F, Novosyadlyy R, et al. Insulin-like growth factor (IGF)-binding protein-1 is highly induced during acute carbon tetrachloride liver injury and potentiates the IGF-I-stimulated activation of rat hepatic stellate cells. Endocrinology 2004;145:3463–72.

59. Sklar MM, Kiess W, Thomas CL, et al. Developmental expression of the tissue insulin-like growth factor II/mannose 6-phosphate receptor in the rat. Measurement by quantitative immunoblotting. J Biol Chem 1989;264:16733–8.

60. Young GP, Taranto TM, Jonas HA, et al. Insulin-like growth factors and the developing and mature rat small intestine: receptors and biological actions. Digestion 1990;46(Suppl 2):240–52.

61. Kurokowa M, Lynch K, Podolsky DK. Effects of growth factors on an intestinal epithelial cell line: transforming growth factor beta inhibits proliferation and stimulates differentiation. Biochem Biophys Res Commun 1987;142:775–82.

62. Conteas CN, McMorrow B, Luk GD. Modulation of epidermal growth factor-induced cell proliferation and receptor binding by insulin in cultured intestinal epithelial cells. Biochem Biophys Res Commun 1989;161:414–9.

63. Duncan MD, Korman LY, Bass BL. Epidermal growth factor primes intestinal epithelial cells for proliferative effect of insulin-like growth factor I. Dig Dis Sci 1994;39:2197–201.

64. Jonas CR, Ziegler TR, Gu LH, et al. Extracellular thiol/disulfide redox state affects proliferation rate in a human colon carcinoma (Caco2) cell line. Free Radic Biol Med 2002;33:1499–506.

65. Lahm H, Suardet L, Laurent PL, et al. Growth regulation and co-stimulation of human colorectal cancer cell lines by insulin-like growth factor I, II and transforming growth factor alpha. Br J Cancer 1992;65:341–6.

66. Kuemmerle JF, Zhou H, Bowers JG. IGF-I stimulates human intestinal smooth muscle cell growth by regulation of G1 phase cell cycle proteins. Am J Physiol Gastrointest Liver Physiol 2004;286:G412–9.

67. Skrtic S, Wallenius K, Gressner AM, et al. Insulin-like growth factor signaling pathways in rat hepatic stellate cells: importance for deoxyribonucleic acid synthesis and hepatocyte growth factor production. Endocrinology 1999;140:5729–35.

68. Burrin DG, Wester TJ, Davis TA, et al. Orally administered IGF-I increases intestinal mucosal growth in formula-fed neonatal pigs. Am J Physiol 1996;270:R1085–91.

69. Trahair JF, Wing SJ, Quinn KJ, et al. Regulation of gastrointestinal growth in fetal sheep by luminally administered insulin-like growth factor-I. J Endocrinol 1997;152:29–38.

70. Potten CS, Owen G, Hewitt D, et al. Stimulation and inhibition of proliferation in the small intestinal crypts of the mouse after in vivo administration of growth factors. Gut 1995;36:864–73.

71. Steeb CB, Trahair JF, Tomas FM, et al. Prolonged administration of IGF peptides enhances growth of gastrointestinal tissues in normal rats. Am J Physiol 1994; 266:G1090–8.

72. Steeb CB, Shoubridge CA, Tivey DR, et al. Systemic infusion of IGF-I or LR(3) IGF-I stimulates visceral organ growth and proliferation of gut tissues in suckling rats. Am J Physiol 1997;272:G522–33.

73. Steeb CB, Trahair JF, Read LC. Administration of insulin-like growth factor-I (IGF-I) peptides for three days stimulates proliferation of the small intestinal epithelium in rats. Gut 1995;37:630–8.

74. Mantell MP, Ziegler TR, Adamson WT, et al. Resection-induced colonic adaptation is augmented by IGF-I and associated with upregulation of colonic IGF-I mRNA. Am J Physiol 1995;269:G974–80.

75. Vanderhoof JA, McCusker RH, Clark R, et al. Truncated and native insulinlike growth factor I enhance mucosal adaptation after jejunoileal resection. Gastroenterology 1992;102:1949–56.

76. Dahly EM, Guo Z, Ney DM. IGF-I augments resection-induced mucosal hyperplasia by altering enterocyte kinetics. Am J Physiol Regul Integr Comp Physiol 2003;285:R800–8.

77. Peterson CA, Ney DM, Hinton PS, et al. Beneficial effects of insulin-like growth factor I on epithelial structure and function in parenterally fed rat jejunum. Gastroenterology 1996;111:1501–8.

78. Inaba T, Saito H, Fukushima R, et al. Insulin-like growth factor 1 has beneficial effects, whereas growth hormone has limited effects on postoperative protein metabolism, gut integrity, and splenic weight in rats with chronic mild liver injury. JPEN J Parenter Enteral Nutr 1997;21:55–62.

79. Chen K, Okuma T, Okamura K, et al. Insulin-like growth factor-I prevents gut atrophy and maintains intestinal integrity in septic rats. JPEN J Parenter Enteral Nutr 1995;19:119–24.

80. Ulshen MH, Dowling RH, Fuller CR, et al. Enhanced growth of small bowel in transgenic mice overexpressing bovine growth hormone. Gastroenterology 1993;104:973–80.

81. Ohneda K, Ulshen MH, Fuller CR, et al. Enhanced growth of small bowel in transgenic mice expressing human insulin-like growth factor I. Gastroenterology 1997;112:444–54.

82. Ward A, Bates P, Fisher R, et al. Disproportionate growth in mice with Igf-2 transgenes. Proc Natl Acad Sci U S A 1994;91:10365–9.

83. Blackburn A, Schmitt A, Schmidt P, et al. Actions and interactions of growth hormone and insulin-like growth factor-II: body and organ growth of transgenic mice. Transgenic Res 1997;6:213–22.

84. Murphy LJ, Rajkumar K, Molner P. Phenotypic manifestations of insulin-like growth factor binding protein-1 (IGFBP-1) and IGFBP-3 overexpression in transgenic mice. Prog Growth Factor Res 1995;6:425–32.

85. Kuemmerle JF, Teng B-Q. Regulation of IGFBP-4 levels in human intestinal smooth muscle cells: confluence-dependent production of an endogenous IGF-I-activated IGFBP-4 protease. Am J Physiol Gastrointest Liver Physiol 2000;279:G975–82.

86. Seguy D, Vahedi K, Kapel N, et al. Low-dose growth hormone in adult home parenteral nutrition-dependent short bowel syndrome patients: a positive study. Gastroenterology 2003;124:293–302.

87. Scolapio JS. Current update of short-bowel syndrome. Curr Opin Gastroenterol 2004;20:143–5.

88. Miller ME, Michaylira CZ, Simmons JG, et al. Suppressor of cytokine signaling-2: a growth hormone-inducible inhibitor of intestinal epithelial cell proliferation. Gastroenterology 2004;127:570–81.

89. Dube PE, Forse CL, Bahrami J, et al. The essential role of insulin-like growth factor-1 in the intestinal tropic effects of glucagon-like peptide-2 in mice. Gastroenterology 2006;131:589–605.

90. Yazbeck R, Howarth GS, Abbott CA. Growth factor based therapies and intestinal disease: is glucagon-like peptide-2 the new way forward? Cytokine Growth Factor Rev 2009;20:175–84.

91. Yazbeck R, Abbott CA, Howarth GS. The use of GLP-2 and related growth factors in intestinal diseases. Curr Opin Investig Drugs 2010;11:440–6.

92. Wilkins HR, Ohneda K, Keku TO, et al. Reduction of spontaneous and irradiation-induced apoptosis in small intestine of IGF-I transgenic mice. Am J Physiol Gastrointest Liver Physiol 2002;283:G457–64.

93. Parrizas M, Saltiel AR, LeRoith D. Insulin-like growth factor 1 inhibits apoptosis using the phosphatidylinositol 3'-kinase and mitogen-activated protein kinase pathways. J Biol Chem 1997;272:154–61.

94. Xin X, Hou YT, Li L, et al. IGF-I increases IGFBP-5 and collagen alpha1(I) mRNAs by the MAPK pathway in rat intestinal smooth muscle cells. Am J Physiol Gastrointest Liver Physiol 2004;286:G777–83.

95. Kuemmerle JF. Endogenous IGF-I protects human intestinal smooth muscle cells from apoptosis by regulation of GSK-3 beta activity. Am J Physiol Gastrointest Liver Physiol 2005;288:G101–10.

96. Knott AW, Juno RJ, Jarboe MD, et al. Smooth muscle overexpression of IGF-I induces a novel adaptive response to small bowel resection. Am J Physiol Gastrointest Liver Physiol 2004;287:G562–70.

97. Theiss AL, Fruchtman S, Lund PK. Growth factors in inflammatory bowel disease: the actions and interactions of growth hormone and insulin-like growth factor-I. Inflamm Bowel Dis 2004;10:871–80.

98. Sanz S, Pucilowska JB, Liu S, et al. Expression of insulin-like growth factor I by activated hepatic stellate cells reduces fibrogenesis and enhances regeneration after liver injury. Gut 2005;54:134–41.

99. Nosho K, Yamamoto H, Taniguchi H, et al. Interplay of insulin-like growth factor-II, insulin-like growth factor-I, insulin-like growth factor-I receptor, COX-2, and matrix metalloproteinase-7, play key roles in the early stage of colorectal carcinogenesis. Clin Cancer Res 2004;10:7950–7.

100. Diehl D, Oesterle D, Eimlinger MW, et al. IGF-II transgenic mice display increased aberrant colon crypt multiplicity and tumor volume after 1,2-dimethylhydrazine treatment. J Carcinog 2006;5:24.

101. Diehl D, Hessel E, Oesterile D, et al. IGFBP-2 overexpression reduces the appearance of dysplastic aberrant crypt foci and inhibits growth of adenomas in chemically induced colorectal carcinogenesis. Int J Cancer 2009;124:2220–5.

102. Natasuizaka M, Ohashi S, Wong GS, et al. Insulin-like growth factor-binding protein-3 promotes transforming growth factor-β1-mediated epithelial-to-mesenchymal transition and motility in transformed human esophageal cells. Carcinogenesis 2010;31:1344–53.

Metabolic Actions of Insulin-Like Growth Factor-I in Normal Physiology and Diabetes

David R. Clemmons, MD

KEYWORDS

- Fat metabolism • Growth • Insulin resistance • Growth hormone

KEY POINTS

- Insulin-like growth factor-I (IGF-I) is an important stimulant of protein synthesis in muscle but it also stimulates free fatty acid uptake and metabolism.
- IGF-I actions are regulated by IGF-binding proteins; in obesity and metabolic syndrome, there is a major dysregulation of IGF-binding protein secretion resulting in alterations in the concentration of free IGF-I and IGF-I actions.
- In Type 1 diabetes, IGF-I synthesis is markedly impaired; in Type 2 diabetes, multiple changes occur in IGF-I actions, including sensitization to its mitogenic actions in some target tissues.

INTRODUCTION

Insulin-like growth factor-I (IGF-I) has significant structural homology with proinsulin. IGF-I, IGF-II and proinsulin evolved from a single precursor molecule approximately 60 million years ago. The function of that single precursor molecule was to provide a chemical signal for cells within primitive organisms to establish that adequate nutrient was present not only for basal metabolic needs but also for protein synthesis and cell proliferation. At the time vertebrates appeared, this system evolved into one with more complexity to be able to store calories as fat. At that time, insulin diverged from IGF-I and the pituitary gland appeared along with growth hormone (GH). The function of these 3 hormones was linked to be able to regulate both nutrient availability during periods of starvation and repletion as well as continuing to provide adequate signals and substrate for growth. As such, the regulation of synthesis and the secretion of these 3 hormones are directly linked to nutrient intake. Because insulin, IGF-I, and IGF-II evolved from a single precursor, they continue to share significant structural homology; however, there are also distinct differences. The primary domains within

This work is supported by a grant from the National Institutes of Health AGO2331.
Conflict of interest: None.
Division of Endocrinology, Department of Medicine, School of Medicine, University of North Carolina, CB# 7170, 8024 Burnett Womack, Chapel Hill, NC 27599-7170, USA
E-mail address: endo@med.unc.edu

Endocrinol Metab Clin N Am 41 (2012) 425–443
doi:10.1016/j.ecl.2012.04.017
0889-8529/12/$ – see front matter © 2012 Elsevier Inc. All rights reserved.

IGF-I and insulin that determine receptor binding have significant amino acid differences that account for major differences in affinity for their respective receptors.[1] Similarly, the IGFs have the unique characteristic of being able to bind to IGF-binding proteins (IGFBPs), which is determined by a specific amino acid sequence in positions, 3, 4, 15, 16 of N terminus of IGF-I molecule and homologous substitutions in IGF-II.[2] These structural differences provide an important distinction for the regulation of IGF-I and insulin bioavailability and, thus indirectly regulate their effects on metabolism.

IGF-I and insulin have distinct receptors. Both receptors are tyrosine kinase–containing receptors and they show 48% amino acid sequence homology.[3] Despite these similarities, the ligand-binding specificity is strict. The affinity of the IGF receptor is 1000 times greater for IGF-I than insulin, and the insulin receptor has a 100-fold greater affinity for insulin compared with IGF-I. Insulin and IGF-I receptor densities vary widely among cell types (ie, mature differentiated hepatocytes and adipocytes have abundant insulin receptors, whereas they have almost no IGF-I receptors). Conversely, cell types, such as vascular smooth muscle cells, have abundant IGF-I receptors and minimal insulin receptors. This difference in receptor distribution accounts for many of the differences in insulin and IGF-I actions. GH has an entirely different structure and its receptor belongs to the cytokine receptor family.[4] GH has a major regulatory influence on the metabolic actions of both IGF-I and insulin and functions in several important ways that are distinct from insulin and IGF-I to modulate nutrient availability that is necessary for both balanced tissue growth and the maintenance of normal intermediary metabolism. Therefore, coordinated regulation of the metabolic actions of these 3 hormones provides an important basis for understanding their individual effects on intermediary metabolism and how they function coordinately to maintain nutrient balance.

NUTRIENT REGULATION OF IGF-I SECRETION

As can be predicted from the phylogenetic development of IGF-I, the primary variable regulating plasma IGF-I concentrations is nutrient intake. Both total caloric and protein intake are important regulatory variables.[5] The effect of caloric intake is such that if caloric intake is reduced by approximately 50%, there is a significant reduction in IGF-I secretion. The effects of protein are more graded in that even small reductions result in changes in IGF-I.[6] For each 25% reduction in protein intake, there is an equivalent reduction in IGF-I. Most IGF-I in plasma (estimated at 80% based on mouse genetic manipulation studies) is derived from hepatic synthesis.[7] Both protein and energy participate in the regulation of hepatic synthesis, with energy regulating IGF-I gene transcription and protein functioning primarily to regulate mRNA stability and translation. A concomitant effect of changes in carbohydrate intake is the indirect effect that occurs as a result of changes in insulin secretion. If carbohydrates are provided at a level of less than the equivalent 700 kcal/d, then even supplemental fat intake will not restore a normal IGF-I. This is because IGF-I synthesis in the liver is also regulated by insulin,[8] which is best demonstrated by measuring serum IGF-I concentrations in untreated patients with Type I diabetes. When they receive insulin they have a substantial increase in serum IGF-I.[9] Studies in experimental animals have also shown that blocking insulin action in the liver lowers serum IGF-I. Therefore, carbohydrate intake functions not only to increase the total amount of energy that is available, thereby increasing IGF-I synthesis, but also by a direct effect of insulin on IGF-I gene transcription, particularly the ability of GH to stimulate IGF-I gene transcription.[8]

GH is the second variable that regulates IGF-I synthesis and secretion, but for the liver to respond to GH with normal IGF-I synthesis adequate nutrition is required. GH is a potent stimulant of IGF-I synthesis and GH administration to GH-deficient animals results in a brisk increase in IGF-I gene transcription in the liver that leads to a major increase in serum IGF-I.[10] The increase in serum IGF-I then feeds back on the pituitary gland to suppress GH secretion and maintain homeostasis. IGFBPs are another variable that regulates serum IGF-I concentrations. There are 6 IGFBPs.[11] IGFBP-3 is the principal binding protein in serum, and its concentration is also increased in response to GH; this change accounts for a significant fraction of the increase in total IGF-I that occurs in response to GH. The increase in IGFBP-3 in response to GH is also modulated by changes in nutrition. When IGF-I is bound to IGFBP-3, the binary complex binds to a third protein termed acid labile subunit (ALS). ALS concentrations are also GH dependent.[12] This ternary complex prolongs the half-life of IGF-I in serum from less than 5 minutes to 16 hours. IGFBP-5 is much less abundant than IGFBP-3, but it also binds to ALS and its concentration increases in response to GH. Thus, changes in IGFBP-3, IGFBP-5, and ALS all function to increase the serum IGF-I concentration by prolonging its half-life. Two other IGFBPs, IGFBP-1 and IGFBP-2, do not bind to ALS and, therefore, only prolong the half-life of IGF-I to periods ranging between 90 minutes and 2 hours. Therefore, they have minimal effects in increasing total serum IGF-I concentrations. However, the regulation of serum concentrations of these proteins is important for regulating IGF-I actions. Under normal circumstances, IGFBP-3 and IGFBP-5 are saturated. Therefore, abrupt changes in IGFBP-1 and IGFBP-2 that are not saturated and that occur as a result of changes in either nutrient intake or insulin secretion can result in major changes in free IGF-I and thereby regulate tissue responsiveness.[13] Other hormones that regulate IGF-I bioactivity include cortisol, which antagonizes the actions of IGF-I and, therefore, can result in an increase in serum concentrations, and thyroxine, which is necessary for normal IGF-I biosynthesis and which can stimulate an increase in IGF-I concentrations in hyperthyroidism. Estrogens function to antagonize the ability of GH to stimulate IGF-I synthesis in the liver and testosterone alters IGF-binding protein concentrations. Additionally, the GH analogue, human placental growth hormone, is an important stimulant of IGF-I synthesis in pregnancy. All of these hormones function coordinately with changes in nutrient intake to modulate the ability of IGF-I to regulate growth and metabolism.

METABOLIC EFFECTS OF IGF-I

Although IGF-I is classically considered an important growth factor because it stimulates the growth of all cell types, it has major metabolic effects. This overarching effect of IGF-I on metabolism is to provide a signal to cells that adequate nutrient is available to avoid apoptosis, enhance cellular protein synthesis, enable cells to undergo hypertrophy in response to an appropriate stimulus, and to allow stimulation of cell division. Therefore, even in cytostatic adult tissues, such as neurons and fused skeletal myoblasts, IGF-I can provide important trophic effects that lead to changes in cellular metabolism. Because IGF-I receptors are ubiquitous, these responses can occur in all cell types. Therefore, the signal induced by IGF-I stimulation of its receptor provides a mechanism for coordinating protein, carbohydrate, or fat metabolism among various cell types. Importantly, each of these processes is regulated coordinately with insulin; in the appropriate target tissue, either insulin or IGF-I may be the primary determinant of each of these processes. Similarly, growth hormone functions to coordinately regulate the ability of each of these hormones to modulate all 3 processes.

PROTEIN METABOLISM

In cells in tissue culture, IGF-I is a potent stimulant of protein synthesis. The phosphoinositide (PI)-3 kinase pathway modulates this response. Following IGF-I receptor activation, the receptor tyrosine kinase, phosphorylates tyrosines on the adaptor protein termed insulin receptor substrate-1 (IRS-1),[14] which provides a binding site for the p85 subunit of PI-3 kinase, which is then activated. Activation of PI-3 kinase results in the coordinate stimulation of AKT, which then leads to the suppression of TSC-2 and the activation of the mammalian target of rapamycin complex 1 (mTORC1). This activation functions to stimulate the phosphorylation of p70S6 kinase and E4B1, a translational repressor. These coordinate actions allow major increases in cellular protein synthesis. The process is modulated by the nutrient-sensitive AMP kinase, which is activated by nutrient restriction and phosphorylates serine 794 on IRS-1, which inhibits its ability to be activated, thus leading to PI-3 kinase inhibition and the inhibition of IGF-I–stimulated protein synthesis.[15] In skeletal muscle, IGF-I stimulates amino acid transport, but it is also a direct stimulant of protein synthesis and an important inhibitor of protein breakdown.[16] The atrogin complex whose assembly can be triggered by a variety of catabolic stimuli, including glucocorticoid excess, is antagonized in the presence of IGF-I stimulation. Conversely, mice that have been genetically altered to constitutively activate this complex are resistant to the anticatabolic effects of IGF-I.[17] This catabolic response is mediated through muscle ring finger protein 1 (MURF1) and muscle atrophy f-box protein (MAF box), which is also termed atrogin. These ligases are E3 ubiquitin ligases and their expression increases during disuse atrophy, following glucocorticoid administration or in response to cytokine stimulation. MAF box upregulation can be antagonized by IGF-I treatment leading to the inhibition of proteosome formation, thus reducing the targeting of proteins for degradation and reducing the rate of catabolism.[18] Insulin can have similar physiologic actions. These effects are mediated in part by the ability of AKT to phosphorylate serine 32 on FOXO3A, which results in the exclusion of FOXO3A from the nucleus. mTOR also blocks MURF1 and MAF box transcription. Studies by O'Connor and coworkers[19] have shown that cytokines that are activated in catabolic states and initiate muscle breakdown through MURF1 and MAF box induction can be antagonized in part by IGF-I actions. Thus, exogenous expression of IGF-I in the skeletal muscle of animals can partially reverse the effect of cytokine or glucocorticoid stimulation on catabolism even in insulin-resistant states.

IGF-I functions both under normal conditions and under conditions of either protein deprivation or when an excess of cytokine stimulation is present to attenuate catabolism. When IGF-I is administered to healthy volunteers, it stimulates protein synthesis; but if catabolism has not been stimulated, it has minimal effects on proteolysis.[20] However, at high concentrations it can suppress proteolysis even within normally fed patients. GH administration also results in an increase in protein synthesis, but the extent to which GH stimulates this response completely independently from IGF-I has not been determined. Of note, the administration of a high concentration of IGF-I (10 mcg/kg/h) to patients with GH receptor mutations resulted in a significant stimulation of protein synthesis.[21] However, the coadministration of GH and IGF-I to normally fed normal patients does not result in a greater response when compared with the individual response to each hormone given separately. However, following caloric deprivation, the administration of GH and IGF-I results in a synergistic increase in protein balance. In adults who are GH deficient, both GH and IGF-I are anabolic and enhance protein synthesis.[22] Insulin can inhibit proteolysis in muscle at very low concentrations, but the concentrations that are required to stimulate protein synthesis are higher. Thus, it would be reasonable to conclude that IGF-I is the major factor maintaining protein synthesis during long intervals between meals, but insulin is a primary factor stimulating anabolism in skeletal muscle following the ingestion of a meal that contains normal protein content.

Both GH and IGF-I have been used experimentally in catabolic illnesses and have been shown to improve nitrogen retention and protein synthesis when administered to patients with severe catabolic conditions, such as burns and renal failure.[23,24] Similarly, patients being treated with high doses of corticosteroids respond to IGF-I with the induction of an anabolic response.[20] IGF-I can also reduce the effect of the loss of gonadal function on protein balance. Young men who were administered a gonadotrophin receptor antagonist who became catabolic responded to either GH or IGF-I with a significant increase in protein synthesis, although it seemed that GH was more potent than IGF-I because it induced an increase in the androgen receptor number in skeletal muscle.[25]

FAT METABOLISM

Although mature adipocytes do not express IGF-I receptors, preadipocytes have abundant IGF-I receptors and IGF-I stimulates preadipocyte differentiation.[26] However, as preadipocytes differentiate they markedly reduce their IGF-I receptor number and insulin receptors become predominant. Thus, in well-formed adipose tissue beds, physiologic concentrations of IGF-I are not effective in stimulating changes in lipid synthesis or lipolysis and IGF-I has effects on primary adipocytes only at high concentrations, which are capable of stimulating glucose transport through the insulin receptor. In contrast, both GH and insulin are potent modulators of these processes. GH has direct effects on mature adipocytes that result in the release of free fatty acids following triglyceride breakdown and in increased free fatty acid oxidation in liver.[27] GH also enhances the lipolytic effect of catecholamines by increasing the adrenergic receptor number in adipocytes. In skeletal muscle, GH increases lipoprotein lipase activity, thus facilitating free fatty acid use. Insulin is a potent stimulant of lipid synthesis and insulin antagonizes triglyceride breakdown. This breakdown occurs in skeletal muscle, liver, and fat. An increase in free fatty acid flux from adipose tissue to liver can result in insulin resistance in the liver, and GH is known to antagonize insulin action through this mechanism.[28] IGF-I is a potent stimulant of free fatty acid uptake and oxidation in skeletal muscle. In an interesting mouse model, Fernandez and colleagues[29] knocked out the IGF-I receptor in skeletal muscle. This model also knocked out the insulin/IGF-I hybrid receptor and to some extent reduced the biosynthesis of insulin receptor homodimers. This action resulted in the development of Type II diabetes over time. That this was related to the loss of the ability of IGF-I to stimulate free fatty acid transport in muscle was strengthened by their observation that the phenotype could be rescued by expressing CD36, a known fatty acid transporter in muscle.[30] This finding led to the conclusion that it is the effect of IGF-I on fatty acid transport in muscle that is mediating this response and that it is so profound that its inhibition can lead to extreme insulin resistance and diabetes. Therefore, an important metabolic effect of IGF-I is to reduce flux of free fatty acids through the liver, which results in an enhancement of the ability of insulin to suppress hepatic glucose output. Supraphysiologic concentrations of IGF-I also suppress insulin secretion, and this may result in the inhibition of insulin's lipogenic effect in fat. Therefore, the 2 major effects that are enhanced by IGF-I are free fatty acid use by muscle which results in decreased free fatty acid flux in the liver and loss of insulin's lipogenic effect in fat. Suppression of GH by IGF-I also results in decreased free fatty flux in the liver and decreases the amount of substrate available for the enhancement of lipid oxidation directly in skeletal muscle, thus reducing the total free fatty acid flux. This mechanism probably functions under normal conditions to regulate glucose homeostasis and GH-induced insulin resistance. The chronic administration of IGF-I to human patients has been shown to decrease fat mass in adults who are GH deficient probably secondary to insulin suppression of insulin-induced lipogenesis. The chronic administration of IGF-I to patients who had GH receptor defects showed increased lipolysis and lipid oxidation rates and loss of total fat mass.[21] The degree of change was similar to the effect of GH when it was administered to patients who were GH deficient.

EFFECTS ON CARBOHYDRATE METABOLISM

An understanding of the effect of IGF-I on carbohydrate metabolism depends on knowledge of its effects in modulating insulin and GH actions. IGF-I reduces serum GH concentrations and it also reduces GH's direct effects on insulin suppression of hepatic gluconeogenesis; by increasing free fatty acid uptake in muscle, it indirectly enhances hepatic insulin action.[31] In both fat and liver, GH stimulates the synthesis of the p85 subunit of PI-3 kinase.[32] This relative increase in p85 leads to the suppression of p110 subunit activity, thus leading to antagonism of insulin action.[33] Therefore, IGF-I may indirectly modulate carbohydrate metabolism through GH suppression and enhancement of insulin action. Following ingestion of a meal, there is a significant increase in free IGF-I. This increase occurs via insulin-induced suppression of IGFBP-1 secretion.[34] The IGFBP-1 gene is transcriptionally regulated by insulin, thus the meal-induced increase in insulin leads to an increase in free IGF-I. This change may be adequate to stimulate fatty acid oxidation in muscle and suppress GH, and these changes may occur at physiologic IGF-I levels. The provision of pharmacologic levels of IGF-I to healthy patients results in further changes in carbohydrate metabolism. IGF-I can directly stimulate glucose transport into muscle through either IGF-I or insulin/IGF-I hybrid receptors,[35,36] although this requires high concentrations of free IGF-I. Additionally, a high concentration of free IGF-I can directly suppress renal gluconeogenesis in mice.[37] Experimental mice in whom the insulin receptor has been deleted show a decrease in blood glucose in response to IGF-I indicating that, in part, its effect can be mediated directly through the stimulation of glucose transport by the IGF-I or the hybrid receptor.[38] Experimental mice in which serum IGF-I is lowered by 80% by deleting expression in the liver have impaired glucose tolerance.[39] However, whether this is a direct effect of reduced IGF-I or caused by an increase in GH, has been difficult to determine because GH levels increase substantially in these mice. Therefore, the extent to which the effect of IGF-I on lowering glucose is caused by the direct effect of IGF-I on glucose transport, the enhancement of FFA metabolism in muscle, or the suppression of GH has been difficult to ascertain. In a comparable study, the author infused a GH receptor antagonist into patients with acromegaly and showed that it improved their insulin sensitivity.[40] The author then repeated the experiment and added an IGF-I infusion. Although IGF-I was infused at supraphysiologic concentrations, these concentrations were capable of further improving insulin sensitivity and lowering glucose even when the activity of GH had been completely suppressed. Simpson and colleagues[41] showed that following suppression of GH with octreotide in patients with Type I diabetes, IGF-I could further lower glucose. This finding suggests that at least at pharmacologic levels, IGF-I does function to enhance insulin sensitivity and lower glucose independently of its ability to suppress GH. However, in individuals who are GH deficient, the administration of a physiologic replacement concentration of IGF-I does not change carbohydrate oxidation; but in patients with GH receptor mutations, it resulted in enhanced carbohydrate oxidation. It also increased hepatic glucose production rates, which was probably caused by the suppression of insulin, but overall normoglycemia was maintained.[32] This finding also supports the conclusion that IGF-I has a glucose-lowering effect secondary to its ability to increase fatty acid oxidation in muscle leading to decreased free fatty acid flux to the liver and enhanced insulin suppression of hepatic glucose output. Thus, the predominant effect of IGF-I on carbohydrate metabolism seems to be secondary to its effects on lipid metabolism. Because suppression of insulin and GH secretion occurs at pharmacologic levels of IGF-I, it is difficult to extrapolate from the results of most published studies and conclude that these effects occur at normal physiologic levels. However, GH suppression would be expected to lead to decreased free fatty acid flux in liver and reduced antagonism of insulin action on gluconeogenesis.

IGF System Component Concentrations and their Utility in Predicting Changes in Carbohydrate and Fat Metabolism

Serum IGF-I concentrations vary widely among healthy humans. Age is a major determinant, and serum levels are low at birth and increase progressively with a peak during puberty, then decrease progressively with the greatest decrease occurring during the second and third decades; but levels continue to decrease throughout the lifespan.[42] These changes parallel the age-dependent changes in GH secretion. Changes in the GH-dependent IGF-binding proteins, IGFBP-3 and IGFBP-5, as well as the acid labile subunit parallel the changes that occur in serum IGF-I; although changes in IGFBP-3 are significantly less sensitive to changes in GH because IGF-II, which is insensitive to changes in GH, is a major determinant of serum IGFBP-3 and to some extent ALS.[43] Other IGF-binding proteins that are non-GH dependent, such as IGFBP-1 and IGFBP-2, have been studied extensively in humans. Insulin is a major suppressor of hepatic IGFBP-1 synthesis, therefore, changes in IGFBP-1 often reflect changes in either insulin secretion or insulin sensitivity.[44] IGFBP-2 changes much less rapidly in response to insulin; however, chronic changes in insulin availability or insulin sensitivity can lead to changes in IGFBP-2.[45] As noted previously, changes in these 2 proteins can have major effects on the plasma concentration of free IGF-I. Acute changes in several nutritional variables regulate IGF-I secretion and plasma concentrations; however, chronic changes in dietary intake that lead to changes in fat mass also regulate IGF-I and GH. In general, when the body mass index increases to greater than 24, there is a substantial increase in serum IGF-I concentrations.[46] Studies have shown that this change occurs as a function of enhanced sensitivity to the ability of GH to stimulate IGF-I synthesis.[47] This change plateaus with a body mass index of 25 and remains constant until the body mass index reaches 36. At that point, although the enhanced sensitivity to GH is maintained, there is a reduction in GH secretion. Therefore, patients who are massively obese have lower 24-hour blood production rates of GH. This effect becomes predominant with a body mass index greater than 37, and serum IGF-I concentrations tend to decrease as a function of increasing weight in this subgroup.[48] There are also changes in binding proteins that occur as a result of obesity, and the net effect is a moderate increase in free IGF-I when the body mass index increases greater than 30.[34] This change in free IGF-I correlates with a lowering of IGFBP-1, which presumably occurs as a result of hyperinsulinemia.

IGF-I AND THE METABOLIC SYNDROME

Several studies have attempted to correlate total plasma IGF-I concentrations with the presence of the metabolic syndrome. In general, patients with a low-normal IGF-I who are obese and meet other criteria for metabolic syndrome tend to have a worse cardiovascular disease outcomes than those with a midnormal to high-normal IGF-I.[49] Clearly, many of these patients have insulin resistance. Whether the degree of resistance or the accompanying changes in inflammatory cytokine secretion is the predominant predictor of a poor outcome has not been definitively determined. There are also studies correlating the lower total serum IGF-I concentrations with increased waist-to-hip ratios or with the development of impaired glucose tolerance both of which predict a worse cardiovascular outcome.[50,51] Therefore, although it seems that a lower serum IGF-I predicts a worse cardiovascular outcome, the exact parameter that is mediating this increased risk has not been determined. Cytokines that are elevated in these patients, such as C-reactive protein (CRP), are known to decrease circulating IGF-I in experimental animals[52] and could contribute to the relationship between low serum IGF-I and the prediction of a poor cardiovascular outcomes.

In patients with Type 1 diabetes, the changes in serum IGF-I are straightforward. In poorly controlled Type 1 diabetes, the lack of adequate insulinization of the liver leads to a major suppression of IGF-I biosynthesis.[53] Thus, the acute administration of insulin to patients with Type 1 diabetes results in a 3.0- to 3.5-fold increase in serum IGF-I because of the restoration of a hepatic synthesis.[9] The administration of insulin via the portal circulation results in a greater increase in serum IGF-I in Type 1 diabetes compared with peripheral insulin administration.[54] Thus, in patients with poorly controlled adolescent Type 1 diabetes, IGF-I can be low enough that optimal growth is not achieved. That this is rate limiting for growth was shown in experimental animals with diabetes and low IGF-I levels in whom a growth response was achieved when the IGF-I levels were normalized.[55] Even though GH concentrations are elevated in these animals, they are refractory to the high GH concentrations because of a low serum IGF-I that is inadequate to sustain normal growth. In addition, in poorly controlled diabetes, there is increased catabolism, particularly in skeletal muscle.[18] In Type 2 diabetes, the range of IGF-I concentrations that has been reported is broad.[56] This finding suggests that because of multiple variables that are interacting to control IGF-I concentrations, such as increases in inflammatory cytokines, decreases in hepatic insulin action caused by insulin resistance, concomitant changes in IGF-binding proteins, and the effects of obesity on IGF-I production, the net effect of all these variables combined is that there is not a uniform abnormality in serum IGF-I concentrations in this disease state.

In contrast to total IGF-I levels, IGFBP levels are significantly altered in Type 2 diabetes; these changes result in changes in free IGF-I.[57] Recent studies from Sweden in patients with prediabetes suggest that IGFBP-1 is initially lower in patients who will subsequently develop Type 2 diabetes.[58] This state is caused by hyperinsulinism, which occurs in the early prediabetic phase of the disease. This hyperinsulinism results in an elevation in free IGF-I; however, as insulin resistance progresses, the liver becomes more resistant to insulin suppression of IGFBP-1 and IGFBP-1 levels increase, which is concomitantly accompanied by a decrease in free IGF-I.[58] Therefore, there may be a natural progression of changes in total IGF-I and free IGF-I that occur as a function of changing insulin secretion and insulin sensitivity over time in Type 2 diabetes. That a change in free IGF-I that occurs as a function of changes in IGFBP-1 could be clinically significant was shown by the administration of IGFBP-1 to experimental animals using concentrations that were sufficient to lower free IGF-I significantly and showing that this resulted in increased serum glucose even in absence of a change in insulin.[59] The administration of insulin to patients with Type 1 diabetes not only results in a major increase in total IGF-I levels but also free IGF-I levels are increased substantially and IGFBP-1 decreases approximately 5-fold.[9] IGFBP-2 is suppressed in obesity, and this may contribute to the increase in free IGF-I.[60] The suppression of IGFBP-2 in patients who are obese may be physiologically relevant because transgenic mice that overexpressed IGFBP-2 are resistant to the development of obesity during high fat feeding, suggesting that this protein may have a direct effect on preadipocyte differentiation.[61] A further confounding variable is IGFBP-3 proteolysis, which occurs in diabetes and results in disproportionate increases in free IGF-I as a function of diabetic control.[62,63]

IGFBP changes also correlate with parameters of metabolic syndrome, and lower IGFBP-1 levels are present in patients with metabolic syndrome with higher CRP. The combination of a high CRP with a low IGFBP-1 value is a strong predictor of the presence of this syndrome.[64,65] Similarly, in middle-aged men, low IGF-I and high CRP along with low testosterone predicted the presence of metabolic syndrome with high probability.[66] Low IGFBP-2 also predicted the presence of metabolic syndrome, and low IGFBP-2 was associated with elevated fasting glucose.[59] Whether these factors reflect insulin resistance and the known effect of inflammatory mediators in suppressing IGF-I concentrations and thereby suppressing IGFBP-1 and IGFBP-2 or whether the primary changes in IGFBP-1 and IGFBP-2 predispose to the development of obesity and insulin resistance has not been resolved. Studies in transgenic mice overexpressing IGFBP-1 show that this induces hyperinsulinemia and glucose intolerance and that the ability of IGFBP-1 to induce these changes depends on its phosphorylation state, which is increased in diabetes.[67] Similarly, following weight loss there is a significant increase in IGFBP-1 and IGFBP-2 both in children and adults, which correlates with an improvement in insulin sensitivity.[68,69] These findings raise the question as to whether changes in IGF-I or IGFBP-1 and IGFBP-2 can predict the development of diabetes. Diet-induced obesity in experimental animals induces resistance to the vasodilatory effects of IGF-I. Likewise, Zucker rats that are extremely obese are resistant to the glucose-lowering effects of IGF-I.[70] Because IGF-I modulates the concentrations of IGFBP-1 and IGFBP-2, it is possible that these values change as a function of early changes in insulin resistance. A recent study used IGFBP-1 concentrations to predict the development of Type 2 diabetes in women in Sweden. Patients with the lowest fasting IGFBP-1 measurements had a high waist circumference and those in the lowest tertile had the highest risk of developing diabetes within 8 years.[58] These patients not only have low fasting IGFBP-1 levels but also have impaired IGFBP-1 suppression after oral glucose loading. Fasting IGFBP-1 values increased over the 8-year interval suggesting that the patients developed hepatic insulin resistance. Plasma IGF-I is associated with insulin sensitivity in patients with prediabetes with different degrees of glucose intolerance. During a 4.5-year follow-up of 615 patients who had IGF-I values in the lower half of the normal range there was an increased predisposition to develop glucose intolerance or Type 2 diabetes and this change was independently associated with IGFBP-1.[71] Maternal IGF-I/IGFBP-1 ratios also predicted the subsequent risk for gestational diabetes, and IGFBP-1 values greater than 68 ng/mL lowered the risk by 57%. A free IGF-I greater than 1 ng/mL lowered the risk by 69%.[72,73] In older individuals (aged >65 years), low IGFBP-1 also predicted an increased risk for glucose intolerance. Patients with a low IGFBP-2 (10th percentile) had an increased hazard ratio for the development of Type 2 diabetes, and those with IGFBP-1 more than the 90th percentile had a reduced risk. After adjustment for all metabolic parameters, the increased relative risk ratio of a low IGFBP-1 remained present. IGFBP-1 also predicted the development of Type 2 diabetes over a 17-year period. Patients in the lowest quintile had an incidence of 12.6%, whereas those in the highest quintile had an incidence of 1.5%.[64] When corrected for age, gender, CRP, and waist circumference, those in the lowest quartile still had an elevated relative risk ratio. Low IGF-II levels also predict weight gain in normal-weight middle-aged patients with Type 2 diabetes. Those in the highest quartile had a 47% decrease in risk of gaining more than 2 kg for a 5-year follow-up period. IGF-I is also negatively correlated with visceral fat mass, suggesting that regional distribution in fat may be predicted by IGF-I concentrations.[74]

GENETIC STUDIES
IGF-I Gene Polymorphisms and Changes in Metabolism

A polymorphism caused by a CA dinucleotide repeat in a microsatellite that is 1 kb upstream from the IGF-I transcription start site results in lower serum IGF-I levels, and some investigators have found this is associated with a lower birth weight.[75] This polymorphism occurs in approximately 11% of the Dutch Caucasian population. A study of 477 Dutch patients with evidence of ischemic heart disease and 808 control subjects demonstrated an increase relative risk of 1.7:1.0 for the presence of ischemic disease in noncarriers of this common polymorphism allele (eg, 192 based pairs). These subjects were also significantly shorter and had an 18% reduction in serum IGF-I.[76] Two other studies conducted in different countries, however, were not able to reproduce this finding. There is a single nucleotide polymorphism at position -202. A polymorphism involving a tandem repeat and the IGF-I promoter was also associated with an increased risk of development of Type 1 diabetes.[77] The CA repeats have also been found in intron-1 in pigs and are associated with lower serum IGF-I concentrations and increased fat deposition.[78] The CA repeat polymorphisms were also analyzed in a group of young adults. Those with the polymorphism had a lower serum concentration and had 1 kg lower birth weight and 8 mm higher systolic blood pressure at age 36 years.[79] The CA repeat polymorphisms were also associated with a lower birth weight and head circumference as well as lower serum IGF-I levels, suggesting that this might predict a later development of cardiovascular disease. IGF-I gene polymorphisms have also been associated with the development of retinopathy and nephropathy in patients with established diabetes.[80,81] Polymorphisms in IGFBP-1 have also been associated with a lower body mass index and the presence of Type 2 diabetes.[82] Four single nucleotide polymorphisms were associated with a lower body mass index that was maintained over time, and there was a negative relationship between plasma IGFBP-1 concentrations and body mass index. Polymorphisms in IGFBP-1 have also been associated with renal protective effects in Type 1 diabetes.[83] An IGFBP-3 gene polymorphism has been described in the promoter region that accounts for an increase in the serum concentrations of this protein.[84] A recent study identified 3 additional polymorphisms and showed that together the 4 polymorphisms account for 6.5% of the variability of IGFBP-3 in the general population.[85]

Response of Patients with Genetic Syndromes of Severe Insulin Resistance to IGF-I

Several subgroups of patients with severe insulin resistance have been administered IGF-I in an attempt to achieve improved glycemic control. Patients with severe type A insulin resistance and mutations in the insulin receptor had major decreases in blood glucose as well as insulin and C-peptide levels when administered recombinant IGF-I.[86] In a subsequent report, 11 patients with various types of insulin receptor mutations were treated for up to 16 months with recombinant human IGF-I. Fasting and postprandial glucose as well as fructosamine and hemoglobin A1C were measured and significantly improved in 6 of 11 of the patients.[87] This degree of improvement was maintained throughout treatment. A subsequent study in patients with severe insulin resistance showed that not only were glucose and insulin concentrations lowered but insulin resistance as measured using a frequently sampled intravenous glucose tolerance test showed significant improvement.[88] This finding was subsequently followed up by another study of 6 patients, 4 of whom had overt diabetes and received 1 month of recombinant IGF-I. Glucose tolerance returned to normal in 3 of the 4 patients with diabetes and the remaining 2 patients showed major reduction in insulin and triglyceride concentrations.[89] Two patients with Rabson-Mendenhall syndrome showed the same benefits in hemoglobin A1C when IGF-I was administered. Children with severe insulin resistance caused by leprechaunism usually die within the first 2 years of life; however, administration of IGF-I to 3 of these patients has resulted in several years of maintenance of normal glucose levels and normal linear growth. The administration of IGF-I to patients with GH receptor mutations who have extremely low IGF-I concentrations showed that normoglycemia was maintained with suppression of insulin concentrations.[90] Hepatic glucose production was increased presumably because of enhanced insulin sensitivity and glucose oxidation rates were decreased. IGF-I has been administered to rare patients with IGF-I gene deletions. In general, these patients have moderate glucose intolerance or overt diabetes and high fasting GH concentrations.[91] The administration of IGF-I has normalized glucose concentrations and, most importantly, normalized insulin sensitivity; however, because GH is also suppressed, it has been impossible to distinguish between the improving insulin resistance caused by suppressing GH as compared with enhancing insulin sensitivity directly by IGF-I.

IGF-I and the Treatment of Type 1 Diabetes

Multiple studies have administered IGF-I to patients with Type 1 diabetes who are also receiving insulin.[92] Many of these studies involved small numbers of patients, although the largest trial had 223 patients. In that trial, the dosages ranged from 20 to 140 mcg/kg/d. In general, hemoglobin A1C was improved and insulin requirements were decreased. In the large study with 223 patients who received IGF-I for 12 weeks, there was a major decrease in insulin requirements and hemoglobin A1C declined by 0.6%.[88] Edema, jaw pain, and tachycardia were present in several patients.[93] Additional patients (n = 4) noted worsening of retinopathy, which resolved during a follow-up period after the administration of IGF-I had ceased. IGF-I is also anabolic in these patients, and in experimental animals with Type 1 diabetes, infusions of IGF-I have been shown to increase long bone growth and protein synthesis.[55] Studies using a hyperinsulinemic clamp have shown that the administration of IGF-I is associated with enhanced insulin sensitivity in Type 1 diabetes. Peripheral insulin stimulated glucose disposal increased by approximately 34% during IGF-I administration.[94] Concomitantly with the improvement in insulin resistance was a lowering of GH. Therefore, the question was raised whether most of the improvement was caused by reduced GH secretion. To address this, 2 types of studies were done. Simpson and colleagues[95] infused octreotide simultaneously with recombinant IGF-I. IGF-I was shown to acutely reduce hepatic glucose production and stimulate peripheral glucose uptake. Glycerol turnover and free fatty acids were unaffected, suggesting to the investigators that the effect was caused by IGF-I enhancement of insulin sensitivity and not a reduction in GH. This finding was further addressed using a GH receptor antagonist. A reduction in the GH effect was clearly achieved with the dosage used, yet there was no improvement in insulin sensitivity, suggesting to the investigators that the effect of IGF-I is also required.[96] When IGF-I was given, insulin sensitivity improved and low-density lipoprotein (LDL), triglycerides, and the LDL to APO-B ratio were significantly decreased. Despite these improvements, significant complications were noted.

Because the administration of high doses IGF-I suppress IGFBP-1 and IGFBP-2, they result in a disproportionate increase in free IGF-I. To try to obviate the effects of excessive free IGF-I in inducing side effects, the combination of IGF-I plus IGFBP-3 has also been administered to patients with Type 1 diabetes.[97] Pharmacologic studies have shown that when this combination is given, the rate of appearance of free IGF-I is substantially reduced, suggesting that it could lead to fewer side effects.[98] The administration of the combination to a group of adults with Type 1 diabetes resulted in a 52% reduction in insulin levels with a 23% reduction in glucose after a 2-week treatment period.[97] The prevalence of side effects was reduced. In another study, 15 adolescents were administered the combination in dosages between 0.1 and 0.8 mg/kg/d. They showed a 41% reduction in overnight insulin requirements and a dose-dependent reduction in hepatic glucose production.[99] Insulin sensitivity was also improved with the 0.4 and 0.8 mg/kg/d dosages. Overnight GH secretion was reduced substantially, suggesting this may be one mechanism by which insulin sensitivity was improved. Therefore, this approach offers a possible future therapeutic option.

IGF-I Administration to Patients with Type 2 Diabetes

Several studies with small numbers of patients were initially performed in patients with Type 2 diabetes. Most of these studies were of short duration.[100] Studies that were 7 days or less showed decreases in glucose, endogenous insulin, C-peptide secretion, and, in some cases, an improved area under the curve after oral glucose administration. In most of these studies, high dosages (eg, 240–360 mcg/kg/d) were administered and were associated with edema, headaches, and arthralgias. A longer study whereby IGF-I was administered to 12 patients for 6 weeks using the dosage of 80 mcg/kg twice a day showed a 3.4-fold enhancement in insulin sensitivity.[101] Similarly, when a 160 mcg/kg/d dosage was administered to patients with Type 2 diabetes and hepatic and peripheral insulin sensitivity were measured, they were shown to be improved after 7 days.[102] These findings suggested that IGF-I was capable of enhancing insulin sensitivity in Type 2 diabetes. Because most of these patients are obese and have very low GH concentrations, it is highly likely this is caused by an effect on free fatty acid metabolism in muscle and suppression of renal gluconeogenesis and not simply suppression of GH secretion.

A large clinical trial in which dosages of 10 to 80 mcg/kg/d were administered to 212 patients for 12 weeks showed that there was a dose-dependent reduction in hemoglobin A1C and mean daily blood glucose.[103] As in previous trials, dosages of IGF-I 40 mg/kg twice a day or greater were accompanied by a significant side-effect profile and the number of side effects increased as the dosage increased. For example, in the 80 mcg/kg twice a day dosage group, the number of patients having significant side effects was approximately 30%. This study was followed by a large trial in which IGF-I was administered to patients with Type 2 diabetes who were being given insulin concomitantly for 12 weeks. Hemoglobin A1C was decreased by an additional 0.8% over that which could be achieved with more intensive insulinization, suggesting that it could be used as an adjunct to insulin therapy in Type 2 diabetes.[104] The administration of IGF-I combined with IGFBP-3 has also been effective in patients with Type 2 diabetes. When 48 patients were treated with this regimen, fasting and postprandial blood glucose decreased significantly by 35% to 40%.[98] These patients were being administered insulin and, therefore, they could be maintained on lower insulin doses. Insulin requirements decreased in the 4 groups by 54% to 82% and fasting glucose decreased by 32% to 37%. The administration of the combination was associated with fewer side effects, but a significant minority of patients had edema, arthralgias, and headaches. This finding suggests that the degree of increase in free IGF-I that has to be achieved to improve glycemic control is such that even when IGF-I is administered with its binding protein to obtain a clinical improvement in insulin sensitivity the concentration of free IGF-I that has to be achieved will induce side effects in a substantial number of patients. These studies suggest that high concentrations of the IGF-I increase insulin sensitivity in Type 2 diabetes but the window between therapeutic utility and toxicity is small.

SUMMARY

IGF-I is ancestrally related to proinsulin and, therefore, retains some physiologic effects that complement the ability of insulin to stimulate glucose uptake. Furthermore, the actions of IGF-I are coordinately regulated with GH, thus enabling organisms to breakdown fat and use this as a substrate to meet the energy needs that are required for growth and to coordinate their effects for stimulation of protein synthesis and an anabolic response. Therefore, IGF-I plays an integral role in coordinating the response to nutrient intake and in initiating the appropriate metabolic changes that enable cells to tolerate a variety of stressful stimuli and resist apoptosis and initiate the tissue repair response that occurs after injury. Furthermore, it plays an important role in facilitating the adaption to major changes in nutrient intake. In this way, IGF-I coordinates the response of the 3 hormones to form a functional unit thereby coordinating nutrient availability and tissue growth. In obesity and metabolic syndrome, as well as in patients with overt diabetes, the metabolic actions of IGF-I are altered significantly. Similarly, its ability to coordinate its functions with those of GH and insulin is impaired in these pathophysiologic states, and this constitutes an important component of the maladaptive response of all 3 hormones to metabolic stress.

REFERENCES

1. Bayne ML, Applebaum J, Chicchi GG, et al. The roles of tyrosines 24, 31, and 60 in the high-affinity binding of insulin-like growth factor-I to the type 1 insulin-like growth factor receptor. J Biol Chem 1990;265:15648.
2. Clemmons DR, Dehoff MH, Busby WH, et al. Competition for binding to insulin-like growth factor (IGF) binding protein-2, 3, 4, and 5 by the IGFs and IGF analogs. Endocrinology 1992;131:890.
3. Ullrich A, Gray A, Tam AW, et al. Insulin-like growth factor I receptor primary structure: comparison with insulin receptor suggests structural determinants that define functional specificity. EMBO J 1986;5:2503–12.
4. Brooks AJ, Waters MJ. The growth hormone receptor: mechanism of activation and clinical implications. Nat Rev Endocrinol 2010;6:515–25.
5. Isley WL, Underwood LE, Clemmons DR. Dietary components that regulate serum somatomedin-C concentrations in humans. J Clin Invest 1983;71:175–82.
6. Underwood LE, Thissen JP, Lemozy S, et al. Hormonal and nutritional regulation of IGF-I and its binding proteins. Horm Res 1994;42:145–51.

7. Yakar S, Liu JL, Stannard B, et al. Normal growth and development in the absence of hepatic insulin-like growth factor I. Proc Natl Acad Sci U S A 1999; 96:7324–9.

8. Phillips LS, Pao CI, Villafuerte BC. Molecular regulation of insulin-like growth factor-I and its principal binding protein, IGFBP-3. Prog Nucleic Acid Res Mol Biol 1998;60:195–265.

9. Bereket A, Lang CH, Blethen AL, et al. Effect of insulin on the insulin-like growth factor system in children with new onset dependent diabetes. J Clin Endocrinol Metab 1995;80:1312–7.

10. Lowe WL, Adamo M, Werner H, et al. Regulation by fasting of insulin-like growth factor I and its receptor: effects on gene expression and binding. J Clin Invest 1989;84:619–26.

11. Holly J, Perks C. The role of insulin-like growth factor binding proteins. Neuroendocrinol 2006;83:154–60.

12. Boisclair YR, Rhoads RP, Ueki I, et al. The acid-labile subunit (ALS) of the 150 kDa IGF-binding protein complex: an important but forgotten component of the circulating IGF system. J Endocrinol 2001;170:63–70.

13. Chen JW, Hojlund K, Beck-Nielsen H, et al. Free rather than total circulating insulin-like growth factor-I determines the feedback on growth hormone release in normal subjects. J Clin Endocrinol Metab 2005;90:366–71.

14. Myers MJ, White MF. Insulin signal transduction and the IRS proteins. Annu Rev Pharmacol 1996;36:615.

15. Ning J, Clemmons DR. AMP-activated protein kinase inhibits IGF-I signaling and protein synthesis in vascular smooth muscle cells via stimulation of insulin receptor substrate 1 S794 and tuberous sclerosis 2 S1345 phosphorylation. Mol Endocrinol 2010;24:1218–29.

16. Adamo ML, Farrar RP. Resistance training, and IGF involvement in the maintenance of muscle mass during the aging process. Ageing Res Rev 2006;5: 310–31.

17. Glass DJ. Skeletal muscle hypertrophy and atrophy signaling pathways. Int J Biochem Cell Biol 2005;37:1974–84.

18. Dehoux M, Van Beneden R, Pasko N, et al. Role of the insulin-like growth factor-I decline in the induction of atrogin-1/MAFbx during fasting and diabetes. Endocrinol 2004;245:4806–12.

19. O'Connor JC, McCusker RH, Strle K, et al. Regulation of IGF-I function by proinflammatory cytokines: at the interface of immunology and endocrinology. Cell Immunol 2008;252:91–110.

20. Mauras N, Beaufrere B. rhIGF-I enhances whole body protein anabolism and significantly diminishes the protein-catabolic effects of prednisone in humans, without a diabetogenic effect. J Clin Endocrinol Metab 1995;80:869–74.

21. Mauras N, Martinez V, Rini J, et al. Recombinant human IGF-I has significant anabolic effects in adults with GH receptor deficiency: studies on protein, glucose and lipid metabolism. J Clin Endocrinol Metab 2000;85:3036–42.

22. Mauras N, O'Brien KO, Welch S, et al. IGF-I and GH treatment in GH deficient humans: differential effects on protein, glucose, lipid and calcium metabolism. J Clin Endocrinol Metab 2000;85:1686–94.

23. Debroy MA, Wolf SE, Zhang XJ, et al. Anabolic effect of insulin-like growth factor in combination with insulin-like growth factor binding protein-3 in severely burned adults. J Trauma 1999;47:904–10.

24. Fouque D, Peng SC, Kopple JD. Impaired metabolic response to recombinant insulin-like growth factor-1 in dialysis patients. Kidney Int 1995;47:876–83.

25. Mauras N, Hayes V, Welch S, et al. Testosterone deficiency in young men: marked alterations in whole body protein kinetics strength and adiposity. J Clin Endocrinol Metab 1998;83:1886–92.
26. Scavo LM, Karase M, Murry M, et al. Insulin-like growth factor-I stimulates both cell growth and lipogenesis during differentiation of human mesenchymal stem cells into adipocytes. J Clin Endocrinol Metab 2004;84:3543–53.
27. DiGirolamo M, Eden S, Enberg O, et al. Specific binding of human growth hormone but not insulin-like growth factors by human adipocytes. FEBS Lett 1986;205:15–9.
28. Mauras N, O'Brien KO, Welch S, et al. Insulin-like growth factor I and growth hormone (GH) treatment in GH-deficient humans: differential effects on protein, glucose, lipid, and calcium metabolism. J Clin Endocrinol Metab 2000;85:1686–94.
29. Fernandez AM, Kim JK, Yakar S, et al. Functional inactivation of the IGF-I and insulin receptors in skeletal muscle causes type 2 diabetes. Genes Dev 2001; 15:1926–34.
30. Heron-Milhavet L, Haluzik M, Yakar S, et al. Muscle-specific overexpression of CD36 reverses the insulin resistance and diabetes of MKR mice. Endocrinol 2004;145:4667–76.
31. Yuen KC, Dunger DB. Therapeutic aspect of growth hormone and insulin-like growth factor-I treatment on visceral fat and insulin sensitivity in adults. Diabetes Obes Metab 2007;9:11–22.
32. del Rincon JP, Lida K, Gaylinn BD, et al. Growth hormone regulation of p85alpha expression and phosphoinositide 3-kinase activity in adipose tissue: mechanism of growth hormone-mediated insulin resistance. Diabetes 2007;56:1638–46.
33. Barbour LA, Mizanoor Rahman S, Gurevich I, et al. Increased p85alpha potent negative regulator of skeletal muscle insulin signaling and induces in vivo insulin resistance associated with growth hormone excess. J Biol Chem 2005;280: 37489–94.
34. Frystyk J. Free insulin-like growth factors—measurements and relationships to growth hormone secretion and glucose homeostasis. Growth Horm IGF Res 2004;14:337–75.
35. Furling D, Marette A, Puymirat J. Insulin-like growth factor I circumvents defective insulin action in human myotonic dystrophy skeletal cells. Endocrinol 1999; 140:4244–50.
36. Henry RR, Abrams L, Nikoulina S, et al. Insulin action and glucose metabolism in nondiabetic control and NIDDM subjects. Diabetes 1995;44:936–46.
37. Pennisi P, Gavrilova O, Setser-Portas J, et al. Recombinant human insulin-like growth factor-I treatment inhibits gluconeogenesis in a transgenic mouse model of type 2 diabetes mellitus. Endocrinol 2006;147:L2619–30.
38. LeRoith D, Kim H, Fernandez AM, et al. Inactivation of muscle insulin and IGF-I receptors and insulin responsiveness. Curr Opin Clin Nutr Metab Care 2002;5:371–5.
39. Yakar S, Liu JL, Fernandez AM, et al. Liver-specific Igf-1 gene deletion leads to muscle insulin insensitivity. Diabetes 2001;50:1110–8.
40. O'Connell T, Clemmons DR. IGF-I/IGF-binding protein-3 combination improves insulin resistance by GH-dependent and independent mechanisms. J Clin Endocrinol Metab 2002;87:4356–60.
41. Simpson H, Savine R, Sonksen P, et al. Growth hormone replacement therapy for adults: into the new millennium. Growth Horm IGF Res 2002;12:12–33.
42. Brabant G, von zur Muhlen A, Wuster C, et al. Serum insulin-like growth factor I reference values for an automated chemiluminescence immunoassay system: results from a multicenter study. Horm Res 2003;60:53–60.

43. Leung KC, Ho KK. Measurement of growth hormone, insulin-like growth factor I and their binding proteins: the clinical aspects. Clin Chim Acta 2001;313: 119–23.

44. Brismar K, Hilding A, Lindgren B. Regulation of IGFBP-1 in humans. Prog Growth Factor Res 1995;6:449–56.

45. Arafat AM, Weickert MO, Frystyk J, et al. The role of insulin-like growth factor (IGF) binding protein-2 in the insulin-mediated decrease in IGF-I bioactivity. J Clin Endocrinol Metab 2009;94:5093–6101.

46. Lukanova A, Soderberg S, Stattin P, et al. Nonlinear relationship of insulin-like growth factor (IGF)-I and IGF-I/IGF-binding protein-3 ratio with indices of adiposity and plasma insulin concentrations (Sweden). Cancer Causes Control 2002;13:509–16.

47. Maccario M, Tassone F, Gauna C, et al. Effects of short-term administration of low-dose rhGH on IGF-I levels in obesity and Cushing's syndrome: indirect evaluation of sensitivity to GH. Eur J Endocrinol 2001;144:251–6.

48. Schneider HJ, Saller B, Klotsche J, et al. Opposite associations of age-dependent insulin-like growth factor-I standard deviation scores with nutritional state in normal weight and obese subjects. Eur J Endocrinol 2006;154: 699–706.

49. Saydah S, Ballard-Barbash R, Potischman N. Association of metabolic syndrome with insulin-like growth factors among adults in the US. Cancer Causes Control 2009;20:1309–16.

50. Martha S, Pantam N, Thungathurthi S, et al. Study of insulin resistance in relation to serum IGf-I levels in subjects with different degrees of glucose tolerance. Int J Diabetes Dev Ctries 2008;28:54–9.

51. Dunger D, Yuen K, Ong K. Insulin-like growth factor I and impaired glucose tolerance. Horm Res 2004;1:10–7.

52. Efstratiadis G, Tiaousis G, Athyros VG, et al. Total serum insulin-like growth factor-1 and C-reactive protein in metabolic syndrome with or without diabetes. Angiology 2006;57:303–11.

53. Maes M, Ketelslegers JM, Underwood LE. Low circulating somatomedin-C/insulin-like growth factor I in insulin-dependent diabetes and malnutrition: growth hormone receptor and post-receptor defects. Acta Endocrinol Suppl 1986;279:86–92.

54. Hanaire-Broutin H, Sallerin-Caute B, Poncet MF, et al. Insulin therapy and GH-IGF-I axis disorders in diabetes: impact and GH-IGF-I axis disorders in diabetes: impact of glycaemic control and hepatic insulinization. Diabetes Metab 1996;22:245–50.

55. Scheiwiller E, Guler HP, Merryweather J, et al. Growth restoration of insulin-deficient diabetic rats by recombinant human insulin-like growth factor I. Nature 1986;323:169–71.

56. Sandhu MS. Insulin-like growth factor-I and risk of type 2 diabetes and coronary heart disease: molecular epidemiology. Endocr Dev 2005;9:44–54.

57. Frystyk J, Skjaerbaek C, Vestbo E, et al. Circulating levels of free insulin-like growth factors in obese subjects: the impact of type 2 diabetes. Diabetes Metab Res Rev 1999;15:314–22.

58. Lewitt MS, Hilding A, Brismar K, et al. IGF-binding protein 1 and abdominal obesity in the development of type 2 diabetes in women. Eur J Endocrinol 2010;163:233–42.

59. Lewitt MS, Denyer GS, Cooney GJ, et al. Insulin-like growth factor-binding protein-1 modulates blood glucose levels. Endocrinol 1991;129:2254–6.

60. Heald AH, Haushal K, Siddals KW, et al. Insulin-like growth factor binding protein-2 (IGFBP-2) is a marker for the metabolic syndrome. Exp Clin Endocrinol Diabetes 2006;114:371–6.

61. Wheatcroft SB, Kearney MT, Shah AM, et al. IGF-binding protein-2 protects against the development of obesity and insulin resistance. Diabetes 2007;56: 285–94.

62. Bang P, Brismar K, Rosenfeld RG. Increased proteolysis of insulin-like growth factor-binding protein-3 (IGFBP-3) in noninsulin-dependent diabetes mellitus serum, with elevation of a 29-kilodalton (kDa) glycosylated IGFBP-3 fragment contained in the approximately 130- to 150 kDa ternary complex. J Clin Endocrinol Metab 1994;78:1119–27.

63. Cheetham TD, Holly JM, Baxter RC. The effects of recombinant human IGF-I administration on concentrations of acid labile subunit, IGF binding protein-3, IGF-I, IGF-II and proteolysis of IGF binding protein-3 in adolescents with insulin-dependent diabetes mellitus. J Endocrinol 1998;157:81–7.

64. Petersson U, Ostegrn CJ, Brudin L, et al. Low levels of insulin-like growth factor binding protein-1 (IGFBP-1) are prospectively associated with the incidence of type 2 diabetes and impaired glucose tolerance (IGT): the Soderakra Cardiovascular Risk Factor Study. Diabetes Metab 2009;35:198–205.

65. Heald AH, Anderson SG, Ivison F, et al. C-reactive protein and the insulin-like growth factor (IGF) system in relation to risk of cardiovascular disease in different ethnic groups. Atherosclerosis 2003;170:79–86.

66. Tong PC, Ho CS, Yeung VT, et al. Association of testosterone, insulin-like growth factor-I, and C-reactive protein with metabolic syndrome in Chinese middle-aged men with a family history of type 2 diabetes. J Clin Endocrinol Metab 2005;90:6418–23.

67. Sakai K, D'Ercole AJ, Murphy LJ, et al. Physiological differences in insulin-like growth factor binding protein-1 (IGFBP-1) phosphorylation in IGFBP-1 transgenic mice. Diabetes 2001;50:32–8.

68. Wabisch M, Blum WF, Muche R, et al. Insulin-like growth factors and their binding proteins before and after weight loss and their associations with hormonal and metabolic parameters in obese adolescent girls. Int J Obes Relat Metab Disord 1996;20:1073–80.

69. Reinehr T, Kleber M, Toschke AM, et al. Longitudinal association between IGFBP-1 levels and parameters of the metabolic syndrome in obese children before and after weight loss. Int J Pediatr Obes 2011;6(3–4):236–43.

70. Jacob RJ, Sherwin RS, Greenawalt K, et al. Simultaneous insulinlike growth factor I and insulin resistance in obese Zucker rats. Diabetes 1992;41: 691–7.

71. Sandhu MS, Heald AH, Gibson JM, et al. Circulating concentrations of insulin-like growth factor-I and development of glucose intolerance: a prospective observational study. Lancet 2002;359:1740–5.

72. Qiu C, Vadachkoria S, Meryman L, et al. Maternal plasma concentrations of IGF-1, IGFBP-1, and C-peptide in early pregnancy and subsequent risk of gestational diabetes mellitus. Am J Obstet Gynecol 2005;193:1691–7.

73. Rajpathak SN, McGinn AP, Strickler HD, et al. Insulin-like growth factor (IGF) axis, inflammation, and glucose intolerance among older adults. Growth Horm IGF Res 2008;19:166–73.

74. Heald AH, Karvestedt L, Anderson SG, et al. Low insulin-like growth factor-II levels predict weight gain in normal weight subjects with type 2 diabetes. Am J Med 2006;119:167 e9–15.

75. Arends N, Johnston L, Hokken-Koelega A, et al. Polymorphism in the IGF-I gene: clinical relevance for short children born small for gestational age (SGA). J Clin Endocrinol 2002;87:2720.

76. Vaessen N, Hautink P, Janssen JA, et al. A polymorphism in the gene for IGF-I: functional properties and risk for type 2 diabetes and myocardial infarction. Diabetes 2001;50:637–42.

77. Eerligh P, Roep BO, Giphart MJ, et al. Insulin-like growth factor 1 promoter polymorphism influences insulin gene variable number of tandem repeat-associated risk for juvenile onset type 1 diabetes. Tissue Antigens 2004;63: 568–71.

78. Estany J, Tor M, Villalba D, et al. Association of CA repeat polymorphism at intron 1 of insulin-like growth factor (IGF-I) gene with circulating IGF-I concentration, growth and fatness in swine. Physiol Genomics 2007;31:236–43.

79. te Velde SJ, van Rossum EF, Voorhoeve PG, et al. An IGF-I promoter polymorphism modifies the relationships between birth weight and risk factors for cardiovascular disease and diabetes at age 36. BMC Endocr Disord 2005;5:5.

80. Rietveld I, Hofman A, Pols HA, et al. An insulin-like growth factor-I gene polymorphism modifies the risk of microalbuminuria in subjects with an abnormal glucose tolerance. Eur J Endocrinol 2006;154:715–21.

81. Rietveld I, Ikram MK, Vingerling JR, et al. An IGF-I gene polymorphism modifies the risk of diabetic retinopathy. Diabetes 2006;55:2387–91.

82. Heald AH, Stephens RH, McElduff P, et al. Polymorphisms in insulin-like growth factor binding protein-1 (IGFBP-1) are associated with altered circulating IGF-I and lower mass index in type-2 diabetes mellitus. Endo Abs 2006;11:413.

83. Stephens RH, McElduff P, Heald AH, et al. Polymorphisms in IGF-binding protein 1 are associated with impaired renal function in type 2 diabetes. Diabetes 2005;54:3547–53.

84. Deal C, Ma J, Wilkin F, et al. Novel promoter polymorphism in insulin-like growth factor-binding protein-3: correlation with serum levels and interaction with known regulators. J Clin Endocrinol Metab 2001;86:124–80.

85. Kaplan RC, Petersen AK, Chen MH, et al. A genome-wide association study identifies novel loci associated with circulating IGF-I and IGFBP-3. Hum Mol Genet 2011;1093:1–11.

86. Zenobi PD, Glatz Y, Keller A, et al. Beneficial metabolic effects of insulin-like growth factor I in patients with severe insulin-resistant diabetes type A. Eur J Endocrinol 1994;131:251–7.

87. Nakae J, Kato M, Murashita M, et al. Long-term effect of recombinant human insulin-like growth factor I on metabolic and growth control in a patient with leprechaunism. J Clin Endocrinol Metab 1998;83:542–9.

88. Morrow LA, O'Brien MB, Moller DE, et al. Recombinant human insulin-like growth factor-I therapy improves glycemic control and insulin action in the type A syndrome of severe insulin resistance. J Clin Endocrinol Metab 1994;79:205–10.

89. Moses AC, Morrow LA, O'Brien M, et al. Insulin-like growth factor I (rhIGF-I) as a therapeutic agent for hyperinsulinemic insulin resistant diabetes mellitus. Diabetes Res Clin Pract 1995;28:S185–94.

90. Savage MO, Burren CP, Blair JC, et al. Growth hormone insensitivity: pathophysiology, diagnosis, clinical variation and future perspectives. Horm Res 2001;2: 32–5.

91. Woods KA, Camacho-Hubner C, Bergman RN, et al. Effects of insulin-like growth factor I (IGF-I) therapy on body composition and insulin resistance in IGF-I gene deletion. J Clin Endocrinol Metab 2000;85:1407–11.

92. Quattrin T, Thrailkill K, Baker L, et al. Improvement in HbA1c without increased hypoglycemia in adolescents and young adults with type 1 diabetes mellitus treated with recombinant human insulin-like growth factor-I and insulin. rhIGF-I in IDDM Study Group. J Pediatr Endocrinol Metab 2001;14:267–77.

93. Quattrin T, Thralkill K, Baker L, et al. Dual hormonal replacement with insulin and recombinant human insulin-like growth factor I in IDDM. Effects on glycemic control, IGF-I levels, and safety profile. Diabetes Care 1997;20:374–80.

94. Carroll PV, Christ ER, Umpleby AM, et al. IGF-I treatment in adults with type diabetes: effects on glucose and protein metabolism in the fasting state and during a hyperinsulinemic-euglycemic amino acid clamp. Diabetes 2000;49: 789–96.

95. Simpson HL, Jackson NC, Shoejaee-Moradie F, et al. Insulin-like growth factor I has a direct effect on glucose and protein metabolism, but no effect on lipid metabolism in type 1 diabetes. J Clin Endocrinol Metab 2004;89:425–32.

96. Williams RM, Amin R, Shojaee-Moradie F, et al. The effects of a specific growth hormone antagonist on overnight insulin requirements and insulin sensitivity in young adults with type 1 diabetes mellitus. Diabetologia 2003;46:1203–10.

97. Clemmons DR, Moses AC, McKay MJ, et al. The combination of insulin-like growth factor I and insulin-like growth factor-binding protein-3 reduces insulin requirements in insulin-dependent type 1 diabetes: evidence for in vivo biological activity. J Clin Endocrinol Metab 2000;85:1518–24.

98. Clemmons DR, Moses AC, Sommer A, et al. Rh/IGF/rhIGFBP-3 administration to patients with type 2 diabetes mellitus reduces insulin requirements while also lowering fasting glucose. Growth Horm IGF Res 2005;15:265–74.

99. Saukkonen T, Shojaee-Moradie F, Williams RM, et al. Effects of recombinant human IGF-I/IGF-binding protein-3 complex on glucose and glycerol metabolism in type 1 diabetes. Diabetes 2006;55:2365–70.

100. Schalch DS, Turman NJ, Marcsisin VS, et al. Short-term effects of recombinant human insulin-like growth factor I on metabolic control of patients with type II diabetes mellitus. J Clin Endocrinol Metab 1993;77:1563–8.

101. Moses AC, Young SC, Morrow LA, et al. Recombinant human insulin-like growth factor I increases insulin sensitivity and improves glycemic control in type II diabetes. Diabetes 1996;45:91–100.

102. Cusi K, DeFronzo R. Recombinant human insulin-like growth factor I treatment for 1 week improves metabolic control in type 2 diabetes by ameliorating hepatic and muscle insulin resistance. J Clin Endocrinol Metab 2000;85:3077–84.

103. Rh in NIDDM Study Group. Evidence from a dose ranging study that recombinant insulin-like growth factor-I (RhIGF-I) effectively and safely improves glycemic control in the noninsulin dependent diabetes mellitus. Diabetes 1996;45:91–100.

104. RhIGF-I co therapy with insulin subgroup. RhIGF-I improves glucose control in insulin requiring type 2 diabetes mellitus reduces insulin requirements while also lowering fasting glucose [abstract: 582]. Proceedings of the 5th Annual Meeting of The American Diabetes Association. San Antonio (TX), June 14, 1997.

Index

Note: Page numbers of article titles are in **boldface** type.

Endocrinol Metab Clin N Am 41 (2012) 445–473
doi:10.1016/S0889-8529(12)00061-8
0889-8529/12/$ – see front matter © 2012 Elsevier Inc. All rights reserved.

endo.theclinics.com

Moving?

Make sure your subscription moves with you!

To notify us of your new address, find your **Clinics Account Number** (located on your mailing label above your name), and contact customer service at:

Email: journalscustomerservice-usa@elsevier.com

800-654-2452 (subscribers in the U.S. & Canada)
314-447-8871 (subscribers outside of the U.S. & Canada)

Fax number: 314-447-8029

Elsevier Health Sciences Division
Subscription Customer Service
3251 Riverport Lane
Maryland Heights, MO 63043

*To ensure uninterrupted delivery of your subscription, please notify us at least 4 weeks in advance of move.

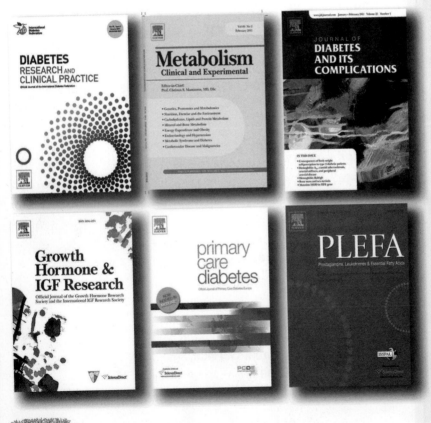